# COMPUTER DIAGNOSIS

## AND

# DIAGNOSTIC METHODS

# COMPUTER DIAGNOSIS AND DIAGNOSTIC METHODS

The Proceedings of the Second
Conference on the Diagnostic Process, 2d , University of Michigan,
held at the University of Michigan                    1971.

*Edited by*

**JOHN A. JACQUEZ, M.D.**

*Professor*
*Department of Physiology*
*The Medical School*
*Associate Professor*
*Department of Biostatistics*
*The School of Public Health*
*The University of Michigan*
*Ann Arbor, Michigan*

RC71
A1
C67
1971
(1972)

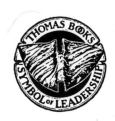

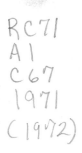

## CHARLES C THOMAS • PUBLISHER
*Springfield* • *Illinois* • *U.S.A.*

*Published and Distributed Throughout the World by*
CHARLES C THOMAS • PUBLISHER
BANNERSTONE HOUSE
301-327 East Lawrence Avenue, Springfield, Illinois, U.S.A.

© 1972, by CHARLES C THOMAS • PUBLISHER
ISBN 0-398-02521-5
Library of Congress Catalog Card Number: 72-75922

*Printed in the United States of America*
*EE-11*

# SESSIONS CHAIRMEN

JOHN ROMANO, M.D., Chairman, Department of Psychiatry, University of Rochester Medical Center, Rochester, New York.

ARNOLD W. PRATT, M.D., Director, Division of Computer Research and Technology, National Institutes of Health, Bethesda, Maryland.

ALLEN NEWELL, Ph.D., Professor, Department of Computer Science, Carnegie-Mellon University, Pittsburgh Pennsylvania.

EUGENE ACKERMAN, Ph.D., Director, Division of Health Computer Sciences, University of Minnesota, Minneapolis, Minnesota.

DONALD A. B. LINDBERG, M.D., Director, Medical Center Computer Program, University of Missouri, Columbia, Missouri.

MORTIMER MENDELSOHN, M.D., Professor, Department of Radiology, University of Pennsylvania, Philadelphia, Pennsylvania.

# CONTRIBUTORS

JOHN B. BAILLIEUL, M.A., Assistant in Computer Science, Department of Medicine, Harvard Medical School, Boston, Massachusetts.

G. OCTO BARNETT, M.D., Director, Laboratory of Computer Science, Massachusetts General Hospital, Associate Professor of Medicine, Harvard Medical School, Boston, Massachusetts.

JEROME CORNFIELD, Ph.D., Research Professor of Biostatistics, Department of Biostatistics, Graduate School of Public Health, University of Pittsburgh, Pittsburgh, Pennsylvania.

ROSALIE A. DUNN, Ph.D., Assistant Professor of Clinical Engineering, George Washington University, Washington, D.C.; Chief, Biostatistics Section, Veterans Administration Research Center for Cardiovascular Data Processing, VA Hospital, Washington, D.C.

WARD EDWARDS, Ph.D., Professor of Psychology and Head, Engineering Psychology Laboratory, Institute of Science and Technology, The University of Michigan, Ann Arbor, Michigan.

RALPH L. ENGLE, JR., M.D., Professor of Medicine and Chief, Division of Medical Systems and Computer Science, Department of Medicine, Cornell University Medical College, New York, New York.

EDWARD S. EPSTEIN, Ph.D., Professor, Department of Meteorology and Oceanography, The University of Michigan, Ann Arbor, Michigan.

BARBARA B. FARQUHAR, A.B., Assistant in Computer Science, Department of Medicine, Harvard Medical School, Boston, Massachusetts.

BETTY J. FLEHINGER, Ph.D., Visiting Associate Professor of Biomathematics, Graduate School of Medical Sciences, Cornell University; Research Staff member, IBM T. J. Watson Research Center, Yorktown Heights, New York.

ALLEN S. GINSBERG, Ph.D., Health Research Project Leader, NYC-RAND Institute, New York, New York.

PAUL J. GLACKMAN, M.S., Research Assistant, Department of Industrial Engineering, The University of Wisconsin, Madison, Wisconsin.

JOHN H. GREIST, M.D., Assistant Professor, Department of Psychiatry, The University of Wisconsin, Madison, Wisconsin.

DAVID H. GUSTAFSON, Ph.D., Associate Professor, Departments of Industrial Engineering and Preventive Medicine, The University of Wisconsin, Madison, Wisconsin.

JOHN A. JACQUEZ, M.D., Professor, Department of Physiology, The Medical School, and Associate Professor, Department of Biostatistics, The School of Public Health, The University of Michigan, Ann Arbor, Michigan.

BENJAMIN KLEINMUNTZ, Ph.D., Professor, Department of Psychology, Carnegie-Mellon University, Pittsburgh, Pennsylvania.

FRANK C. LARSON, M.D., Professor, Departments of Medicine and Pathology, Director of Clinical Laboratories, University Hospital, University of Wisconsin, Madison, Wisconsin.

ROBERT S. LEDLEY, M.A., D.D.S., President, National Biomedical Research Foundation, Georgetown University Medical Center, Washington, D.C.

MARTIN LIPKIN, M.D., Associate Professor of Medicine, Cornell University Medical College, New York City, New York.

ROBERT L. LUDKE, M.S., Research Assistant, Department of Industrial Engineering, The University of Wisconsin, Madison, Wisconsin.

LEE B. LUSTED, M.D., Professor, Department of Radiology, The University of Chicago, Chicago, Illinois.

JOHN E. OVERALL, Ph.D., Research Professor, Department of Neurology and Psychiatry, The University of Texas Medical Branch, Galveston, Texas.

HUBERT V. PIPBERGER, M.D., Professor of Medicine and Clinical Engineering, George Washington University, Washington, D.C.; Chief, Veterans Administration Research Center for Cardiovascular Data Processing, VA Hospital, Washington, D.C.

JUDITH M. S. PREWITT, M.S., M.A., Mathematician, Division of Computer Research and Technology, National Institutes of Health, Bethesda, Maryland.

T. ALLEN PRYOR, M.S., Department of Biophysics and Bioengineering, Latter-Day Saints Hospital, Salt Lake City, Utah.

LEONARD J. SAVAGE, Professor, Department of Statistics, Yale University, New Haven, Connecticut.

WARNER V. SLACK, M.D., Department of Medicine, Beth Israel Hospital, Boston, Massachusetts.

JOHN A. SWETS, Ph.D., Senior Vice President, General Manager of Research, Development, and Consulting, Bolt Beranek and Newman Inc., Cambridge, Massachusetts.

HOMER R. WARNER, M.D., Ph.D., Department of Biophysics and Bioengineering, Latter-day Saints Hospital, Salt Lake City, Utah.

JACK ZLOTNICK, Analytic Services Inc., Falls Church, Virginia.

# PREFACE

THE FIRST UNIVERSITY of Michigan conference on the Diagnostic Process was held at the Medical School of the University of Michigan in 1963. At that time many were excited about the possible applications of computers in diagnosis and medical data processing. It seemed to me that the constellation of problems and activities involved in medical diagnosis deserved attention as aspects of one overall activity, the diagnostic process, and that it was important whether or not computers were involved. Important activities in the diagnostic process include the classification of disease, study of significance of the history, the physical, and of specific signs and symptoms in diagnosis, the medical record and its importance for management of a patient, the study of how individual physicians diagnose disease, comparative studies of the performance of different formulae for diagnosis and of course computer-assisted diagnosis. That first conference was small and the discussion was lively. It was an exciting time. Computers were bringing many changes to the sciences and their technologies, and there was every reason to expect similar changes in medicine and particularly in hospital operations. So we were concerned with defining the major problems and pointing the way to future research. But our American society was approaching that peak of assertive self-confidence that is as much the fruit of previous accomplishments as it is a measure of present power. The weaknesses that became apparent in our social fabric in the following few years have influenced both our investment in research and development and our views of the role of computers.

There have been many changes since that conference. Computing has matured as a science and a profession and the helter-skelter growth of the early years is past. There have been advances in statistical methodology and more importantly the views and philosophy of the Bayesians and subjective probabilists have gained greatly. We have accumulated quite a few experiences in the application of algorithmic methods of diagnosis and in particular Bayes' Theorem and the methods of multiple regression have been tried with a number of medical data bases. More importantly, with the rapid changes in our society, the traditional patterns of delivery of medical care are showing strains and all indications are that the near future will see some marked changes in these patterns. All of the pressures are in the direction of centralization, toward larger group practices and the operation of group health systems, and away from the practice of medicine by individual physicians and even small groups. This and the increasing cost of medical services may well lead to more need for computer-based medical information systems that include computer-assisted patient interviewing and computer-assisted screening and diagnosis. The second University of Michigan conference on the diagnostic process was organized to review the present status of algorithmic methods of diagnosis and the role of computer assisted diagnosis in patient management. This publication will hopefully play the role of a status report and of a forecast of things to come.

The organization of this conference owes much to the encouragement and prodding of Dr. Helen Gee, Scientist-Administrator of the Computer Research Study Section of the National Institutes of Health. My friends and colleagues on the Computer Research Study Section helped choose topics and speakers for the meeting and many attended the conference and enlivened the discussions. I particularly want to thank the chairmen of the different sessions, Drs. John Romano, Arnold W. Pratt, Allen Newell, Eugene Ackerman, Donald A. B. Lindberg, and Mortimer Mendelsohn for their efforts. The discussions were often spirited and long and were particularly appreciated by the graduate students from the University of Michigan who attended the conference. It is unfortunate that discussions could not be included in the present volume. The papers in this volume are in the order in which they were presented. However, three talks are missing because the speakers did not submit manuscripts and Dr. Ledley could not present his paper at the conference because of illness.

The running of a conference involves many people and many chores that must be done. I want to thank the National Institutes of Health which provided partial support for this conference through a grant, GM 17630. I owe a special thanks to my secretaries, Mrs. Dorothy Erby and Mrs. Dorothy Koeff. Mrs. Erby played a significant role in the organization and actual running of the conference, Mrs. Koeff in the preparation of manuscripts for publication. The Department of Postgraduate Medicine at the University of Michigan provided facilities and staff for the actual running of the conference. Finally I want to thank Mrs. Betty Woodward of Charles C Thomas, Publisher, whose editorial skill and patience helped me through the process of publication.

Professor Savage died on November 1, 1971 while this book was in press. He played a major role in laying the foundations of modern Subjective Probability and in promoting the Bayesian viewpoint in general. His paper and his searching comments during the discussions contributed greatly to the success of this conference. We will miss him.

JOHN A. JACQUEZ

# CONTENTS

# COMPUTER DIAGNOSIS
## AND
# DIAGNOSTIC METHODS

# Chapter 1

# PATIENT POWER: A PATIENT-ORIENTED VALUE SYSTEM*

WARNER V. SLACK

A GREAT DEAL OF TIME and effort has been devoted to the study of the diagnostic process, but the value system, which provides direction for the process, has been largely ignored. What there is in the way of a value system in the clinical transaction is physician-oriented. It is generally assumed that patients agree with their doctors on what would be good and bad outcomes of the transaction (and that if they do not agree, they ought to), and that medical decisions—loaded as they are with value judgments—are rightfully the responsibility of the physician. The "Golden Rule" has been the primary philosophy in clinical medicine, with physicians caring for patients as they themselves would want to be cared for. Actually, of course, people vary in how they evaluate the good and bad of matters related to their health, and I think that the set of values of the individual patient (not of the doctor) should direct the clinical process. The Golden Rule philosophy works for the patient only when the values of the doctor coincide with those of the patient. The patient is in danger of being treated unfairly whenever his values are contrary to those of his physician. Sometimes, of course, there is communication of values between patient and doctor, with the latter respecting and operating on the basis of his patient's values. The stubborn patient can refuse to yield to the dictates of his doctor—signing out of the hospital "against medical advice" is an example of such behavior. But generally, with the major decisions in clinical medicine, the doctor's values prevail whether

* Supported in part by U. S. Public Health Service research grants RR–00249–05 and HS–00283–03.

or not they coincide with those of his patient, and the "good" patient is the one who acquiesces.

A component of the value system directing the traditional diagnostic process (particularly in academic situations) has been what Bross [1] calls the "doctrine of scientific optimism": empirical discovery (in this instance, to find out what the medical problem is) necessarily leads to good for people. Doctors are highly motivated to make a diagnosis, and this is often pursued without consideration for the wants of the patient. And at least sometimes, doctors are more optimistic about diagnostic discovery in others than they would be in themselves.

How then can it be made certain that what is good for the patient in his own opinion is in fact what directs the diagnostic process? The answer is to separate medical decisions based on values from those based on medical expertise and have patients make the former and doctors make the latter. If the patient is incapable of making value judgments (because he is too young or too sick), the person closest to the patient or most familiar with his values should decide. Certainly it should be the patient's right to abdicate his decision-making responsibility to whomever he pleases. In emergency situations, of course, the doctor might have to act on the basis of his own values.

Traditionally, the patient does make the first (and sometimes diagnostically the most difficult) decision—that is, when to go to a doctor. But subsequently, his decision-making opportunities are limited. Questions pertaining to the medical history are asked, the physical examination and laboratory tests are performed, and treatment is initiated, all on a "doctor-knows-best" basis. The approach I am advocating is to have the physician work in a partnership with the patient. In a step-by-step manner, advancing through the diagnostic process, the physician will communicate possible plans of action, and the patient will decide what should be done. Possible medical procedures will be presented to the patient together with the following information: if the action is taken, the likelihood of discovery of medical problems and, in turn, of the possibility of altering these problems; the likelihood of pain (with estimated severity), incapacitation (with estimated degree and duration) and death; and financial burden (with estimated costs being presented). In addition, the chance of problems progressing because of lack of detection and treatment, if the action is *not* taken, will be communicated to the patient together with whatever ignorance there is about outcomes of the action. The patient will apply his value judgments to the information and thereby direct the medical process. The medical chart, traditionally closed to the patient, will be declassified at last and become a document developed jointly by patient and doctor.

The history of the present illness, the review of systems by interview, the components of the physical examination, the diagnostic laboratory procedures and the various available therapeutic approaches will all be treated as medical actions with the physician providing expert information about them, and the patient, on the basis of his own values, judging which actions will be taken. For example, the patient might decide against the review-of-systems interview after weighing the importance of his time against what is known of the actual medical yield of the routine review of systems. Again, the patient might decide to undergo a general physical examination for the possible detection of unexpected abnormalities but decide against a rectal examination because the net gain expected would not be worth the discomfort. A decision as complex as whether or not to have surgery would involve evaluation by the patient of each of the possible outcomes of the procedure. Actually, this sort of breakdown of the diagnostic process with a step-by-step evaluation of what is being done would be helpful no matter whose value system is being used. All too often in medicine, major clinical decisions are made without consideration of the many value judgments involved.

Rogers [2] has developed a "client centered" approach in psychotherapy. Implementation of the patient-oriented value system in general medicine will be difficult, but it can be done. Doctors will have to analyze and communicate more about what is known and not known regarding the outcomes of medical procedures, and patients in turn will have to assume the responsibility for the direction of their health care. Patients will *not* have to learn clinical medicine but they will have to know what to expect from the various plans of action offered by the doctor.

The process will be more time-consuming than when the physician is the sole or primary decision-maker—a disadvantage in these days of physician shortage. But the computer could be helpful here. Experience has been gained over the past five years with the use of computers programmed to interact with patients for the purpose of conducting medical interviews.[3-7] Programmed to branch to new question or statement frames contingent upon responses to current frames, the computer can model the physician in obtaining history data in detail and in exerting control over the interviewing process. Standardization (with responses in computer-processable form, available for use in patient care and research analysis) and economy of physicians' time are advantages of this technic. A reasonable extension of this patient-machine interaction would be the development of programs that present medical options to patients en route through the interview (together with the likelihood of various outcomes) and have the patient provide the direction.

When possible, the patient's value judgments should be made in the context of the clinical transaction. It might be argued that because the noncompliance of patients with physicians' "orders" is so common in traditional medicine, patients would fail to comply with the medical regimens they had decided upon for themselves. However, there is evidence from the work of "self-help" groups (for example, Alcoholics Anonymous) and experience with reinforcement technics with teenage delinquents [8] to support the contention that behavior change is more probable when the decision to change is the responsibility of the person involved and not that of an authority figure—the doctor. Adherence to a pill-taking routine, for example, might be more probable if, after judging the facts, the patient instead of the doctor had made the decision about the medication.

It is possible, however, that with complex decisions, patients will need assistance in generating optimum strategy. A computer-based decision-maker—provided with the patient's values—could be helpful in such a situation. Under these circumstances the patient would initially be interviewed in detail about his values, which would be applied subsequently to the decision-making process. The use of values in the analysis of clinical decision-making has been reported.[9]

The patient's role, like that of the doctor's, is a learned one; part of this role has been to accept without argument the value judgments of physicians. That many patients seem to want doctors to make decisions for them is, I think, a function of conditioning. However, reliance on doctors can be unlearned, and, in my opinion, the resulting self-reliance would eventually add considerable dignity to the patient role. In fact, it might well be that the hostility so commonly directed by laymen to organized medicine as a whole results from the subservience of the role assumed by individual laymen as patients.

## REFERENCES

1. Bross, I. D. F.: *Design for Decision*. New York, The Macmillan Company, 1963.
2. Rogers, C.: *Client Centered Therapy*. Boston, Houghton-Mifflin, 1951.
3. Slack, W. V.; Hicks, G. P.; Reed, C. E.; *et al.*: A computer-based medical history system. *N Engl J Med, 274:*194–198, 1966.
4. Mayne, J. G.; Weksel, W.; Sholtz, P. N.: Toward automating the medical history. *Mayo Clin Proc, 43:*1, 1968.
5. Slack, W. V.: Medical interviewing by computer. *South Med Bull, 57:*39–44, 1969.
6. Grossman, J.; Barnett, G. O.; Swedlow, D.: The collection of medical history data using a real-time computer system. *Proc Conf Eng Med Biol, 10:*39.1, 1968.
7. Slack, W. V.; Van Cura, L. J.: Patient reaction to computer-based medical interviewing. *Comput Biomed Res, 1:*527, 1968.
8. Slack, C. W.: Experimenter-subject psychotherapy: a new method of introducing intensive office treatment for unreachable cases. *Ment Hyg, 44:*238–256, 1960.
9. Ginsberg, A. S.: Decision analysis in clinical patient management with an application to the pleural effusion problem. Ph.D. thesis in Industrial Engineering, Stanford University, 1969.

## Chapter 2

# SIGNAL DETECTION IN MEDICAL DIAGNOSIS

### John A. Swets

A PHYSICIAN LOOKS FOR LESIONS, listens for murmurs, feels for masses. These activities fall under the heading of "detecting weak signals." My message here is that, as with most humans in most situations, the detection of a weak signal by a physician depends not only upon his *sensitivity* but also upon his *decision bias.*

The decision bias, in turn, depends upon the *subjective probability* of the signal in question and upon the *utilities* of the various possible decision outcomes. If, for example, several kinds of evidence suggest a certain disease, the physician is more likely to detect a particular signal if it is usually associated with that disease than if it is inconsistent with the mounting evidence. Probabilities being equal, a physician is more likely to detect a signal that indicates a very serious disease than one that indicates a trivial disorder.

In short, the physician looking for a symptom on the way to a diagnosis is faced with a decision problem like that posed by the larger issue of what diagnosis he should make. When the signal is weak, the matter is not so simple as either "seeing" it or "not seeing" it; rather the observer must assess his degree of confidence that the signal exists, and then make a judgment about whether to proceed as if the signal is there or not there. And when the sensory information is ambiguous, other kinds of information—like probabilities and utilities—naturally enters the picture.

Psychologists have been aware since psychology began of the operation of some judgmental factor in detection, but it was less than 20 years ago that statisticians showed them what to do about it. The theory of statistical decision provides a means of separating the effects of sensory and decision processes, and a technique for measuring the two variables independently. To be fair to history, I should add that psychologists became aware of the relevance of decision theory to detection while working with engineers interested in electronic detectors.

An earlier article [3] presented an introduction to detection-viewed-as-a-decision-process that is appropriate for this volume, and the following sections of this paper reproduce that introduction. Two books published since [2,4] may be consulted for a large body of data that supports this conception of human signal detection. A categorized list of references at the conclusion of this paper gives many of the more important articles of the past few years; the articles selected for citation under each category are those related to signal detection in medical diagnosis.

## STATISTICAL DECISION THEORY

Consider the following game of chance. Three dice are thrown. Two of the dice are ordinary dice. The third die is unusual in that on each of three of its sides it has three spots, whereas on its remaining three sides it has no spots at all. You, as the player of the game, do not observe the throws of the dice. You are simply informed, after each throw, of the total number of spots showing on the three dice. You are then asked to state whether the third die, the unusual one, showed a 3 or a 0. If you are correct—that is, if you assert a 3 showed when it did in fact, or if you assert a 0 showed when it did in fact—you win a dollar. If you are incorrect —that is, if you make either of the two possible types of errors— you lose a dollar.

How do you play the game? Certainly you will want a few minutes to make some computations before you begin. You will want to know the probability of occurrence of each of the possible totals 2 through 12 in the event that the third die shows a 0, and you will want to know the probability of occurrence of each of the possible totals 5 through 15 in the event that the third die shows a 3. Let us ignore the exact values of these probabilities, and grant that the two probability distributions in question will look much like those sketched in Fig. 2–1.

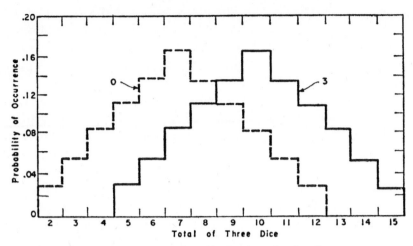

Figure 2–1. The probability distributions for the dice game.

Realizing that you will play the game many times, you will want to establish a policy which defines the circumstances under which you will make each of the two decisions. We can think of this as a *criterion* or a cutoff point along the axis representing the total number of spots showing on the three dice. That is, you will want to choose a number on this axis such that whenever it is equaled or exceeded you will state that a 3 showed on the third die, and such that whenever the total number of spots showing is less than this number, you will state that a 0 showed on the third die. For the game as described, with the a priori probabilities of a 3 and a 0 equal, and with equal values and costs associated with the four possible decision outcomes, it is intuitively clear that the optimal cutoff point is that point where the two curves cross. You will maximize your winnings if you choose this point as the cutoff point and adhere to it.

Now, what if the game is changed? What, for example, if the third die has three spots on five of its sides, and a 0 on only one? Certainly you will now be more willing to state, following each throw, that the third die showed a 3. You will not, however, simply state more often that a 3 occurred without regard to the total showing on the three dice. Rather, you will lower your cutoff point: you will accept a smaller total than before as representing a throw in which the third die showed a 3. Conversely, if the third die has three spots on only one of its sides and 0's on five sides, you will do well to raise your cutoff point—to require a higher total than before for stating that a 3 occurred.

Similarly, your behavior will change if the values and costs associated with the various decision outcomes are changed. If it costs you five dollars every time you state that a 3 showed when in fact it did not, and if you win five dollars every time you state that a 0 showed when in fact it did (the other value and the other cost in the game remaining at one dollar), you will raise your cutoff to a point somewhere above the point where the two distributions cross. Or if, instead, the premium is placed on being correct when a 3 occurred, rather than when a 0 occurred as in the immediately preceding example, you will assume a cutoff somewhere below the point where the two distributions cross.

Again, your behavior will change if the amount of overlap of the two distributions is changed. You will assume a different cutoff than you did in the game as first described if the three sides of the third die showing spots now show four spots rather than three.

This game is simply an example of the type of situation for which the theory of statistical decision was developed. It is intended only to recall the frame of reference of this theory. Statistical decision theory—or the special case of it which is relevant here, the theory of testing statistical hypotheses—specifies the optimal behavior in a situation where one must choose between two alternative statistical hypotheses on the basis of an observed event. In particular, it specifies the optimal cutoff, along the continuum on which the observed events are arranged, as a function of (*a*) the a priori probabilities of the two hypotheses, (*b*) the values and costs associated with the various decision outcomes, and (*c*) the amount of overlap of the distributions that constitute the hypotheses.

According to the mathematical theory of signal detectability, the problem of detecting signals that are weak relative to the background of interference is like the one faced by the player of our dice game. In short, the detection problem is a problem in statistical decision; it requires testing statistical hypotheses. In the theory of signal detectability, this analogy is developed in terms of an idealized observer. It is our thesis that this conception of the detection process may apply to the human observer as well. The next several pages present an analysis of the detection process that will make the bases for this reasoning apparent.

## FUNDAMENTAL DETECTION PROBLEM

In the fundamental detection problem, an observation is made of events occurring in a fixed interval of time, and a decision is made, based on this observation, whether the interval contained only the background interference or a signal as well. The interference, which is random, we shall refer to as *noise* and denote as *N;* the other alternative we shall term *signal plus noise, SN.* In the fundamental problem, only these two alternatives exist— noise is always present, whereas the signal may or may not be present during a specified observation interval. Actually, the observer, who has advance knowledge of the ensemble of signals to be presented, says either "yes, a signal was present" or "no, no signal was present" following each observation. It is important to note that the signal is always observed in a background of noise; some may be introduced by the experimenter or by the external situation, but some is inherent in the sensory processes.

## REPRESENTATION OF SENSORY INFORMATION

We shall, in the following, use the term *observation* to refer to the sensory datum on which the decision is based. We assume that this observation may be represented as varying continuously along a single dimension. Although there is no need to be concrete, it may be helpful to think of the observation as some measure of neural activity, perhaps as the number of impulses arriving at a given point in the cortex within a given time. We assume further that any observation may arise, with specific probabilities either from noise alone or from signal plus noise. We may portray these assumptions graphically, for a signal of a given amplitude, as in Fig. 2–2. The observation is labeled $x$ and plotted on the abscissa. The left-hand distribution, labeled $f_N(x)$, represents the probability density that $x$ will result given the occurrence of noise alone. The right-hand distribution, $f_{SN}(x)$, is the probability density function of $x$ given the occurrence of signal plus noise.

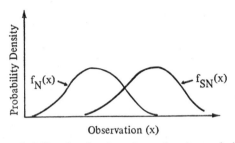

Figure 2–2. The probability density functions of noise and signal plus noise.

(Probability density functions are used, rather than probability functions, since $x$ is assumed to be continuous.) Since the observations will tend to be of greater magnitude when a signal is presented, the mean of the *SN* distribution will be greater than the mean of the *N* distribution. In general, the greater the amplitude of the signal, the greater will be the separation of these means.

## OBSERVATION AS A VALUE OF LIKELIHOOD RATIO

It will be well to question at this point our assumption that the observation may be represented along a single axis. Can we, without serious violation, regard the observation as unidimensional, in spite of the fact that the response of the visual system probably has many dimensions? The answer to this question will involve some concepts that are basic to the theory.

One reasonable answer is that when the signal and interference are alike in character, only the magnitude of the total response of the receiving system is available as an indicator of signal existence. Consequently, no matter how complex the sensory information is in fact, the observations may be represented in theory as having a single dimension. Although this answer is quite acceptable when concerned only with the visual case, we prefer to advance a different answer, one that is applicable also to audition experiments, where, for example, the signal may be a segment of a sinusoid presented in a background of white noise.

So let us assume that the response of the sensory system does have several dimensions, and proceed to represent it as a point in an $m$-dimensional space. Call this point $y$. For every such point in this space there is some probability density that it resulted from noise alone, $f_N(y)$, and, similarly, some probability density that it was due to signal plus noise, $f_{SN}(y)$. Therefore, there exists a likelihood ratio for each point in the space, $\lambda(y) = f_{SN}(y) / f_N(y)$, expressing the likelihood that the point $y$ arose from $SN$ relative to the likelihood that it arose from $N$. Since any point in the space, *i.e.*, any sensory datum, may be thus represented as a real, nonzero number, these points may be considered to lie along a single axis. We may then, if we choose, identify the observation $x$ with $\lambda(y)$; the decision axis becomes likelihood ratio.*

Having established that we may identify the observation $x$ with $\lambda(y)$, let us note that we may equally well identify $x$ with any monotonic transformation of $\lambda(y)$. It can be shown that we lose nothing by distorting the linear continuum as long as order is maintained. As a matter of fact we may gain if, in particular, we identify $x$ with some transformation of $\lambda(y)$ that results in Gaussian density functions on $x$. We have assumed the existence of such a transformation in the representation of the density functions, $f_{SN}(x)$ and $f_N(x)$, in Fig. 2–2. We shall see shortly that the assumption of normality simplifies the problem greatly. A further assumption incorporated into the picture of Fig. 2–2, one made quite tentatively, is that the two density functions are of equal variance. This is equivalent to the assumption that the $SN$ function is a simple translation of the $N$ function, or that adding a signal to the noise merely adds a constant to the $N$ function. Both the Gaussian and equal variance assumptions are subject to experimental test.

To summarize the last few paragraphs, we have assumed that an observation may be characterized by a value of likelihood ratio, $\lambda(y)$, i.e. the likelihood that the response of the sensory system $y$ arose from $SN$ relative to the likelihood that it arose from $N$. This permits us to view the observations as lying along a single axis. We then assumed the existence of a particular transformation of $\lambda(y)$ such that on the resulting variable, $x$, the density functions

---

* Thus the assumption of a unidimensional decision axis is independent of the character of the signal and noise. Rather, it depends upon the fact that just two decision alternatives are considered. More generally, it can be shown that the number of dimensions required to represent the observation is $M-1$, where $M$ is the number of decision alternatives considered by the observer.

are normal. We regard the observer as basing his decisions on the variable $x$.

## DEFINITION OF THE CRITERION

If the representation depicted in Fig. 2–2 is realistic, then the problem posed for an observer attempting to detect signals in noise is indeed similar to the one faced by the player of our dice game. On the basis of an observation, one that varies only in magnitude, he must decide between two alternative hypotheses. He must decide from which hypothesis the observation resulted; he must state that the observation is a member of the one distribution or the other. As did the player of the dice game, the observer must establish a policy that defines the circumstances under which the observation will be regarded as resulting from each of the two possible events. He establishes a criterion, a cutoff $x_c$ on the continuum of observations, to which he can relate any given observation $x_i$. If he finds for the $i$th observation, $x_i$, that $x_i > x_c$, he says "yes"; if $x_i < x_c$, he says "no." Since the observer is assumed to be capable of locating a criterion at any point along the continuum of observations, it is of interest to examine the various factors that, according to the theory, will influence his choice of a particular criterion. To do so requires some additional notation.

In the language of statistical decision theory the observer chooses a subset of all of the observations, namely the Critical Region $A$, such that an observation in this subset leads him to accept the Hypothesis $SN$, to say that a signal was present. All other observations are in the complementary Subset $B$; these lead to rejection of the Hypothesis $SN$, or, equivalently, since the two hypotheses are mutually exclusive and exhaustive, to the acceptance of the Hypothesis $N$. The Critical Region $A$, with reference to Fig. 2–2, consists of the values of $x$ to the right of some criterion value $x_c$.

As in the case of the dice game, a decision will have one of four outcomes: the observer may say "yes" or "no" and may in either case be *correct* or *incorrect*. The decision outcome, in other words, may be a *hit* $(SN \cdot A$, the joint occurrence of the Hypothesis $SN$ and an observation in the Region $A)$, a *miss* $(SN \cdot B)$, a *correct rejection* $(N \cdot B)$, or a *false alarm* $(N \cdot A)$. If the a priori probability of signal occurrence and the parameters of the distributions of Fig. 2–2 are fixed, the choice of a criterion value $x_c$ completely determines the probability of each of these outcomes.

Clearly, the four probabilities are interdependent. For example, an increase in the probability of a hit, $p(SN \cdot A)$, can be achieved only by accepting an increase in the probability of a false alarm, $p(N \cdot A)$, and decreases in the other probabilities, $p(SN \cdot B)$ and $p(N \cdot B)$. Thus a given criterion yields a particular balance among the probabilities of the four possible outcomes; conversely, the balance desired by an observer in any instance will determine the optimal location of his criterion. Now the observer may desire the balance that maximizes the expected value of a decision in a situation where the four possible outcomes of a decision have individual values, as did the player of the dice game. In this case, the location of the best criterion is determined by the same parameters that determined it in the dice game. The observer, however, may desire a balance that maximizes some other quantity —i.e., a balance that is optimum according to some other definition of optimum—in which case a different criterion will be appropriate. He may, for example, want to maximize $p(SN \cdot A)$ while satisfying a restriction on $p(N \cdot A)$, as we typically do when as experimenters we assume an .05 or .01 level of confidence. Alternatively, he may want to maximize the number of correct decisions. Again, he may prefer a criterion that will maximize the reduction in uncertainty.

In statistical decision theory, and in the theory of signal detectability, the optimal criterion under each of these definitions of optimum is specified in terms of the likelihood ratio. That is to say, it can be shown that, if we define the observation in terms of the likelihood ratio, $\lambda(x) = f_{SN}(x) / f_N(x)$, then the optimal criterion can always be specified by some value $\beta$ of $\lambda(x)$. In other words, the Critical Region $A$ that corresponds to the criterion contains all observations with likelihood ratio greater than or equal to $\beta$, and none of those with likelihood ratio less than $\beta$.

We shall illustrate this manner of specifying the optimal criterion for just one of the definitions of optimum proposed above, namely, the maximization of the total expected value of a decision in a situation where the four possible outcomes of a decision have individual values associated with them. This is the definition of optimum that we assumed in the dice game. For this purpose we shall need the concept of *conditional probability* as opposed to the *probability of joint occurrence* introduced above. It should be stated that conditional probabilities will have a place in our discussion beyond their use in this illustration; the ones we shall introduce are, as a matter of fact, the fundamental quantities in evaluating the observer's performance.

There are two conditional probabilities of principal interest. These are the conditional probabilities of the observer saying "yes": $p_{SN}(A)$, the probability of a Yes decision *conditional upon*, or *given*, the occurrence of a signal, and $p_N(A)$, the probability of a Yes decision given the occurrence of noise alone. These two are sufficient, for the other two are simply their complements: $p_{SN}(B) = 1 - p_{SN}(A)$ and $p_N(B) = 1 - p_N(A)$. The conditional and joint probabilities are related as follows:

$$p_{SN}(A) = \frac{p(SN \cdot A)}{p(SN)}$$

$$p_N(A) = \frac{p(N \cdot A)}{p(N)} \tag{1}$$

where: $p(SN)$ is the a priori probability of signal occurrence and $p(N) = 1 - p(SN)$ is the a priori probability of occurrence of noise alone.

Equation 1 makes apparent the convenience of using conditional rather than joint probabilities—conditional probabilities are independent of the a priori probability of occurrence of the signal and of noise alone. With reference to Fig. 2–2, we may define $p_{SN}(A)$, or the conditional probability of a hit, as the integral of $f_{SN}(x)$ over the Critical Region $A$, and $p_N(A)$, the conditional probability of a false alarm, as the integral of $f_N(x)$ over $A$. That is, $p_N(A)$ and $p_{SN}(A)$ represent, respectively, the areas under the two curves of Fig. 2–2 to the right of some criterion value of $x$.

To pursue our illustration of how an optimal criterion may be specified by a critical value of likelihood ratio $\beta$, let us note that the expected value of a decision (denoted $EV$) is defined in statistical decision theory as the sum, over the potential outcomes of a decision, of the products of probability of outcome and the desirability of outcome. Thus, using the notation $V$ for *positive* individual values and $K$ for costs or *negative* individual values, we have the following equation:

$$EV = V_{SN \cdot A}p(SN \cdot A) + V_{N \cdot B}p(N \cdot B) \\ - K_{SN \cdot B}p(SN \cdot B) - K_{N \cdot A}p(N \cdot A) \qquad (2)$$

Now if a priori and conditional probabilities are substituted for the joint probabilities in Equation 2 following Equation 1, for example, $p(SN)p_{SN}(A)$ *for* $p(SN \cdot A)$, then collecting terms yields the result that maximizing $EV$ is equivalent to maximizing:

$$p_{SN}(A) - \beta p_N(A) \qquad (3)$$

where

$$\beta = \frac{p(N)}{p(SN)} \cdot \frac{(V_{N \cdot B} + K_{N \cdot A})}{(V_{SN \cdot A} + K_{SN \cdot B})} \qquad (4)$$

It can be shown that this value of $\beta$ is equal to the value of likelihood ratio, $\lambda(x)$, that corresponds to the optimal criterion. From Equation 3 it may be seen that the value $\beta$ simply weights the hits and false alarms, and from Equation 4 we see that $\beta$ is determined by the a priori probabilities of occurrence of signal and of noise alone and by the values associated with the individual decision outcomes. It should be noted that Equation 3 applies to all definitions of optimum. Equation 4 shows the determinants of $\beta$ in only the special case of the expected-value definition of optimum.

Return for a moment to Fig. 2–2, keeping in mind the result that $\beta$ is a critical value of $\lambda(x) = f_{SN}(x) / f_N(x)$. It should be clear that the optimal cutoff $x_c$ along the $x$ axis is at the point on this axis where the ratio of the ordinate value of $f_{SN}(x)$ to the ordinate value of $f_N(x)$ is a certain number, namely $\beta$. In the symmetrical case, where the two a priori probabilities are equal and the four individual values are equal, $\beta = 1$ and the optimal value of $x_c$ is the point where $f_{SN}(x) = f_N(x)$, where the two curves cross. If the four values are equal but $p(SN) = 5/6$ and $p(N) = 1/6$, another case described in connection with the dice game, then $\beta = 1/5$ and the optimal value of $x_c$ is shifted a certain distance to the left. This shift may be seen intuitively to be in the proper direction —a higher value of $p(SN)$ should lead to a greater willingness to accept the Hypothesis *SN*, i.e. a more lenient cutoff. To consider one more example from the dice game, if $p(SN) = p(N)$ = 0.5, if $V_{N \cdot B}$ and $K_{N \cdot A}$ are set at five dollars and $V_{SN \cdot A}$ and $K_{SN \cdot B}$ are equal to one dollar, then $\beta = 5$ and the optimal value of $x_c$ shifts a certain distance to the right. Again intuitively, if it is more important to be correct when the Hypothesis *N* is true, a high, or strict, criterion should be adopted.

In any case, $\beta$ specifies the optimal weighting of hits relative to false alarms: $x_c$ should always be located at the point on the *x* axis corresponding to $\beta$. As we pointed out in discussing the dice game, just where this value of $x_c$ will be with reference to the *x* axis depends not only upon the a priori probabilities and the values but also upon the overlap of the two density functions, in short, upon the signal strength. We shall define a measure of signal strength within the next few pages. For now, it is important to note that for any detection goal to which the observer may subscribe, and for any set of parameters that may characterize a detection situation (such as a priori probabilities and values associated with decision outcomes), the optimal criterion may be specified in terms of a single number, $\beta$, a critical value of likelihood ratio.*

## RECEIVER OPERATING CHARACTERISTIC

Whatever criterion the observer actually uses, even if it is not one of the optimal criteria, can also be described by a single number, by some value of likelihood ratio. Let us proceed to a consideration of how the observer's performance may be evaluated with respect to the location of his criterion, and, at the same time we shall see how his performance may be evaluated with respect to his sensory capabilities.

As we have noted, the fundamental quantities in the evaluation

---

* We have reached a point in the discussion where we can justify the statement made earlier that the decision axis may be equally well regarded as likelihood ratio or as any monotonic transformation of likelihood ratio. Any distortion of the linear continuum of likelihood ratio, that maintains order, is equivalent to likelihood ratio in terms of determining a criterion. The decisions made are the same whether the criterion is set at likelihood ratio equal to $\beta$ or at the value that corresponds to $\beta$ of some new variable. To illustrate, if a criterion leads to a Yes response whenever $\lambda(y) > 2$, if $x = [\lambda(y)]^2$ the decisions will be the same if the observer says "yes" whenever $x > 4$.

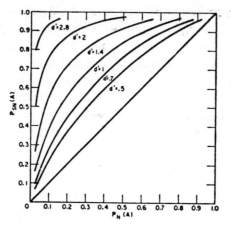

Figure 2–3. The receiver-operating-characteristic curves. (These curves show $P_{SN}(A)$ vs $P_N(A)$ with d' as the parameter. They are based on the assumptions that the probability density functions, $f_N(x)$ and $f_{SN}(x)$, are normal and of equal variance.)

of performance are $p_N(A)$ and $p_{SN}(A)$, these quantities representing, respectively, the areas under the two curves of Fig. 2–2 to the right of some criterion value of x. If we set up a graph of $p_{SN}(A)$ versus $p_N(A)$ and trace on it the curve resulting as we move the decision criterion along the decision axis of Fig. 2–2, we sketch one of the arcs shown in Fig. 2–3. Ignore, for a moment, all but one of these arcs. If the decision criterion is set way at the left in Fig. 2–2, we obtain a point in the upper right-hand corner of Fig. 2–3: both $p_{SN}(A)$ and $p_N(A)$ are unity. If the criterion is set at the right end of the decision axis in Fig. 2–2, the point at the other extreme of Fig. 2–3, $p_{SN}(A) = p_N(A) = 0$, is obtained. In between these extremes lie the criterion values of more practical interest. It should be noted that the exact form of the curve shown in Fig. 2–3 is not the only form which might result, but it is the form which will result if the observer chooses a criterion in terms of likelihood ratio, and the probability density functions are normal and of equal variance.

This curve is a form of the *operating characteristic* as it is known in statistics; in the context of the detection problem it is usually referred to as the *receiver operating characteristic,* or ROC, curve. The optimal "operating level" may be seen from

Equation 3 to be at the point of the ROC curve where its slope is $\beta$. That is, the expression $p_{SN}(A) - \beta p_N(A)$ defines a utility line of slope $\beta$, and the point of tangency of this line to the ROC curve is the optimal operating level. Thus the theory specifies the appropriate hit probability and false alarm probability for any definition of optimum and any set of parameters characterizing the detection situation.

It is now apparent how the observer's choice of a criterion in a given experiment may be indexed. The proportions obtained in an experiment are used as estimates of the probabilities, $p_N(A)$ and $p_{SN}(A)$; thus, the observer's behavior yields a point on an ROC curve. The slope of the curve at this point corresponds to the value of likelihood ratio at which he has located his criterion. Thus we work backward from the ROC curve to infer the criterion that is employed by the observer.

There is, of course, a family of ROC curves, as shown in Fig. 2–3, a given curve corresponding to a given separation between the means of the density functions $f_N(x)$ and $f_{SN}(x)$. The parameter of these curves has been called $d'$, where $d'$ is defined as the difference between the means of the two density functions expressed in terms of their standard deviation, i.e.:

$$d' = \frac{M_{f_{SN}(x)} - M_{f_N(x)}}{\sigma_{f_N(x)}} \tag{5}$$

Since the separation between the means of the two density functions is a function of signal amplitude, $d'$ is an index of the detectability of a given signal for a given observer.

Recalling our assumptions that the density functions $f_N(x)$ and $f_{SN}(x)$ are normal and of equal variance, we may see from Equation 5 that the quantity denoted $d'$ is simply the familiar normal deviate, or $x/\sigma$ measure. From the pair of values $p_N(A)$ and $p_{SN}(A)$ that are obtained experimentally, one may proceed to a published table of areas under the normal curve to determine a value of $d'$. A simpler computational procedure is achieved by plotting the points $[p_N(A), p_{SN}(A)]$ on graph paper having a probability scale and a normal deviate scale on both axes.

We see now that the four-fold table of the responses that are made to a particular stimulus may be treated as having two independent parameters—the experiment yields measures of two independent aspects of the observer's performance. The variable $d'$ is a measure of the observer's sensory capabilities, or of the effective signal strength. This may be thought of as the object of interest in classical psychophysics. The criterion $\beta$ that is employed by the observer, which determines the $p_N(A)$ and $p_{SN}(A)$ for some fixed $d'$, reflects the effect of variables which have been variously called the set, attitude, or motives of the observer. It is the ability to distinguish between these two aspects of detection performance that comprises one of the main advantages of the theory proposed here. These two aspects of behavior are confounded in an experiment in which the dependent variable is the intensity of the signal that is required for a threshold response.

## REFERENCES

**General Survey**

1. Green, D. M.: Application of detection theory in psychophysics. *Proc IEEE, 58*:713–723, 1970.
2. Green, D. M. and Swets, J. A.: *Signal Detection Theory and Psychophysics.* New York, Wiley, 1966.
3. Swets, J. A.; Tanner, W. P., Jr.; and Birdsall, T. G.: Decision processes in perception. *Psychol Rev, 68*:301–340, 1961.
4. Swets, J. A. (Ed.): *Signal Detection and Recognition by Human Observers.* New York, Wiley, 1964.
5. Swets, J. A.: Theory of signal detection in psychology. In *Encyclopedia of Science and Technology.* New York, McGraw-Hill, 1971, pp. 354–355.

**Medical Diagnosis**

6. Kundel, H. L.; Revesz, G.; and Stauffer, H. M.: The electro-optical processing of radiographic images. *Radiol Clin North Am, 3*:447–460, 1969.
7. Ling, D.; Ling, A. H.; and Doehring, D. G.: Stimulus, response, and observer variables in the auditory screening of newborn infants. *J Speech Hear Res, 13*:9–18, 1970.
8. Lusted, L. B.: *Introduction to Medical Decision Making.* Springfield, Thomas, 1968.
9. Lusted, L. B.: Perception of the roentgen image: applications of signal detectability theory. *Radiol Clin North Am, 3*:435–445, 1969.
10. Lusted, L. B.: Signal detectability and medical decision-making. *Science, 171*:1217–1219, 1971.

11. Lusted, L. B.: Decision-making studies in patient management. *N Engl J Med, 284*:416–424, 1971.

## Methods and Measures

12. Abrahamson, I. G. and Levitt, H.: Statistical analysis of data from experiments in human signal detection. *J Math Psychol, 6*:391–417, 1969.
13. Dorosh, M. E.; Tong, J. E.; and Boissonneault, D. R.: White noise, instructions, and two-flash fusion with two signal-detection procedures. *Psychonal Sci, 20*:98–99, 1970.
14. Nachmias, J.: Effects of presentation probability and number of response alternatives on simple visual detection. *Percept Psychophys, 3*:151–155, 1968.
15. Pollack, I. and Hsieh, R.: Sampling variability of the area under the ROC-curve and of $d'_e$. *Psychol Bull, 71*:161–173, 1969.
16. Shipley, E. F.: A signal detection theory analysis of a category judgment experiment. *Percept Psychophys, 7*:38–42, 1970.
17. Watson, C. S. and Clopton, B. M.: Motivated changes of auditory sensitivity in a simple detection task. *Percept Psychophys, 5*:281–287, 1969.

## Vision

18. Allan, L. G.: Visual position discrimination: A model relating temporal and spatial factors. *Percept Psychophys, 4*:267–278, 1968.
19. Baron, J.: Temporal ROC curves and the psychological moment. *Psyconal Sci, 15*:299–300, 1969.
20. Campbell, F. W.; Nachmias, J.; and Jukes, J.: Spatial-frequency discrimination in human vision. *J Opt Soc Am, 60*:555–559, (No. 4) 1970.
21. Glorioso, R. M. and Levy, R. M.: Operator behavior in a dynamic visual signal detection task. *Percept Psychophys, 4*:5–9, 1968.
22. Halpern, J. and Ulehla, J. Z.: The effect of multiple responses and certainty estimates on the integration of visual information. *Percept Psychophys, 7*:129–132, 1970.
23. Handel, S. and Christ, R. E.: Detection and identification of geometric forms using peripheral and central viewing. *Percept Psychophys, 6*: 47–49, 1969.
24. Keller, W. and Kinchla, R. A.: Visual movement discrimination. *Percept Psychophys, 3*:233–236, 1968.
25. Leshowitz, B.; Taub, H. B. and Raab, D. H.: Visual detection of signals in the presence of continuous and pulsed backgrounds. *Percept Psycophys, 4*:207–213, 1968.
26. Lowe, G.: Interval of time uncertainty in visual detection. *Percept Psychophys, 2*:278–280, 1967.
27. Nachmias, J. and Kocher, E. C.: Vision detection and discrimination of luminance increments. *J Opt Soc Am, 60*:382–389, 1970.

28. Thijssen, J. M.: *Differential Luminance Sensitivity of the Human Visual System*. Drukkerij Gebr. Janssen N. V., Nijmegen, 1969.
29. Ulehla, J. Z.; Halpern, J.; and Cerf, A.: Integration of information in a visual discrimination task. *Percept Psychophys, 4:*1–4, 1968.
30. White, M. J.: Signal-detection analysis of laterality differences: Some preliminary data, free of recall and report-sequence characteristics. *J Exp Psychol, 83:*174–176, 1970.
31. Wickelgren, W. A.: Strength theories of disjunctive visual detection. *Percept Phychophys, 2:*331–337, 1967.
32. Winnick, W. A. and Bruder, G. E.: Signal detection approach to the study of retinal locus in tachistoscopic recognition. *J Exp Psychol, 78:* 528–531, 1968.

### Audition

33. Henning, B. G.: Frequency discrimination in noise. *J Acoust Soc Am, 41:* 774–777, 1967.
34. Henning, B. G.: A model for auditory discrimination and detection. *J Acoust Soc Am, 42:*1325–1334, 1967.
35. Ronken, D. A.: Monaural detection of a phase difference between clicks. *J Acoust Soc Am, 47:*1091–1099, 1970.

### Vision and Audition

36. Fidell, S.: Sensory function in multimodal signal detection. *J Acoust Soc Am, 47:*1009–1015, 1970.
37. Gunn, W. J. and Loeb, M.: Correlation of performance in detecting visual and auditory signals. *Am J Psychol, 80:*236–242, 1966.
38. Kinchla, R. A.; Townsend, J.; Yellott, J. I., Jr. and Atkinson, R. C.: Influence of correlated visual cues on auditory signal detection. *Percept Psychophys, 1:*67–73, 1966.

### Minor Senses

39. Boyer, W. N.; Cross, H. A.; Guyot, G. W. and Washington, D. M.: A TSD determination of a DL using two-point tactual stimuli applied to the back. *Psychon Sci, 21:*195–196, 1970.
40. Cross, H. A.; Boyer, W. N. and Guyot, G. W.: Determination of a DL using two-point tactual stimuli: A signal-detection approach. *Psych Sci, 21:*198–199, 1970.
41. Gescheider, G. A.; Barton, G.; Bruce, M. R.; Goldberg, J. H. and Greenspan, M. J.: Effects of simultaneous auditory stimulation on the detection of tactile stimuli. *J Exp Psychol, 81:*120–125, 1969.
42. Rollman, G. B.: Detection models: Experimental tests with electrocutaneous stimuli. *Percept Psychophys, 5:*377–380, 1969.
43. Semb, G.: The detectability of the odor of butanol. *Percept Psychophys, 4:*335–340, 1969.

44. Steinmetz, G.; Pryor, G. T. and Stone, H.: Effect of blank samples on absolute odor threshold determinations. *Percept Psychophys, 6:*142–144, 1969.
45. Swets, J. A.; Markowitz, J. and Franzen, O.: Vibrotactile signal detection. *Percept Psychophys, 6:*83–88, 1969.

## Recognition

46. Alexander, L. T. and Cooperband, A. S.: Visual detection of compound motion. *J Exp Psychol, 71:*816–821, 1966.
47. Hershman, R. L. and Lichtenstein, M.: Detection and localization: An extension of the theory of signal detectability. *J Acoust Soc Am, 42:* 446–452, 1967.
48. Hershman, R. L. and Lichtenstein, M.: Signal detection and localization by real observers. *Percept Psychophys, 6:*53–57, 1969.
49. Lindner, W. A.: Recognition performance as a function of detection criterion in a simultaneous detection-recognition task. *J Acoust Soc Am, 44:*204–211, 1968.
50. Tanner, T. A., Jr.; Rauk, J. A.; and Atkinson, R. C.: Signal recognition as influenced by information feedback. *J Math Psychol, 2:*259–274, 1970.

## Reaction Time

51. Bindra, D.; Williams, J. A. and Wise, J. S.: Judgments of sameness and difference: Experiments on decision time. *Science, 150:*1625–1627, 1965.
52. Carterette, E. D.; Friedman, M. P. and Cosmides, R.: Reaction-time distributions in the detection of weak signals in noise. *J Acoust Soc Am, 38:*531–542, 1965.
53. Gescheider, G. A.; Wright, J. H. and Evans, M. B.: Reaction time in the detection of vibrotactile signals. *J Exp Psychol, 77:*501–504, 1968.
54. Gescheider, G. A.; Wright, J. H.; Weber, B. J.; Kirchner, B. M. and Milligan, E. A.: Reaction time as a function of the intensity and probability of occurrence of vibrotactile signals. *Percept Psychophys, 5:* 18–20, 1969.
55. Link, S. W. and Tindall, A. D.: Speed and accuracy in comparative judgments of line length. *Percept Psychophys, 9:*284–288, 1971.
56. Murray, H. G.: Stimulus intensity and reaction time: Evaluation of a decision-theory model. *J Exp Psychol, 84:*383–391, 1970.
57. Pachella, R. G. and Pew, R. W.: Speed-accuracy tradeoff in reaction time: Effect of discrete criterion times. *J Exp Psychol, 76:*19–24, 1968.

## Vigilance

58. Davenport, W. G.: Auditory vigilance: The effects of costs and values on signals. *Aust J Psychol, 20:*213–218, 1968.

59. Davenport, W. G.: Vibrotactile vigilance: The effects of costs and values on signals. *Percept Psychophys, 5:*25–28, 1969.
60. Hatfield, J. L. and Loeb, M.: Sense mode and coupling in a vigilance task. *Percept Psychophys, 4:*29–36, 1968.
61. Hatfield, J. and Soderquist, D. R.: Practice effects and signal detection indices in an auditory vigilance task. *J Acoust Soc Am, 46:*1458, 1969.
62. Hatfield, J. L. and Soderquist, D. R.: Coupling effects and performance in vigilance tasks. *Hum Factors, 12:*351–359, 1970.
63. Levine, J. M.: The effects of values and costs on the detection and identification of signals in auditory vigilance. *Hum Factors, 8:*525–537, 1966.
64. Loeb, M. and Alluisi, E. A.: Influence of display, task, and organismic variables on indices of monitoring behavior. *Acta Psychol, 33:*343–366, 1970.
65. Milosevic, S.: Detection du signal en fonction due critere de reponse. *Le Travail Humain, 32:*81–86, 1969.
66. Taylor, M. M.: Detectability theory and the interpretation of vigilance data. *Acta Psychol, 27:*390–399, 1967.

## Attention

67. Franzén, O.; Markowitz, J. and Swets, J. A.: Spatially-limited attention to vibrotactile stimulation. *Percept Psychophys, 7:*193–196, 1970.
68. Kinchla, R. A.: Temporal and channel uncertainty in detection: A multiple-observation analysis. *Percept Psychophys, 5:*129–136, 1969.
69. Lindsay, P. H.; Taylor, M. M. and Forbes, S. M.: Attention and multidimensional discrimination. *Percept Psychophys, 4:*113–117, 1968.
70. Moray, N. and O'Brien, T.: Signal-detection theory applied to selective listening. *J Acoust Soc Am, 42:*765–772, 1967.
71. Swets, J. A. and Kristofferson, A. B.: Attention. *Ann Rev Psychol, 21:*339–366, 1970.
72. Taylor, M. M.; Lindsay, P. H. and Forbes, S. M.: Quantification of shared-capacity processing in auditory and visual discrimination. *Acta Psychol, 27:*223–232, 1967.

## Memory

73. Allen, L. R. and Garton, R. F.: Detection and criterion change associated with different test contexts in recognition memory. *Percept Psychophys, 6:*1–4, 1969.
74. Bernbach, H. A.: Decision processes in memory. *Psychol Rev, 74:*462–480, 1967.
75. Donaldson, W. and Murdock, B. B., Jr.: Criterion change in continuous recognition memory. *J Exp Psychol, 76:*325–330, 1968.
76. Gibson, K. L.: Criterion shifts and the determination of the memory operating characteristics. *Psycon Sci., 9:*207–208, 1967.

77. Lockhart, R. S. and Murdock, B. B., Jr.: Memory and the theory of signal detection. *Psychol Bull, 74:*100–109, 1970.

78. Massaro, D. W.: The role of the decision system in sensory and memory judgments. *Percept Psychophys, 5:*270–272, 1969.

79. Swets, J. A.: Signal detection as a model of information retrieval. In F. Bresson and M. deMontmollin (Eds.) : *The Simulation of Human Behavior.* Dunod, Paris, 1969, pp. 253–264.

80. Wickelgren, W. A.: Sparing of short-term memory in an amnesic patient: implications for strength theory of memory. *Neuropsychologica, 6:* 235–244, 1968.

81. Young, R. K.; Saegert, J. and Lindsley, D.: Retention as a function of meaningfulness. *J Exp Psychol, 78:*89–94, 1968.

### Conceptual Judgment

82. Ulehla, J. Z.; Canges, L. and Wackwitz, F.: Signal detectability theory applied to conceptual discrimination. *Psychon Sci, 8:*221–222, 1967.

83. Ulehla, J. Z.; Little, K. B. and Weyl, T. C.: Operating characteristics and realisms of certainty estimates. *Psychon Sci, 9:*77–78, 1967.

### Personality

84. Clark, C. W.: The psyche in psychophysics: A sensory-decision theory analysis of the effect of instructions on flicker sensitivity and response bias. *Psychol Bull, 65:*358–366, 1966.

85. Poortinga, Y. H.: Signal-detection experiments as tests for risk-taking: A pilot study. *Psychon Sci, 14:*185–188, 1969.

86. Price, R. H.: Signal-detection methods in personality and perception. *Psychol Bull, 66:*55–62, 1966.

87. Price, R. H. and Eriksen, C. W.: Size constancy in schizophrenia: A re-analysis. *J Abnorm Psychol, 71:*155–160, 1966.

88. Stephens, S. D. G.: Auditory threshold variance, signal detection theory and personality. *Intern Audiol, 7:*131–137, 1969.

89. Strickland, B. R. and Rodwan, A. S.: Relation of certain personality variables to decision-making in perception. *Percept Psychophys, 18:*353–359, 1964.

### Extended Theory

90. Kinchla, R. A. and Allan, L. G.: A theory of visual movement perception. *Psychol Rev, 76:*537–558, 1969.

91. Thijssen, J. M. and Vendrik, A. J. H.: Internal noise and transducer function in sensory detection experiments: Evaluation of psychometric curves and of ROC curves. *Percept Psychophys, 3:*387–400, 1968.

92. Treisman, M. and Watts, T. R.: Relation between signal detectability theory and the traditional procedures for measuring sensory thresholds: Estimating d′ from results given by the method of constant stimuli. *Psychol Bull, 66:*438–454, 1966.

93. Treisman, M. and Leshowitz, B.: The effects of duration, area, and background intensity on the visual intensity difference threshold given by the forced-choice procedure: Derivations from a statistical decision model for sensory discrimination. *Percept Psychophys, 6:*281–296, 1969.

94. Wickelgren, W. A.: Unidimensional strength theory and component analysis of noise in absolute and comparative judgments. *J Math Psychol, 5:*102–122, 1968.

## Chapter 3

# OBSERVER ERROR, SIGNAL DETECTABILITY AND MEDICAL DECISION-MAKING

### Lee B. Lusted

Decision ANALYSIS HAS received little formal attention in medicine. Physicians are professional decision-makers and they are concerned every day with decision-making processes but in recent years interest in the methodology of diagnosis has declined in the face of an emphasis on the accumulation of new medical knowledge. Now, however, questions are being raised about the proliferation of medical information and the delivery of health care. These questions are more concerned with methodology than they are with information content per se and it is at this point that decision-making studies become important.

Decision analysis using the tools of probability and preference theory and supported by computer data processing is demonstrated below for a specific study in the accuracy of interpretation of chest x-rays for active tuberculosis.

## INTRODUCTION

Many radiologists were disturbed by Knowles' articles,[1] "Radiology—A Case Study in Technology and Manpower" which appeared in the *New England Journal of Medicine* on June 5 and 12, 1969. In his concluding paragraph, Knowles said, in part the following:

> For example, one could and should ask how many renal arteriograms in patients with hypertension have resulted directly in the surgical or medical cure of the patient's hypertension. Or one could ask how many lung scans have altered the diagnosis, treatment or prognosis of the patient thought to have a pulmonary embolus. Such studies might conceivably put a discriminatory brake on the use of a technology seemingly run wild. As one looks at the costs of developing modern radiotherapeutic facilities, one must ask what the benefit of radiother-

apy is as contrasted with the cost although in this instance even to ask the question, in an affluent, developed country will bring criticism raining down around the shoulders of the questioner.

What can a radiologist answer? Do the same questions about the relative value and costs of diagnostic tests and treatment apply to all areas of medicine? Probably they do because the questions are parts of two larger problems; namely (a) the unmanaged proliferation of medical data and (b) the distribution of health care.

As Kuhn [2] points out, two characteristics of a scientific revolution are professional insecurity and social pressure for reform. Professional insecurity is a result of a breakdown in the traditional way of doing business and social pressure for reform builds up because existing institutions have ceased to meet adequately the problems posed by society.

Under conditions of scientific revolution an environment often is created which is favorable for seeking completely new solutions to old problems. It is in this context that I propose to consider decision-making studies with computer assistance as useful keys to the puzzles presented by Knowles. I shall discuss two standard tools of decision-making; namely, probability and preference theory. Probability is a measure of uncertainty about data or a decision, and preference is used as a measure of value.

## A STUDY OF VALUES AND COSTS USING SIGNAL DETECTABILITY AND DECISION THEORY

Studies to answer Knowles' questions about the necessity for some types of roentgenographic examinations and about whether such studies "might conceivably put a discriminatory brake on the use of a technology seemingly run wild" will require a consideration of relative values and costs. As a first step in the development of appropriate investigations I cite a study from diagnostic radiology to show how decision analysis can be used to explore relationships of values and costs. The example uses a chest x-ray interpretation for the presence of active tuberculosis as the theme and an analysis is given in terms of signal detectability and decision theory.

Accurate interpretation of a roentgenogram depends upon

visual perception by the radiologist of the images recorded on film or some other medium. The images so recorded may be considered a signal or a group of signals, and the radiologist observes these signals against a background of shadows which introduce noise. The radiologist in his role as a decision-maker uses the signals to choose among alternative diagnoses and this decision situation often occurs under conditions of uncertainty.

## Some Comments About Signal Detectability

The general theory of signal detectability is based largely on probability theory and was developed most fully in the early 1950's by mathematicians and engineers at the University of Michigan, at Harvard University, and at the Massachusetts Institute of Technology. Much of the theoretical material arose from an analysis of radar and information systems. For example, an observer watches a radar screen and he is asked to detect a signal on the television type screen which indicates the presence of an airplane. This signal might be a small "blip" or a bright spot of light. The signal is always observed against a background of noise caused by electronic noises in the radar receiver, by extraneous radar echoes from the ground surface, sea surface, nearby buildings and so forth.

The evaluation of a radar system or other systems which detect signals requires a standard with which the system performance can be compared. Therefore, a concept of central importance in detection theory is that of an ideal or optimal detector. Such a concept is applicable to human performance but few sensory psychologists knew about detection theory in the late 1940's and early 1950's. However, it was not long until several investigators [3] realized that the concept of an ideal detector could serve as a standard of reference by which human performance could be evaluated and which could provide a means of comparing human performance with a variety of different non-optimal detection devices.

Detection theory with an emphasis on decision-making was used in experiments on vision and on audition in the 1950's. In an experiment on vision an observer is asked to observe an illuminated screen upon which a signal of pulsed light is projected. The observer is to state during each observation time interval whether a signal is or is not present. This type of study, and a wide variety of subsequent studies, demonstrated that a host of factors which affect the observer's attitude are compressed into a single variable called the *decision criterion*. This finding is an important contribution of modern detection theory.

The main purpose for using decision theory is to separate the detectability of a signal, a sensory process, from the decision criteria of the observer, a response or decision process. Detection theory is a normative theory and the ultimate defense of the general aspects of procedures which are described by detection theory is a pragmatic one—they work.

## Chest X-Ray Interpretation as a Signal Recognition Study

Let us perform an experiment similar to those designed by Yerushalmy [4,5] to study the accuracy of chest film interpretation for the presence of active tuberculosis. You are one of ten physicians participating in the study and you will be asked to make a diagnosis about the presence or absence of active disease on a series of 70 mm chest photofluorograms selected from a large population (over 14,000) of college students. You will be asked to provide an average of 3000 film readings according to a randomized scheme so that you will provide ten independent interpretations of each film.

The photofluorograms are all "proven cases." We record for your interpretations the number of cases of tuberculosis which you diagnose correctly (true positive); the number of cases which are actually negative but which you call positive (false positive); the number of negative cases which you diagnose correctly (true negative) and finally, the number of cases which are truly positive for tuberculosis but which you call negative (false negative).

We now find your observer error rate and we call this your attitude about the diagnostic criteria for tuberculosis.

Your true positive (T.P.) percentage is

$$\text{T.P. (\%)} = \frac{\text{No. true positives you read}}{\text{No. true positives you read} + \text{No. false negatives you read}} \times 100$$

Your false negative (F.N.) percentage is

$$\text{F.N. (\%)} = \frac{\text{No. false negatives you read}}{\text{No. true positives you read} + \text{No. false negatives you read}} \times 100$$

Note that the percentage of true positives plus the percentage of false negatives add to 100 percent.

T.P. (%) + F.N. (%) = 100 Percent Diseased Patients Tested

Your true negative (T.N.) percentage is

$$\text{T.N. (\%)} = \frac{\text{No. true negatives you read}}{\text{No. true negatives you read} + \text{No. false positives you read}} \times 100 \quad \text{Specificity}$$

Your false positive (F.P.) percentage is

$$\text{F.P. (\%)} = \frac{\text{No. false positives you read}}{\text{No. true negatives you read} + \text{No. false positives you read}} \times 100$$

Note that the percentage of true negatives plus the percentage of false positives add to 100 percent.

T.N. (%) + F.P. (%) = 100 Percent Negative Patients Tested

The four possible outcomes for your diagnosis may be displayed in a matrix as shown below. This is called a *decision matrix* in decision theory studies.

*Your Diagnosis*

| | | Positive | Negative | |
|---|---|---|---|---|
| **Disease Category** | Positive | % True Positive | % False Negative | = 100% Diseased Patients Tested |
| | Negative | % False Positive | % True Negative | = 100% Negative Patients Tested |

Your error rate is indicated by the percentage of false positives and false negatives. In this study you and the other nine physicians each have an error rate.

A convenient means of displaying the error rates for the study is a graph of percent false negative versus percent false positive as shown in Fig. 3–1. Each physician generates a point which represents his percent F.N. and percent F.P. errors for each series of films he interprets. Fig. 3–1 shows the results obtained in a large

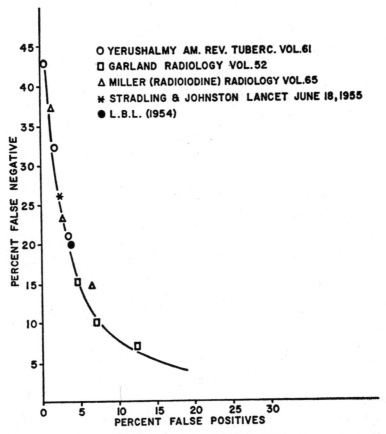

Figure 3–1. Operating characteristic curve for the interpretation of chest photofluorograms for pulmonary tuberculosis. A reciprocal relationship is demonstrated between the percentage of false negative and false positive interpretations. The radiologist has a choice of operating point on the curve which depends on how he views the relative "cost" of false negative vs false positive errors (i.e. how optimistic or how pessimistic he wishes to be) .

number of studies by Yerushalmy,[5] by Garland,[6] and by other investigators. Note the interesting reciprocal relationship between the percent false negative and percent false positive errors. Note also that a smooth curve can be drawn through the points. I participated in one of Yerushalmy's studies and my error rate was 20 percent false negatives and 4 percent false positives.[7]

The curve shown in Fig. 3–1 is called a receiver operating characteristic curve (ROC) in detection theory. I will use interchangeably the terms ROC curve, receiver operating characteristic curve, and operating characteristic curve. The convention in detection theory is to plot an ROC curve in terms of percent false positive versus percent true positive responses. By the use of the decision matrix it is easy to convert the ROC curve in Fig. 3–1 to a conventional ROC curve shown in Fig. 3–2. The two curves mean exactly the same thing.

The decision matrix shown previously has only two degrees of freedom and not four. That is, only two numbers can be entered freely in the matrix and the other two numbers will follow. For example, from the percent false negatives the percent true positives is obtained as follows:

$$100\% - F.N.(\%) = T.P.(\%)$$

A physical interpretation of the decision matrix percentages is shown in the right-hand diagram in Fig. 3–2. Note that the area under the right-hand Gaussian distribution curve is divided into two parts by the vertical line, namely, a true positive area (T.P.%) and an area to the left of the vertical line which represents a false negative area (F.N.%). These two areas add to 100 percent. Likewise the left-hand Gaussian distribution curve is divided into two areas; namely, a true negative area (T.N.%) and an area to the right of the vertical line which represents the false positive area (F.P.%). These two areas add to 100 percent.

The diagnostic attitude of each physician is specified uniquely for a particular series of chest film interpretations by a particular T.P.(%)–F.P.(%) point. This point on the ROC curve corresponds to a position on the X axis of the vertical line which divides the two overlapping population curves into a subgroup relationship of T.P., F.N., T.N., and F.P. Each physician sets the vertical

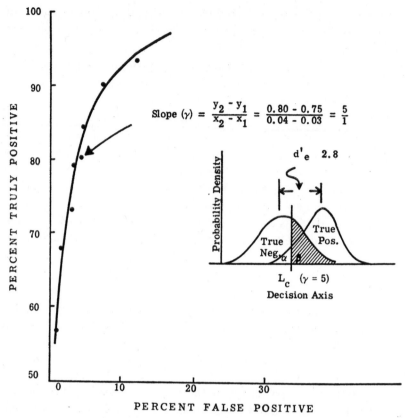

Figure 3–2. Operating characteristic curve for the interpretation of chest photofluorograms for the presence of pulmonary tuberculosis. The data of Fig. 3–1 have been replotted as percent false positive vs percent true positive. The measure d′ which represents the diagnostic criteria can be obtained from tables given by Swets (see Reference 3) in terms of T.P. (%) vs F.P. (%). The data have been used to reconstruct the possible appearance of normal probability density distribution functions for the negative population and positive tuberculosis population.

line according to his attitude for a combination of T.P. (%) –F.P. (%) which he prefers. How he does this is not clear at present and we leave this as a subject for future investigation. Since you and your colleagues very likely will have different values of T.P. (%) –F.P. (%) , then a plot of the ten points for the ten physicians will generate an ROC curve which should look something like the curve in Fig. 3–2.

## Why a Receiver Operating Characteristic (ROC) Curve Is a Useful Device

A receiver operating characteristic curve provides a natural distinction between the inherent detectability of a signal which in this study is a roentgen image, and the judgment or diagnosis of the observer (the physician). The unique feature of this presentation is that the results are completely independent of any assumptions one might make about the statistical distribution of the sensory events produced by the signal plus noise or by noise alone. The results are "distribution free."

It is very difficult for a human observer to maintain a constant decision attitude over any prolonged period of time. This is a factor which contributes to the finding that a radiologist will disagree with his own film interpretations about one out of five times on a second reading of the same films. Although the radiologist cannot maintain a constant decision attitude, that is, he cannot maintain a constant spot of operation on the ROC curve, he can use consistent decision rules for a diagnosis. This consistency is demonstrated as long as he produces a true positive, false positive interpretation result which lies on or very near the ROC curve for a particular type of roentgenographic examination. He can move up or down on the ROC curve and use consistent decision rules. However, if he moves off of the ROC curve he has changed his decision rules, and to be consistent about his diagnoses he cannot permit this to happen.

How can the radiologist decide what interpretation attitude to adopt? Should he be pessimistic, optimistic, or somewhat in between? It is important for the radiologist to know what his attitude is because when the signal has been specified, that is, when the radiographic image has been completed, the errors in interpretation he is willing to accept are a result of his interpretation attitude. What percent false positives is he willing to accept? This question can be answered in terms of values vs. costs and at the present time each radiologist must decide this for himself. A method which demonstrates a relationship among values and costs is discussed next.

## Estimation of Values and Costs of a Decision from an ROC Curve

The expected values for the four possible outcomes of a decision which were discussed previously can be used to study the relative importance which the radiologist attaches to the values of his correct decisions compared with the costs of his errors. Expected value is expressed mathematically as the sum of the products of probability times value for each of the four decision outcomes.

A radiologist who has participated in a film interpretation study and has found a percent true positive, percent false positive ratio for his diagnoses has given a likelihood ratio point on an ROC curve which corrresponds to a position of the vertical line on the decision axis. This likelihood ratio represents an optimal decision criterion for this radiologist in this study. We use the ratio to develop his expected value relationship.

The likelihood ratio of a point on an ROC curve is the slope of the curve at that point. The likelihood ratio for the ROC curve in Fig. 3–2 at my point of operation is 5 (slope of the curve is 5).

The slope which represents an optimum decision rule criterion is used as shown below to study my attitude on values and costs of the four decision outcomes.

$$5 = \frac{p(TN)}{p(TP)} \cdot \frac{V_{TN} + K_{FP}}{V_{TP} + K_{FN}}$$

where $p(TN)$ = probability of a true negative diagnosis
$p(TP)$ = probability of a true positive diagnosis
$V_{TN}$ = Value (for the radiologist) of a true negative diagnosis
$V_{TP}$ = Value (for the radiologist) of a true positive diagnosis
$K_{FP}$ = Cost (for the radiologist) of a false positive diagnosis
$K_{FN}$ = Cost (for the radiologist) of a false negative diagnosis

In the study by Yerushalmy [4] the probabilities of true negative and true positive give the following:

$$\frac{P(TN)}{P(TP)} = 2000$$

*(handwritten margin note: where on curve, how diff form prev?)*

so

$$5 = 2000 \cdot \frac{V_{TN} + K_{FP}}{V_{TP} + K_{FN}}$$

This may be rewritten as follows:

$$\frac{5}{2000} = \frac{1}{400} \approx \frac{V_{TN} + K_{FP}}{V_{TP} + K_{FN}}$$

With the help of this expression I wish to explore my attitude about the costs of false negative and false positive errors for this particular diagnosis of active tuberculosis. I begin by asking some questions about my attitude concerning the values of true positive and true negative diagnoses. The list of questions is a sample and is not meant to be exhaustive. The reader may develop additional questions.

| *Questions about Values* | *My attitude about Relative Value of True Positive vs. True Negative Diagnoses* $\dfrac{V_{TP}}{V_{TN}}$ |
|---|---|
| *Subjective Values* | |
| 1. Value to my self-esteem of correct diagnosis | 1 |
| 2. Value to referring physicians of correct diagnosis | 1 |
| 3. Value to my reputation with referring physicians | 1 |
| 4. Value to patient of correct diagnosis | $< 1$ |
| 5. Value to my reputation with patients | 1 |
| 6. Value to society of correct diagnosis | $> 1$ |
| *Objective Values* | |
| 1. My professional fee | 1 |
| 2. Cost in dollars to the patient | $> 1$ |

From this argument I conclude that for me for this particular diagnosis $V_{TP} \approx V_{TN}$ and I arbitrarily will set $V_{TP} \approx V_{TN} \approx 1$ unit.

Then I rewrite the previous expression as $\dfrac{1}{400} \approx \dfrac{1 + K_{FP}}{1 + K_{FN}}$.

Now I ask myself if the cost for me of a false postive or a false negative diagnosis is very much greater than the value I attached to the correct diagnosis. For this argument I conclude that it is

and so I rewrite the expression again $\dfrac{1}{400} \approx \dfrac{K_{FP}}{K_{FN}}$ or $K_{FN} \approx 400 K_{FP}$.

This expression can be interpreted in decision analysis terms to mean that for me in this particular diagnostic test the cost or loss of a false negative diagnosis must be 400 times the cost or loss of a false positive diagnosis to warrant a positive diagnosis of tuberculosis. That is, the consequences of ignoring tuberculosis when it is present must be at least 400 times as serious as the consequences of further testing or treatment of tuberculosis when the patient does not in fact have tuberculosis. I am willing to trade the cost of 1 false negative for the cost of 400 false positive diagnoses.

The development of operating characteristic curves seems to be the best method at present to study the relationship of values and costs of a roentgen diagnostic decision. By a change in attitude it is possible to change my point of operation on the ROC curve. If I adopt an attitude of "better safe than sorry" I tend to call a doubtful lesion positive. This attitude moves my point of operation up and left on the ROC curve. The slope of the curve is decreasing and the preceding argument shows that I am now willing to trade the cost of 1 false negative 800 or 1,000 false positive diagnoses. Eventually the cost of false negative and false positive diagnoses will be related to dollars. This is a subject for future study.

Operating characteristic curve analysis appears to be a useful device in two areas of diagnostic radiology which currently are receiving much attention; namely, (a) the training of radiologists' assistants to screen radiographs and (b) evaluation of relative diagnostic usefulness of complex technical systems.

### Training Radiologists' Assistants to Screen Mammograms

The use of paramedical personnel to assist physicians has been accepted to the extent that training programs have been started to train personnel in several specialty areas such as radiology, pediatrics, and obstetrics.

In radiology the assistant might be expected to increase the effectiveness and efficiency of the radiologist by screening certain types of roentgenographic examinations such as chest x-rays or mammograms (x-rays of the breast). The assistant separates the mammograms into two groups; a group of negative cases and a group of positive cases which would be interpreted by the radiologist. This could reduce the number of cases seen by the radiologist by 50 to 70 percent.

How is the screening performance of the assistant to be evaluated? One method makes use of operating characteristic curves. Alcorn and O'Donnell [8,9] have published reports of a program to train nonradiologic personnel to act as mammogram screeners. In Fig. 3–3, Curve A shows an ROC curve taken from the data of

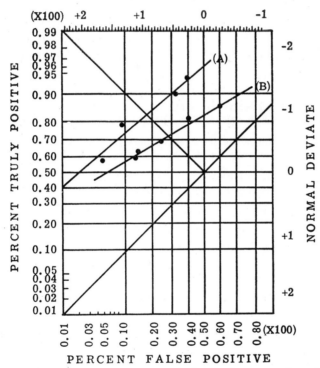

Figure 3–3. Operating characteristic curves for the interpretation of mammograms plotted on normal-normal coordinates (codex #41,453). Curve A has been constructed from data of Egan.[10] Curve B is from the data of Alcorn and O'Donnell [8,9] and represents the ROC curve for mammogram interpretation by six nonradiologic personnel who were being trained to be mammogram screeners.

Two parameters may be extracted from each curve, the slope and the sensitivity index $d^1_e$—where $d^1_e$ is defined as twice the normal deviate of the intersection of the ROC curve and the negative diagonal.

Egan [10] for the interpretation of mammograms for the presence of breast cancer. This curve represents the performance of radiologists who are skilled in the interpretation of mammograms. Curve B in Fig. 3-3 shows the diagnostic performance of the six radiologists assistants in Alcorn and O'Donnell's program. The six participants included two medical secretaries, two x-ray technologists who had experience with mammography, and two senior x-ray technologists not experienced in mammography.

Alcorn and O'Donnell have proceeded to develop decision trees and flow charts to use in training the assistants, and they report improved performance from the use of these materials. Alcorn hopes the assistants can reach a performance of 90 percent true positive and 10 percent false positive. He would be willing then to give them the responsibility for clinical mammogram screening.

## EVALUATION OF THE RELATIVE DIAGNOSTIC USEFULNESS OF A COMPLEX TECHNICAL SYSTEM

Operating characteristic curves may be used to evaluate the performance of a technical device which modifies the conventional roentgenogram. For example, suppose that we are considering the installation of a closed loop television system between the radiology department and several surgery rooms for transmission of roentgen images. One way to evaluate the performance of the television system is to use a proven case series of roentgenograms and to develop an ROC curve for radiologist diagnostic performance. The same series of films are read twice by the same radiologists; first, viewed directly and then viewed on the television monitor. If the ROC curves obtained under both conditions are identical or nearly identical, then the conclusion is that the television system is not introducing factors which affect the radiologist's diagnostic performance. Kundel, Revesz, and Stauffer [11] are studying this type of evaluation process in their laboratory.

Suppose, however, that the radiologists view the roentgenograms directly and obtain an ROC curve similar to Curve A, Fig. 3-3, and that after viewing the films on the television monitor an ROC curve similar to Curve B, Fig. 3-3, is obtained. Then the conclusion is that the television system has affected adversely the performance of the radiologists, and the radiologist will have to decide whether he is willing to accept this decreased performance compared with whatever advantages might accrue from the use of the system. Kundel, Revesz and Stauffer [11] give the following observer performance data on the effect of using a television chain to transmit a radiographic image of the chest. Some of the chest films showed lung nodules as found in lung cancer.

| Viewing Mode | Number of Observers | False Negative | False Positive | Index of Detectability d' |
|---|---|---|---|---|
| Direct Viewing | 21 | 0.14 | 0.24 | 1.91 |
| Unprocessed Television | 3 | 0.34 | 0.30 | 0.98 |
| Television Contrast Enhancement | 10 | 0.24 | 0.26 | 1.41 |

The television systems seem to degrade the radiologist's diagnostic performance. The same argument about performance testing can be applied to any technic which is being considered as an image enhancement process. The same argument also can be applied to compare the relative effectiveness of two roentgen diagnostic procedures. When a goal is stated in decision-making terms, that is, a diagnostic performance goal is given in terms of the accuracy (percent true positive diagnosis) and the errors (percent false positive diagnosis) which we are willing to accept, then it is possible to evaluate the relative usefulness of different roentgen technics or technical devices. Evaluation of imaging systems in terms of observer performance rather than in terms of physical constants of the system or in terms of modulation transfer function [12] represents a significant change from the present point of view. I think this change is essential for the evaluation of new equipment and technics to be used in diagnostic radiology.

## REFERENCES

1. Knowles, J. H.: Radiology—A case study in technology and manpower. *N Engl J Med, 280:*1271–1278, 1323–1329, 1969.
2. Kuhn, T. S.: *The Structure of Scientific Revolutions.* Chicago, Univ Chicago Press, 1962, p. 91 (paperback).
3. Swets, J. A. (Ed.) : *Signal Detection and Recognition by Human Observers.* New York, Wiley, 1964.
4. Yerushalmy, J.: Reliability of chest radiography in the diagnosis of pulmonary lesions. *Am J Surg, 84:*231–240, 1955.

5. Yerushalmy, J.: The statistical assessment of the variability in observer perception and description of roentgenographic pulmonary shadows. *Radiol Clin North Am, 7:*381–392, 1969.

6. Garland, L. H.: Studies in the accuracy of diagnostic procedures. *Am J Roentgenol, 821:*25–38, 1959.

7. Lusted, L. B.: *Introduction to Medical Decision Making.* Springfield, Thomas, 1968, p. 122.

8. Alcorn, F. S., and O'Donnell, E.: Mammogram screeners: Modified program learning for nonradiologic personnel. *Radiology, 90:*336–339, 1968.

9. Alcorn, F. S., and O'Donnell, E.: The training of nonphysician personnel for use in a mammography program. *Cancer, 23:*879, 1969.

10. Egan, R. L.: *Mammography.* Springfield, Thomas, 1964.

11. Kundel, H. L., Revesz, G., and Stauffer, H. M.: The electro-optical processing of radiographic images. *Radiol Clin North Am, 7:*447–460, 1969.

12. Rossmann, K.: Point spread-function, line spread-function, and modulation transfer function. *Radiology, 93:*257–272, 1969.

Chapter 4

# MEDICAL INFORMATION PROCESSING BY COMPUTER*

BENJAMIN KLEINMUNTZ

ANY SCIENTIFIC FIELD that deals with large amounts of data to be analyzed, coordinated and compiled at rapid rates invites the application of high speed data processing techniques. The area of medical information processing is just such a field. Accordingly, scientists have used electronic digital computer technology in this area for a number of years. The computer as an aid in medical information processing has been cast in two quite distinct but complementary roles: as an instrument of computation and as a noncomputational device. Sometimes the machine assumes both roles and this will be apparent in the following sections.

## PATIENT FILES (COMPUTATIONAL)

Hospital patient files are made up of a collection of many people's records. For any given patient, the record contains information about him for the duration of his stay in the hospital. Public Health statisticians or administrators and investigators interested in conducting epidemiological studies are frequently concerned with some aspect of the total population of patients. For example, questions involving the incidence of a given diagnosis (in a geographic region or within a hospital), and the association of certain symptoms with particular diseases, can be answered only by referring to the population of patient records.

The efficient search of these records has been made possible by automating hospital record-keeping. Such automation requires a

* This research was supported in part by the National Institute of Mental Health, Grant Nos. MH 07722–07 and MH NS 19427–01.

method of standardizing the amount and type of information that is notated on each patient's record. Standardization can be achieved by developing a uniform format in terms of which each physician can input patient data. Along these lines, one investigator [3,12] has developed special computer programs that secure their input information from the user by means of dialogue. These input programs are Socratic in that the computer elicits answers from the clinician, who in turn may address the computer—either orally or with a minimum of button-pushing, or by means of other learned responses. The input device may be located near the computer, or at a remote station.

So that a substantial data base or dictionary may be compiled in computer memory, the cooperation of a large number of hospital personnel is required. Thus it is not sufficient just to have the physician read-in the system signs; it is also necessary to enlist the help of nurses, aides, and pharmacologists. Once such cooperation is attained and the files are compiled, any statistical analysis that can be performed by a clerk can be executed by the computer. Data analysis procedures are available in the form of extensive libraries of "canned" statistical programs.

Statistical analyses of medical records could help in making a clinical diagnosis. The computer, for example, might be presented with the case of a patient exhibiting low grade fever, sore throat, and persistent headaches. By comparing the given symptoms, plus additional history and laboratory test findings with similar file cases, the computer might find that in 75 percent of the cases in which this configuration of symptoms and signs occurred the diagnosis is a sure case of mononucleosis, the other cases being distributed in other diagnostic categories. Obviously the physician might arrive at the same diagnosis without the aid of a computer, but in cases in which the combination of symptoms presents a complex diagnostic problem, it might be helpful to have immediate access to a large file of medical case histories.

The computer is a valuable aid to the physician also because it can be programmed to take into account the relative frequency of kinds of various diseases and it can arrive at an estimated probability for each of the possibility of diseases that the patient might have. In practice, diagnosis is never a simple, single-step affair.

Several stages are involved because each increment of new data about a patient modifies the existing diagnostic picture. The advantage of the computer for this form of sequential decision-making lies in its facility for immediate information retrieval and rapid computational capabilities. The drawback of the computer for medical diagnosis, obviously, is that it cannot do a physical examination, read a medical chart or convert narrative information for its use. All information from these sources must be transcribed onto a checklist.

## ON-LINE CLINICAL DATA PROCESSING (COMPUTATIONAL)

The speed with which a digital computer performs analyses enables these machines to process data while they are being collected. Therefore in addition to searching files, as above, computers can be used to perform simultaneous computations as the data are being input. Such computers are called *on-line* machines, as distinguished from those that are *off-line,* where input-output chores are performed by separate auxiliary equipment. In the early stages of computer technology, off-line machines were necessary because input and output mechanisms, being electromechanical, were much slower than the completely electronic storage, processing, and control units of the computer. But lately, computer processing has been synchronized with such auxiliary equipment, performing many operations between successive inputs. Thus, between successive inputs (inputting data is still relatively slow), the computer has time to perform a number of calculations.

The main advantage of on-line computation is that it tends to provide the user with immediate feedback. A fast computer, for example, could calculate the auto- and cross-correlation * of an electrocardiogram (ECG) or of an electroencephalogram (EEG) while the record is being taken, thus providing valuable diagnostic information. On-line computation of symptom and sign data,

---

* The auto-correlation function, which is a relatively recent form of mathematical computation, provides a test of periodicity in a time series recording such as the electroencephalogram. When a periodic signal is present, even though hidden to the eye, this function will identify its periodicity. Cross-correlations permit comparisons of wave or phase characteristics between pairs of EEG recordings.

either with a direct patient "hookup" † or by having the session on-line,‡ permits the computer to provide immediate advice about possible further tests to be performed on the individual patients.

This advantage of on-line clinical data acquisition can perhaps be best illustrated by referring to some work going on in electroencephalography.[1,7] It is in this area of investigation that considerable attention is being given to problems besetting scientists who wish to collect electrophysiological data and to receive almost simultaneous feedback in the form of the data's analysis.

Electroencephalography has its origins in the observation by Caton, in 1875, that spontaneous electrical activity can be obtained from the brain of animals. The relation of this activity to cerebral function was demonstrated by the observation that sensory stimulation could alter the ongoing electrical findings. It was not until 1929 that a German psychiatrist, Hans Berger, demonstrated that the electrical activity of the brain could be recorded from man. The recording of such activity through the intact human skull came to be termed electroencephalography, and after considerable controversy began to be used in clinical medicine.

Clinical electroencephalography concerns itself mainly with interpreting the EEG for the purpose of aiding the diagnosis of central nervous system disorders. The clinical electroencephalographer examines the record of a patient's EEG for signs of irregularity in the continuously oscillating brain waveforms. This examination consists of a visual analysis and search for specific amplitude, frequency, and waveform variations that conform to empirically agreed upon signs of pathology (see Fig. 4–1).

Experimental neurophysiology, in contrast to its clinical counterpart, is more concerned with evoking particular waveforms and manipulating the brain structures that underly the pattern of this electrical activity. And it is here that most of the interesting computer analyses have been conducted. Unfortunately most wave-

---

† Direct hookups require a special purpose machine called an analog computer. These machines are equipped to accept electrophysiological data (ECG and EEG) directly.

‡ Facilitation of ongoing interactions between man and the on-line computer requires the ability to have the computer accept and execute several programs concurrently in "a time sharing" fashion.

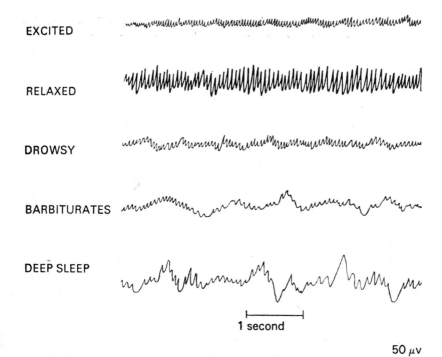

EXCITED

RELAXED

DROWSY

BARBITURATES

DEEP SLEEP

1 second

50 μv

Figure 4–1. Normal EEG waveforms taken from the intact human skull during various states of the organism.

forms that are currently of greatest interest to the experimental neurophysiologist are of little value to the clinician. But the future of these computer analyses and its applications to EEG recording and interpreting holds considerable promise for the clinician.

Typically the experimentalist records EEG data on special-purpose magnetic tapes and these data are converted from ana-logue to digital computers—or they are "digitized." * This procedure can occur off-line as well as on-line; but when it is off-line the lag between EEG recording and its analysis may be anywhere from several hours to many days. However, all the steps

---

* Voltage waveforms such as are obtained in EEG recording cannot be directly read into a digital computer, since they do not contain digits. Also EEG inputs occur as a function of time. Therefore, these data must be converted into digital form, with special attention to preserving the time function.

involved in EEG recording, digitization, and interpretation can be synchronized for on-line computation. The advantage of on-line computation, of course lies in the immediate feedback that is thus provided. One such on-line procedure has already been used in the operating room during brain surgery.[14] Here the full benefit of immediate feedback can be seen. The surgeon is given access to an instrument that permits him to operate on the basis of results that are emerging as he works.

As promising as on-line computer analysis of the EEG may seem at the present time, it is essential to emphasize that such computation is far from being generally available to clinicians for some time to come. It is of considerable interest, also, to note that although the computer has been successfully used to analyze EEG recordings and to classify persons on the basis of these analyses,[53] no machine has yet captured the human's skill in recognizing the multitudes of different wave forms. Such pattern recognition is truly still the human's forté.*

## FETAL CARDIAC DATA ACQUISITION
## (COMPUTATIONAL)

A number of investigators are working on automating acquisition and processing of fetal heart rate (FHR) and fetal electrocardiogram (FECG) variables. These measurements have been of great interest to electrocardiographers, especially when they are obtained during vaginal [18,29] and caesarian delivery.[19] FHR and FECG irregularities are among the first signs of fetal distress.

Automating FHR and FECG data acquisition allows continuous data recording, and potentially could provide the attending surgeon with "a quick look" appraisal. Such an appraisal may dictate that immediate delivery of the fetus is essential, or it may signify that conditions are normal. Stethoscopic sampling of the FHR, which is presently the most commonly used technique, does not provide a complete picture of these measurements, since it is impossible to record these data continuously throughout labor and delivery. Moreover, with continuous recording techniques, it

---

* For a report on the advantages and limitations of an on-line data acquisition system in the clinical laboratory and in an intensive care ward, the reader is referred to an essay by Hicks, *et al.*[17] and Osborn, *et al.*[38] respectively.

would be possible to correlate FHR and FECG patterns with various operative procedures, and with different phases of childbirth. But such automation, and the accompanying advantages, are far from being operational at the present time. Unfortunately, current costs, limited computer programming sophistication, and hardware considerations still present problems that await solution prior to realizing such computer systems.

### HEART AUSCULTATION BY COMPUTER (COMPUTATIONAL)

Physicians differ widely in their perception and interpretation of heart murmurs obtained by clinical auscultation. Heart auscultation is typically performed by placing a stethoscope on the left lateral position of the patient and listening to the precordium for valvular heart anomalies. Because the diagnosis of heart disease depends on the outcome of auscultation, a group of investigators [50] conducted a study in which they tested the accuracy of this method. They demonstrated that experienced physicians differentiate normal from abnormal heart conditions by the method of auscultation with success rates of 4 percent false positive and 37 percent false negative.

These investigators then conducted an automated analysis of phonocardiograms. The first step in this procedure was to tape record the heart sounds by means of a special-purpose audiovisual recorder.* These tapes were next transcribed onto a continuous (analog) linear tape and were converted for the digital computer. The digitized recording was then submitted to numerous multivariate statistical analyses by computer. The overall success rate was significantly higher (7 percent false positive and false negative) than clinical and tape-recorded heart auscultations.

The prospects for the future are good for providing the surgeon with continuous heart auscultation data during his operative procedure. And these data, when considered together with other electrophysiological recordings, all being analyzed and interpreted almost simultaneously, should add to the clinician's diagnostic

---

* The same physicians who performed the clinical auscultations listened to these recordings. Their success rate was about equal to that obtained after they had performed the clinical auscultations.

accuracy. The costs for such on-line systems are considerable, however, and large time-sharing computers to process these data are still not readily available for routine use. In the meantime, many computations can be performed off-line; and if the diagnostic success rate continues to be consistently higher than that of clinical auscultation, then the computer is an important clinical adjunct even in its present form.

## HUMAN METABOLISM DATA ACQUISITION BY COMPUTER (COMPUTATIONAL)

The observation of recurring patterns in the metabolism of humans, particularly as reflected in the urine composition, plays an important part in diagnosing the state of the organism at any point in time. Metabolism patterns are affected by many factors, particularly normal diurnal periodicities, normal schedules, and numerous other environmental changes, such as room temperature and position in bed. The problem of acquiring metabolism data from spinal-cord injured quadriplegics is currently being investigated in a multidisciplinary project at the Highland View Hospital in Cleveland.[20] Although this project is oriented toward manipulating experimental variables, the value of such data acquisition for clinical decision-making should be apparent.

The system is designed so that urine data are collected from a continuous-flow indwelling catheter; and bladder temperature, peripheral temperature, pulse, respiration, and muscle activity are measured by telemetry. Although the system is still not completely automated, such automatic data collection is clearly within view.

The biochemical analysis is automated and consists of transporting the urine sample out of the patient's room to a large cold room where it is weighed and measured for the presence of sodium, potassium, creatinine, chlorine, and nitrogen. The data are presented in analog form and then digitized for computer analysis. Clearly the objective of a fully automated system will be to provide the physician with an arrangement whereby he can obtain almost immediate feedback. From an instrumentation point of view, the major problems encountered in fully automating this system consist mainly of integrating it with the patient, while at the same time designing it to input data that satisfy the requirements of the digital computer. When these human and hardware problems are resolved, the physician will have access to one other tool to aid him in arriving at an accurate diagnosis.*

## PATTERN RECOGNITION
## (COMPUTATIONAL AND NONCOMPUTATIONAL)

A pattern is a form which is characterized by a definite arrangement or interrelation of parts. The letters A, B, and C, for example, are alphabetic patterns. ECG and EEG tracings are also patterns. There are two main aspects in programming a computer to recognize patterns: the perceptual and the cognitive. The first of these—beyond which present-day computer technology has not made notable progress—consists of programming the computer to recognize that the same class name should be assigned to different manifestations of the same pattern or form. For example, small circles and large circles must be recognized as circles; and short A's, tall A's, fat A's, and sloppy A's must be recognized as an A. Perceptions of this kind are trivial for humans, once they have been taught to differentiate one pattern from another and to assign class names to various patterns. And an electroencephalographer has no more difficulty differentiating between, let us say, alpha and delta rhythms than does a child in discriminating between the letters A and B.

The second, or cognitive, aspect of pattern-recognition programming is concerned with interpreting the identified forms. That is to say, many beginning medical students can learn to differentiate between an EEG alpha and delta rhythm and can be taught to recognize unusual waveforms such as "spike" or "dome" discharges, but they may need many years of additional experience to interpret (or to learn to attach correct clinical significance) to these recognized patterns. Moreover, understanding the in-context meaning of particular waveform occurrences within an individual's EEG record requires a form of cognitive pattern recognition which is more complex than just perceptual identification.

Generally speaking, even perceptual pattern recognition by computers has proved more difficult than was initially anticipated.

---

* For reports on computer-based monitoring systems and comprehensive patient monitoring concepts, the reader should see articles by Warner [54] and Stacy.[47]

This skill of the human to recognize patterns, upon close investigation, turns out to involve many complex processes. One reason for the difficulty in programming the computer to recognize patterns lies in the difficulty the human has in explicating his ongoing process. A human who abstracts a pattern often is unaware of the basis of his classification. Asked to define the pattern he has recognized, the human may point to examples of similar patterns instead of explicating its characteristics. Thus, if pressed the human says he recognized the letter A, or a particular circle, because it resembles an A or a circle. In other words the human's pattern recognition is a consequence of experience or learning, and if asked to introspect about the process he says that he is matching the new pattern with one that he has in mind.

The simplest automatic pattern-recognizing programs are based on a straight-forward matching notion.[16] They compare the new input with a stored ideal version of each alternative, and the closest match compares the input with a stencil of each letter; the most closely fitting stencil indicates the choice.

But there are difficulties in this simple matching procedure. For while it seems reasonable to store perfect patterns and to retrieve and match these ideals with new inputs, the question of handling inputs of imperfect patterns or variations of the ideal patterns presents a problem. Occasionally this problem can be surmounted. Devices for reading printed numbers from checks get around the problem by creating artificial differences in size and shape between numerals to accentuate the differences. And plausibly, ECG or EEG tracings could be thus accentuated. However, the imperfections and variations are often so large that there is minimal correspondence between inputs and stored ideals. Generally, therefore, pattern recognition by computer has favored methods that analyze inputs.

The strategy usually followed in analyzing inputs has been to select several attributes of the alternative patterns and to characterize the inputs, as well as the alternative patterns, in terms of these attributes. Thus an attribute of hand-lettered characters, for instance, might be number of curves. Each pattern has a particular value of each attribute [for example, R has one curve (and two straight lines) ]. The combination of an attribute and its value is called a *property,* so that R has the property of one curve and two straight lines. In practice, to recognize a given pattern, the computer compares the observed properties of the input object with the stored distributions of values for that pattern. The machine then computes the likelihood that the input object is an instance of stored pattern. There are two such programs that use the strategy of analyzing inputs, which are of potential use in recognizing patterns such as are obtained in medical settings. These are MAUDE (Morse Automatic Decoder), described by Gold [13] and *Pandemonium,* used and described by Doyle,[8] by Selfridge and Neisser [43] and by Kleinmuntz.[27,28]

Many other, more complex pattern-recognition computer programs are being developed [11,51,52] and applications of these programs for medicine are apparent. For example, once the computer learns to recognize patterns of shadows and spots on x-rays, it could be programmed to differentiate diseased from nondiseased chest x-rays.* Likewise, once the machine learns to recognize EEG patterns ( for example, alpha rhythm, spikes, domes, *petit mal* variants) it can be taught to undertake the next, or interpretive, phase of EEG reading. And if the error rates can be minimized for both the perceptual and the cognitive performances of these programs, then perhaps computers can become valuable consultants in these areas. The rather unhurried pace of progress in pattern recognition, however, suggests that these future developments are far from imminent.

## LOGICAL REASONING IN MEDICAL DIAGNOSIS (COMPUTATIONAL AND NONCOMPUTATIONAL)

Using a combination of symbolic logic (propositional calculus) and probability theory, two investigators [30,31] demonstrated that the computer could be an aid to the physician in arriving at a diagnosis and in choosing an optimum treatment plan.

The use of logic for this purpose is closely related to the concept of symptom-disease complexes (SDC). According to these

---

* Sterling and Perry [48] recently described an interesting pattern-recognition program, which is designed to visualize radiation-dose distributions used during radiotherapy. Basically the program provides the therapist patterns of dose distributions resulting from the configurations of treatment conditions.

| S₁ | 111 | 101 | 0 | 0 |
|---|---|---|---|---|
| S₂ | 111 | 000 | 1 | 0 |
| D₁ | 110 | 110 | 1 | 0 |
| D₂ | 101 | 101 | 0 | 0 |

$D_1$ and $D_2$.

workers, a symptom complex is a list of the symptoms that a patient *does* and *does not* possess; a disease complex is a similar list of diseases. An SDC is a list of both symptoms and diseases that a patient *does* and *does not* have. As an example of this, consider Fig. 4–2 where two symptoms, $S_1$ and $S_2$, and two diseases $D_1$ and $D_2$ are presented. Each column represents an SDC, where a unit in the row signifies that the patient has the corresponding symptom or disease, and zero signifies that the patient does not have the symptom or disease. Thus the column in the rectangle of Fig. 4–2 represents the SDC of the patient having $S_1$, not having $S_2$, having $D_1$, and having $D_2$. The columns of this figure represent all conceivable (by applying the truth tables of symbolic logic) SDCs that can be formed from two symptoms and two diseases.

Ledley [30] uses the phrase "all conceivable SDCs," but then points out that not all of these are possible or actually occur. That is to say, "all conceivable SDCs" as computed by the truth table method does not necessarily correspond to what is possible according to medical knowledge. The effect of medical knowledge on the shape of the truth table matrix is to reduce the totality of all conceivable SDCs to those that are compatible with the assertions embodied in the medical knowledge. Fig. 4–3 represents all possible SDCs for the situation in which application of knowledge has reduced the logical basis of possibilities.

| S₁ | 1111 | 1 | 111 | 0000 | 0000 |
|---|---|---|---|---|---|
| S₂ | 1111 | 0 | 000 | 1111 | 0000 |
| D₁ | 1100 | 1 | 100 | 1100 | 1100 |
| D₂ | 1010 | 1 | 010 | 1010 | 1010 |

Figure 4–2. Logical basis for two symptoms, $S_1$ and $S_2$, and two diseases, Figure 4–3. Reduced logical basis resulting from applying medical knowledge to the truth table of Fig. 2. The rectangle is the case of a patient having $\overline{S}_1 \bullet S_2$ (see text).

The preceding description is somewhat abstract (and over-simplified), and therefore it may be helpful to clarify it with an illustration. Using the reduced logical basis of SDCs presented in Fig. 4–3, suppose a particular patient presents the following symptom complex: He does not have $S_1$, but does have $S_2$, written symbolically, this is as follows:

$$\overline{S}_1 \cdot S_2$$

where the "—" bar represents NOT and the dot "." represents AND. To make the diagnosis, consider Fig. 4–3, which contains the reduced basis of all possible SDCs for those columns that include the symptom complex $\overline{S}_1 S_2$. There is one such column (rectangle), and this informs the diagnostician that the patient with this symptom complex has disease complex $D_1 \overline{D}_2$. In other words, the diagnosis is that the patient has $D_1$, but not $D_2$. These truth table matrices are stored in the computer, and the machine is programmed to search, detect, and print-out the diagnosis in the form of the logical possibilities. Although a computer is not essential for this storage and retrieval exercise, considerable time and effort are conserved by the use of the machine.

Although such computer analysis may seem elegant at first glance, the fact of the matter is that SDCs are not all-or-none affairs. The problem of diagnosis really revolves about the following question: Given the patient's present symptom-complex, what is the probability that he has a particular disease complex? The answer to this question requires the application of statistical decision theory. Such application often presents a computational burden that is cumbersome for humans and is a job best left to computers.

## COMPUTER SIMULATION OF CLINICAL DIAGNOSIS (NONCOMPUTATIONAL)

Up to this point, the use of computers in medical settings had its primary emphasis on getting a task done. That task is arriving at a diagnosis. An entirely different research strategy has been followed by some investigators [4] who are more interested in studying the diagnostic decision process of physicians than they are in developing a computer program that accurately classifies diseases. Some of this research will be discussed in detail here.

It was within the context of complex information processing by computers developed by Newell *et al.*,[36,37] that we undertook a number of studies involving the diagnostic problem solving of clinical neurologists.[25,26,56] The two fundamental assumptions guiding these studies were (a) that clinical decision making is a special instance of problem solving and (b) that problem solving behavior can be studied by computers as a complex information processing phenomenon.

The distinction between the complex information processing approach and numerous statistical decision theory strategies is that the former's goal is to parallel rather closely the consistencies, inconsistencies, errors, and shortcuts of the human diagnostician, whereas the statistical approaches are intended to produce a decision-making system that is an optimal or best possible system. Thus the main distinction is that the latter strategy strives for optimality and the former for accuracy in reproducing thinking. The advantage of the complex information processing approach is that its emphasis is on simulating the human clinician and as such may yield information that may be useful for modeling him, which in turn could be used as a teaching device.

To learn about neurologists' diagnostic search strategies, we devised a scheme which allowed the clinician to "think aloud." This was a method comparable to the one we used successfully in Q-sorting MMPI profiles,[24] but yet appropriate to the neurology problem. A variant of the childhood game of "Twenty Questions" fulfilled these requirements. The game is played by having one player, called the experimenter, think of a disease, while the other player, or subject, tries to diagnose the disease the experimenter has in mind. The experimenter can play any of a number of roles: He can pretend, for example, that he is a patient suffering from symptoms x, y, and z; or he could assume the role of the neurologist who is thinking of a particular disorder that is characterized by symptoms x, y, and z. The diagnostician's job in either case is to inquire about the presence of certain symptoms, signs, or biographical data and he may, if he chooses, ask for certain laboratory test results. It is necessary that the experimenter be an experienced neurologist so that he can answer the subject's questions. He must be able to recognize the appropriateness of many symptoms, signs, and laboratory tests that might possibly be relevant for a particular disease.

These games are tape-recorded, and the end product, after appropriate editing, can be represented by a tree structure (see Fig. 4–4) in which each point, or node, in the tree has exactly one connection to a point closer to the top or root of the tree. The starting point at the top, or the root, of the tree is the sub-

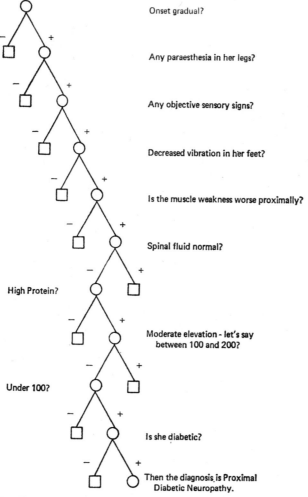

Figure 4–4. Fifty-seven year old white female with aching and weakness in the lower extremities.

ject's first question. All subsequent questions are the tests that are performed at the various nodes of the tree. Each nodal point, then, represents the question asked by the subject or diagnostician; if the experimenter's reply is negative, then there is a branch to the left; if a positive reply is obtained, there is a branch to the right. Unless a diagnosis has been reached each node is connected to exactly two lower nodes and through them to any number of still lower nodes. A path is a collection of lines from the root of the tree to a terminal node and is the schematic representation of the search strategy used by the neurologist to arrive at a diagnosis. In other words, the tree structure is a representation of the diagnostician's solution path from a certain set of givens to the diagnosis.

In order to illustrate this procedure, we present one such game in detail in Fig. 4–4. The diagnostician was given the information that he is to diagnose the case of a 57-year-old white female with aching and weakness in the lower extremities.

Inspection of this tree structure discloses that from the point at which the diagnostician asked the first question ("Was this gradual in onset?") until a diagnosis was reached, there were exactly eleven questions or test nodes and ten binary branchings. Of the latter, seven were positive and the remainder were negative branchings. But more important than these descriptive features of the diagram is the fact that we have the diagnostician's solution path, which presumably is related to the way he might function when confronted with a patient exhibiting similar symptoms.

In order to gain a further glimpse of this neurologist's reasoning process, he was instructed during a subsequent session to state his reasons for asking each of his questions. Table 4–I contains the same information that was presented in Fig. 4–4 with the addition of the neurologist's stated reasons. Having the neurologist articulate his reasoning provided us with a rich "thinking aloud" protocol, while at the same time it allowed us to secure a test-retest reliability estimate of the size and structure of the tree structure.

There are numerous promising possibilities open to us in the way these data could be best utilized. The most obvious of these

TABLE 4-I

PROTOCOL OF A DIAGNOSTICIAN'S QUESTIONS AND STATED REASONS OF A DISEASE CHARACTERIZED BY ACHING AND WEAKNESS IN THE LOWER EXTREMITIES IN A 57-YEAR-OLD WHITE FEMALE *

| Question and Answer at Test node | | Stated Reason |
|---|---|---|
| Gradual in onset? | (Yes) | It is very important to narrow it down to one of two categories. That is between degenerate or tumor disorders and infections and vascular diseases. |
| Any paraesthesia in her legs? | (Yes) | This is just to implicate the sensory tracts. |
| Any objective sensory signs? | (Yes) | This includes decreased position sense which is a posterior column sign usually. |
| Decreased vibration sense in her feet too? | (Yes) | Both carried in the same column, and I'm just reaffirming this. |
| Is her muscle weakness worse proximally? | (Yes) | Different diseases give you different proximal vs distal weakness. |
| Did the lady have normal spinal fluid? | (No) | I want to see if there is increased protein and cells in the fluid and therefore if she has tumor vs inflammatory disease. |
| High protein? | (Yes) | This is just one of the constituents cells, protein and perhaps glucose. |
| Between 100 and 200? | (No) | If it is markedly increased, it could be a tumor. |
| Under 100? | (Yes) | Normal is up to 45. Therefore, let's think of diabetes. |
| Is she diabetic? | (Yes) | |
| Ok, the diagnosis is proximal diabetic neuropathy. | (Yes) | |

*Note:* See also Fig. 4-4.

uses is to collect a larger number of protocols from one neurologist. These protocols would serve as a data-base, which could be stored in the computer, and, along with the clinician's heuristics, would represent one neurologist's method of diagnostic problem-solving. Ideally, the neurologist selected for such representation would be a highly proficient one. But one need not be so delimited. Conceivably, proficient and nonproficient diagnosticians could be simulated and then their strategies compared.

Individual differences among diagnosticians could also be ascertained by our laboratory procedures. That there are individual differences among diagnosticians in their ability to attain correct decisions is obvious. Not so obvious, however, are ways and means to measure those differences. Using the tree structure approach to diagnostic problem solving, we have been able to demonstrate graphically the existence of individual differences among diagnosticians. A comparison of the trees yielded by experienced and inexperienced neurologists, for example, disclosed that the latters' structures contain many more nodes, more naive questions and search strategies that yield considerably less information per question than those of experienced neurologists.

Finally, we can mention a third possible use to which our tree structure approach could be put. Based on the data collected from all proficient neurologists who participated in the diagnostic games, sufficient information has been collected to construct a medical model which resembles optimal diagnostic problem solving. Using the data base of this model, as well as the heuristics for accessing this data base as inputs to a computer, we can utilize the computer as a tutor to students who will sit opposite it. Thus, upon command the machine will print out a set of givens (i.e. fever and headache in a 12-year-old), and the student can play the role of the diagnostician. Or the problem can be turned around. Rather than having the computer serve as a tutor and the subjects sitting opposite it, we can arrange the situation so that the computer attempts to achieve a diagnosis, and the expert neurologist will answer its questions. This is perhaps closer to the situation as it may ultimately exist where the machine acts as a backup diagnostician for the human clinician who may consult it for provisional diagnoses during his own work-up of a patient. In either case, whether the computer is tutor or diagnostician, the implications for its use in medical education, a topic which we will develop further below, is obvious.

## COMPUTER-BASED MEDICAL INSTRUCTION (NONCOMPUTATIONAL)

The idea of programmed and computer-based instruction has its roots in research with "teaching machines." Programmed instruction is an educational technique in which a series of instructional materials or items is presented to the student who must select a correct alternative or fill in a missing answer. The distinguishing feature from conventional instruction is that the program is designed to provide the student immediate feedback from which he can determine whether his answer was right or wrong. The device by which programmed instruction is conducted is called the *Teaching Machine*. The latter may range in complexity from textbooks with special page format (to allow feedback), to elaborate electromechanical machines in which the program may be under the control of a digital computer.

Programmed instruction is among other things a response to the challenge of providing for individual differences among learners. A properly programmed tutoring device provides each student with the opportunity to work at his own pace, at the same time allowing him to make as few or as many errors as are necessary for him to learn the material completely. Moreover, such automated instruction relieves the human teacher of his routine, repetitive, and drillmaster role, thus permitting him to concentrate more on the motivational, social, and inspirational aspects of teaching.

The application of data processing and computer technology to the functioning of such programmed instruction is a relatively recent development [42,44] when compared to the idea of an automatic tutor.[41,45] This idea has only recently materialized in the installation of computer-linked typewriter input stations in classrooms and laboratories for faculty and student use. Among the more significant computer-based instructional programs currently being developed outside the medical field are the following:[15] A program that teaches students to count in the binary-number system and to add, subtract, multiply, and divide and, further, to convert from decimal numbers to binary ones and from binary to decimal numbers; [42] a special program of feedback messages designed to provide computer programmers with knowledge of where they made errors in their programs; [39,40] an elementary school mathematics program; [49] and PLATO (Programmed Logic for Automatic Teaching Operations), a general-purpose teaching machine system. Since the PLATO system is most closely related to computer-aided research currently being conducted in medical education, we will dwell in some detail on this program [2,5] before discussing computer-aided medical instruction.

At the Coordinated Science Laboratory of the engineering department at the University of Illinois, a group of scientists have been developing PLATO. The PLATO system utilizes a computer as the central control element for teaching a number of students simultaneously, while allowing each student to proceed through the lesson material independently. The system provides for communication in two directions. Each student is provided with an electronic key set as a means for responding to the computer's queries and a television screen for viewing information selected by the computer. There are two sources of information which are usually displayed on the student's television screen: a bank of slides prestored in an electronic slide selector under the control of the computer and a computer-controlled storage tube that permits plotting (at each of many student stations) diagrams, symbols, and words on the student's storage tube.

PLATO has two systems of teaching methods, a "tutorial logic" and an "inquiry logic." The first of these is designed to lead the student through a fixed sequence of topics and provides branching contingencies that depend on the student's speed of learning. The system first presents facts and examples, as is illustrated in Fig. 4–5, and then poses problems covering the material presented. The student selects answers and, when he is ready, asks PLATO for feedback. When he finds the problems too difficult he may choose to branch to easier material. The lesson material is organized in two sequences: the main sequence consisting of the minimum material that must be used by all the students, and the "help" sequence that is designed for students who have difficulty with questions in the main sequence.

The student begins by viewing test material in the main sequence. When he has completed reading a page of text, he pushes the button labeled CONTINUE (see Fig. 4–5) and thus proceeds to the next page, or he can return to the preceding page of text by pushing the botton labeled REVERSE. Generally, students

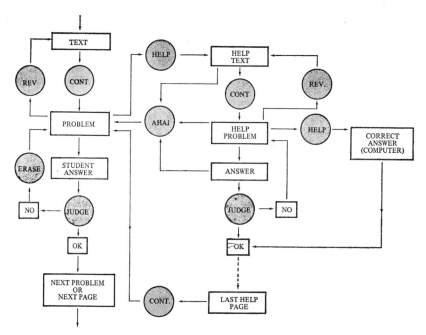

Figure 4–5. A flow-chart of the tutorial teaching logic. See text for a key to the abbreviations. (From Bitzer, 1965)

proceed through the lesson material by using the following logic buttons provided to them on a keyset: RENEW, ERASE, AHA, JUDGE, REVERSE, HELP AND CONTINUE.

Questions are answered by having the student type the appropriate responses with the use of buttons similarly labeled to those of a typewriter.

His answer appears on a cathode ray tube almost simultaneously. The student then may push the JUDGE button, and the computer determines the acceptability of the answer by printing out OK or NO next to the answer. By using the ERASE button, the student can remove incorrect answers. He can push the HELP button if he has difficulty with the question, and this would take him into a help sequence that pertains to the question.

The lesson materials are prepared for the tutorial logic by arranging them in a set of slides with at least one help slide for each question in the main sequence. Also, a parameter tape is prepared which contains the answers to the questions, their location on the slide page, and the order in which the slides are logically connected. Finally, error categories must be specified (for error detection) and a list made of monitored problems and their criteria for evaluation.

The inquiry-teaching logic system permits dialogues between the student and the computer. This system came about as a result of an interest in giving the student even more control of the way he learns than the tutorial system permits. The inquiry system allows the student to ask questions of the computer. Typically, in a lesson by this system, general problems are presented to the student. To solve them he must request and organize appropriate information from the computer. The student may be asked to demonstrate his achievement by answering questions and he may also ask questions within a given range of possibilities in order to obtain information.

The innovation of the inquiry logic is that this system provides the student a syntax by which he can ask questions about the lesson he is studying. Thus, for example, in the tutorial logic the student communicates with the computer either with one of control requests (that is, "Turn the page"; "Give me help"; "Judge my answer"), or composes short answers that usually must match one of the alternative stored responses. If he types a question such as "What is a coefficient?" the computer might respond with a NO, since it treats his response as an answer. The inquiry logic system, on the other hand, provides the student with the syntax and hence with the opportunity to ask such questions.

This syntax essentially requires that the student ask questions in a specific coded format that permits retrieval of information stored in the computer. One example given by the originators of the system [5] is as follows: The student in a teaching program for nurses who would like the answer to the question "What's the effect of administering nitroglycerine on the heart rate of the patient?" must type the coded format for the following sequence of phrases: "Return patient to original state"; "Give drugs"; "Select nitroglycerine"; "Check condition of patient, vital signs, pulse rate" (at this point the computer answers the question originally posed).

Similarly several researchers at Bolt, Beranek, and Newman [10] have developed a computer teaching system and applied it to a problem in teaching medical diagnosis. This system is designed to enable the medical student to augment his experience and his diagnostic skill.

The Bolt, Beranek, and Newman computer program, called the *Socratic System* because of its inquiry format, states a problem (that is, a medical history and a request for a diagnosis) to a student and engages him in "conversation" while he solves the problem. The conversation, of course, is accomplished through the use of an electric typewriter* connected to, and controlled by, the computer. The student types a question or an assertion and the machine types back a response—an answer, a comment, or another question. This conversation is executed by supplying the student with a list specifying the vocabulary for the problem. During the session, the student's questions and declarations must be selected from the terms on this list.

The vocabulary can be extensive, and the student is allowed considerable freedom in his approach to solving the problem. He can specify the information he wants and can make assertions regarding the solutions. The system records the information given to the student and answers each of his questions by typing one or more replies from a prespecified set of responses. At any point in time, the computer response depends on what has just been said and on everything that preceded it. Thus the system carries on a tutorial dialogue with the student, one in which interesting contingencies may be developed.

Computer-aided teaching of medical diagnosis, which also has been tried in at least two other studies [9,21] raises many interesting possibilities for introducing programmed instructional techniques into the medical school curriculum. The clinical experience of medical students is necessarily restricted by the variety of case material available to them and their limited exposure to live

---

* For a discussion of some of the problems to be faced in designing a computer-based tutor to deal with written and spoken language, see **Reference 46**.

patients. Thus, a student may not see any cases of a particular disease during his school years, and some cases he will encounter in his later practice of medicine may differ significantly from the classical or textbook cases. The student's "probability matrix," built up from his personal experience with a limited number of cases, may differ considerably from a matrix that is based on a large number of cases. Practice with programs like the one previously described may permit students to enlarge their probability matrices.

These computer programs, then, are capable of generating a vast number of hypothetical patients beckoning to be "examined" by inexperienced medical students. The limited usefulness of these programs must nevertheless be recognized. The medical student is not able to view the "acutely prostrated" patient; he gains no experience in obtaining heart auscultation; and generally, he conceptualizes, rather than practices, medicine. Moreover, the artificial setting of the man-machine interaction does not drive home the lesson of the "real-life" consequences of performing an inappropriate procedure, nor does it confront the neophyte physician with the reality of the discomforts—physical and economic— that accompany his selection of particular laboratory tests or exploratory procedures. But then again, these disadvantages must be weighed against the advantages of the added experience he gains that may otherwise be unavailable to him.

## SUMMARY AND CONCLUSION

The use of the computer for medical information processing was introduced about a decade ago. Considerable inroads have now been made toward its applications to the problems in medicine. The future of the computer as an information machine and decision-maker in clinical areas is limited only by human ingenuity. There seems to be no lack of such ingenuity in developing the software and hardware that are essential for its usefulness to the clinician. How far or how quickly these developments will advance is difficult to predict; but some of the promising present uses suggest that an interesting decade is ahead.

Present uses of the computer, both as a computational and noncomputational device include the following: Automated search of patients' files; on-line clinical data processing; fetal heart rate and fetal electrocardiogram data acquisition; heart auscultation by computer; metabolism data acquisition; pattern recognition by computer; medical diagnosis using the logic of the propositional calculus; computer simulation of diagnostic problem solving; and computer-based medical instruction.

## REFERENCES

1. Adey, W. R.: Computer analysis in neurophysiology. In R. W. Stacy and B. D. Waxman (Eds.): *Computers in Biomedical Research,* Vol. 1. New York, Academic Press, 1965, pp. 223–263.

2. Alpert, D. and Bitzer, D. L.: Advances in computer-based education. *Science, 167*:1582–1590, 1970.

3. Baruch, J. J.: Hospital automation via computer time-sharing. In R. W. Stacy and B. D. Waxman (Eds.): *Computers in Biomedical Research,* Vol. 2. New York, Academic Press, 1965, pp. 291–312.

4. Bellman, R., Friend, M. B., and Kurland, L.: Simulation of the initial psychiatric interview. *Behav Sci, 11*:389–399, 1966.

5. Bitzer, D. L. and Easley, J. A. Jr.: Plato: A computer controlled teaching system. In M. A. Sass and W. D. Wilkinson (Eds.): *Symposium on Computer Augmentation of Human Reasoning.* Washington, D. C., Spartan Books, 1965, pp. 89–103.

6. Brazier, M. A. B.: Introductory comments. *Electroencephalogr Clin Neurophysiol 20* (Suppl): 2–6, 1961.

7. Brazier, M. A. B.: The application of computers to electroencephalography. In Stacy, R. W., and Waxman, B. D. (Eds.): *Computers in Biomedical Research,* Vol. 1. New York, Academic Press, 1965, pp. 295–315.

8. Doyle, W.: Recognition of sloppy, hand-printed characters. *Proc West Joint Computer Conf, 17*:133–142, 1960.

9. Entwisle, G. and Entwisle, D. R.: The use of a digital computer as a teaching machine. *J Med Educ, 38*:805–812, 1963.

10. Feurzeig, W., Munter, P., Swets, J. and Breen, M.: Computer-aided teaching in medical diagnosis. *J Med Educ, 39*:746–754, 1964.

11. Fogel, L. J., Owens, A. J. and Walsh, M. J.: *Artificial Intelligence Through Simulated Evolution.* New York, Wiley, 1966.

12. Frey, H. S.: An on-line graphic inquiry system for analysis of tumor registry data. In Stacy, R. W. and Waxman, B. D. (Eds.): *Computers in Biomedical Research,* Volume 3. New York, Academic Press, 1969, pp. 87ff.

13. Gold, B.: Machine recognition of hand-sent Morse code. *IRE Transactions on Information Theory, 2:* (pt. 5), 17–24, 1959.

14. Goldring, S., Kelly, D. L. Jr. and O'Leary, J. L.: Somatosensory cortex of man as revealed by computer processing of periphally evoked cortical potentials. *Trans Am Neurol Assoc, 89:*108–111, 1964.

15. Goodlad, J. I., O'Toole, J. F. Jr. and Tyler, L. L.: *Computers and Information Systems in Education.* New York, Harcourt, 1966.

16. Green, B. F. Jr.: *Digital Computers in Research: An Introduction for Behavioral and Social Scientists.* New York, McGraw-Hill, 1963.

17. Hicks, G. P., Evenson, M. A., Gieschen, M. M. and Laison, F. C.: On-line data acquisition in the clinical laboratory. In Stacy, R. W. and Waxman, B. D. (Eds.): *Computers in biomedical research,* Vol. 3. New York, Academic Press, 1969, pp. 15ff.

18. Hon, E. H.: Computer aids in evaluating fetal distress. In R. W. Stacy and Waxman, B. D. (Eds.): *Computers in Biomedical Research,* Vol. 1. New York, Academic Press, 1965, pp. 409–437.

19. Kendall, B. and Farrell, D. M.: Observation of fetal heart rate during caesarian section. In K. Enslein and J. F. Winslow (Eds.): *Data Acquisition and Processing in Biology and Medicine,* Vol. 4. London, Pergamon Press, 1966, pp. 203–211.

20. King, P. and Apple, H.: Computer-oriented study of human metabolism. In K. Enslein and J. F. Kinslow (Eds.): *Data Acquisition and Processing in Biology and Medicine,* Vol. 4. London, Pergamon Press, 1967, pp. 23–36.

21. Kirsch, A. D.: A computerized medical training game as a teaching aid. In K. Enslein (Ed.), *Data Acquisition and Processing in Biology and Medicine,* Vol. 2. New York, Macmillan, 1964, pp. 139–147.

22. Kleinmuntz, B.: A portrait of the computer as a young clinician. *Behav Sci, 8:*154–156 (a), 1963.

23. Kleinmuntz, B.: MMPI decision rules for the identification of college maladjustment: A digital computer approach. *Psychol Monogr, 77:* (Whole No. 577, *14*) (b), 1963.

24. Kleinmuntz, B.: Personality test interpretation by digital computer. *Science, 139:*416–418 (c), 1963.

25. Kleinmuntz, B.: Diagnosic problem solving by computer. *Jap Psychol Res, 7:*189–194, 1965.

26. Kleinmuntz, B.: *Formal Representation of Human Judgment.* New York, Wiley, 1968.

27. Kleinmuntz, B.: *Clinical Information Processing by Computer: An essay and Selected Readings.* New York, Holt, Rinehart and Winston, 1969.

28. Kleinmuntz, B.: Clinical information processing by computer. In *New Directions in Psychology 4,* New York, Holt, Rinehart and Winston, 1970, pp. 123ff.

29. Larks, S. D. and Larks, G. G.: Acquisition and processing of fetal cardiac data: Electrical axis of the fetal heart. In K. Enslein and J. F.

Kinslow (Eds.): *Data acquisition and processing in biology and medicine,* Vol. 4. London, Pergamon Press, 1966, pp. 191–202.

30. Ledley, R. W.: Advances in biomedical science and diagnosis. In H. Borko (Ed.): *Computer Applications in the Behavioral Sciences.* Englewood Cliffs, N. J., Prentice-Hall, 1962, pp. 490–521.

31. Ledley, R. S. and Lusted, L. B.: Reasoning foundations of medical diagnosis. *Science, 130:*9–22, 1959.

32. Lusted, L. B.: Computer techniques in medical diagnosis. In R. W. Stacy and B. Waxman (Eds.): *Computers in Biomedical Research,* Vol. 1. New York, Academic Press, 1965, pp. 319–338.

33. Lusted, L. B.: *Introduction to Medical Decision Making.* Springfield, Thomas, 1968.

34. Newell, A., Shaw, J. C. and Simon, H. A.: Empirical explorations of the Logic Theory Machine. *Proc West Joint Computer Conference, 11:*218–230, 1957.

35. Newell, A., Shaw, J. C. and Simon, H. A.: The elements of a theory of human problem solving. *Psychol Rev, 65:*151–166, 1958.

36. Newell, A. and Simon, H. A.: Computer simulation of human thinking. *Science, 134:*2011–2017, 1961.

37. Newell, A. and Simon, H. A.: An information processing theory of human problem solving. (Manuscript in preparation, to be published 1971)

38. Osborn, J. J., Beaumont, J. O., Raison, J. C. A. and Abbott, R. P.: Computation for quantitative on-line measurements in an intensive care ward. In Stacy, R. W. and Waxman, B. D. (Eds.): *Computers in biomedical research,* Vol. 3. New York, Academic Press, 1969, pp. 207ff.

39. Perlis, A. G.: Research and development in programming study assignments. *Progress Report.* Computer Center, Carnegie Institute of Technology, July 1959.

40. Perlis, A. G.: Personal communication, 1963.

41. Pressey, S. L.: A simple apparatus which gives tests and scores and teaches. *School and Society, 23:*586, 1926.

42. Rath, G. J., Andersen, N. S. and Brainerd, R. C.: The IBM research center teaching machine project. In E. H. Galanter (Ed.): *Automatic Teaching: The State of the Art.* New York, Wiley, 1959, pp. 117–130.

43. Selfridge, O. and Neisser, U.: Pattern recognition by machine. In E. A. Feigenbaum and J. Feldman (Eds.): *Computers and Thought.* New York, McGraw-Hill, 1963, pp. 237–250.

44. Silberman, H. F. and Coulson, J. E.: Automated teaching. In H. Borko (Ed.): *Computer Applications in the Behavioral Science.* Englewood Cliffs, N.J., Prentice-Hall, 1962, pp. 308–355.

45. Skinner, B. F.: Teaching machines. *Science, 128:*969–977, 1958.

46. Spolsky, B.: Some problems of computer-based instruction. *Behav Sci,* *11:*487–496, 1966.
47. Stacy, R. W.: The comprehensive patient-monitoring concept. In Stacy, R. W. and Waxman, B. D. (Eds.) : *Computers in Biomedical Research,* Vol. 3. New York, Academic Press, 1969, pp. 253ff.
48. Sterling, T. D. and Perry, H.: Computation of radiation dosages. In R. W. Stacy and B. Waxman (Eds.): *Computers in Biomedical Research,* Vol. 1. New York, Academic Press, 1965, pp. 439–464.
49. Suppes, P.: *Computer-Assisted Instruction in the Schools: Potentialities, Problems, Prospects.* Stanford, Calif., Institute for Mathematical Studies in the Social Sciences, Stanford University Press, 1965.
50. Taranta, A., Spagnolo, M., Snyder, R., Gerbarg, D. S. and Hofler, J. J.: Auscultation of the heart by physicians and by computer. In K. Enslein (Ed.) : *Data Acquisition and Processing in Biology and Medicine,* Vol. 3. New York, Macmillan, 1964, pp. 23–52.
51. Uhr, L.: *Pattern Recognition.* New York, Wiley, 1966.
52. Uhr, L.: Pattern recognition, concept formation and learning. (Manuscript in preparation; personal communication, 1970)
53. Walter, D. O., Kado, R. T., Rhodes, J. M. and Adey, W. R.: Electroencephalographic baselines in astronaut candidates estimated by computation and pattern recognition techniques. (Unpublished paper by the Space Biology Laboratory of UCLA, 1967)
54. Warner, H. R.: Computer-based patient monitoring. In Stacy, R. W. and Waxman, B. D. (Eds.) : *Computers in biomedical research,* Vol. 3. New York, Academic Press, 1969, pp. 239ff.
55. Weizenbaum, J.: ELIZA-A Computer program for the study of natural language communication between man and machine. *Communications of the ACM, 9:*36–45, 1966.
56. Wortman, P. M.: Representation and strategy in diagnostic problem solving. *Hum Factors, 8:*48–53, 1966.

## Chapter 5

# EMPIRICAL APPROACHES TO CLASSIFICATION

JOHN E. OVERALL

CLASSIFICATION IS THE PROCESS of organizing into meaningful relationships the members of a heterogeneous population of objects, individuals, or diseases. *Classes* are groups of objects, individuals, or diseases which are so similar to one another that for many practical purposes they can be treated alike. Classification research is concerned with defining the underlying classes or sub-types in a mixed population. In contrast to most of the discussions at this conference, in which concern centers around the application of computer techniques to diagnostic decision-making, the present paper is concerned with the potential use of computers in defining the classification categories into which individuals are to be assigned. Whereas numerous familiar classification schemes in medicine and the biological sciences have been developed by subjective logic, powerful analytic methods and computer algorithms can now be brought to bear on this problem. We will be considering in this paper methods that can be used to develop diagnostic schemes, while later speakers will be concerned with accurate assignment of individuals once the diagnostic scheme has been specified.

Computer classification methods have two major types of application in medical research. One is concerned with similarity relationships between *diseases,* and the other is concerned with identifying homogeneous sub-types of *individuals.* The classification of *diseases* has long been recognized as an important problem in medicine. For example, the *Standard Nomenclature of Diseases and Operations* of the American Medical Association represents a classification of diseases according to topography and etiology. The *International Classification of Diseases* is an alternative

73

scheme that was developed with greater emphasis on coding that is useful for statistical tabulations. It seems reasonable to expect that in the near future computer-based analytic methods will be employed to optimize the classification of disease entities with regard to a variety of practical criteria.

The other important application for classification methodology in medical research has to do with identification of underlying latent groupings among *individuals* rather than diseases. Many diseases cannot be observed directly so that their presence must be inferred from patterns of observable manifestations. Individuals suffering from the same disorder tend to have similar patterns of manifest indicators (signs, symptoms and laboratory tests). Individuals suffering from different disorders tend to have less similar patterns. Empirical classification methods can be used to identify homogeneous groups and, thereby, to provide a basis for inferences concerning the number and nature of underlying disorders present in a heterogeneous population.

In the past, medical disorders have been classified largely as specific disease processes. From a practical point of view, it may be more meaningful to classify patients according to the nature of optimum therapeutic intervention because surely there are more diseases than there are effective treatments. It is not infrequent in modern medicine that a new laboratory procedure lays bare a multidimensional spectrum of differences among patients who were previously thought to be suffering from a single disorder. For example, until recently hyperlipidemia (elevated serum lipids including cholesterol) was considered to be a unitary disorder and was treated almost solely by restriction of dietary fats. When researchers applied methods of electrophoresis to human plasma, a number of different lipid molecules were discovered to make up the total plasma lipids in varying proportions.[2] Depending on the pattern of lipid components, five distinct *types* of hyperlipoproteinemias are now recognized. Given that a new laboratory technique has resulted in identification of multiple quantitative variables that exist at varying levels in different individuals, empirical classification methods can be used to answer the following questions: What are the most frequently occurring patterns and how do they differ from one another? Among serum lipid patterns, for example, are there really five distinct types, or is Type II really only a mixture of Types I and III? Is Type IV really a homogeneous unitary type, or does it actually consist of two or more sub-types that may have different etiologic and metabolic significance?

The medically trained individual recognizes an important distinction between classification and diagnosis. The term diagnosis implies a specified disease with defined etiology and morphology. Different diseases are known to result from different causal agents, to have different mechanisms of action, and to involve different physical systems or bodily functions. Medical diagnosis is the process of specifying the disease from which a patient suffers. Classification, on the other hand, involves establishing orderly relationships among individuals (or diseases) according to similarities on specified attributes.

While it is important to recognize a distinction between methods for the development of a *classification* system and the methods required for *assignment* of individuals among classification categories, the relevance of one problem for the other should not be overlooked. Empirically derived classification schemes involve grouping of individuals (or diseases) according to similarities and differences on specified attributes. Each class is composed of individuals or diseases that are relatively similar to one another and relatively dissimilar to members of other classes. The information required to assign individuals among such empirically defined classes is implied in the information that was used in development of the classification scheme. As a consequence, great care must be exercised in the selection of variables upon which an empirically derived classification system is to be based.

In some areas of medicine, but particularly in psychiatry and psychology, the number and nature of underlying disorders is not well established. Empirical classification methods can be used to identify homogeneous groups of individuals, say groups of psychiatric patients, who are similar on relevant indicators of psychopathology. Assuming that the original composite sample is representative, the homogeneous subgroups can be accepted as representing different classes in the general (psychiatric) population. Because patients within each class tend to be similar, while patients within different classes tend to be relatively dissimilar, the classes are highly discriminable and constitute categories into which individual patients can be assigned with minimum error.

The "theory of types" assumes a distinct pattern or profile to be associated with each different disorder. Except for more or less random errors in nature, all patients of a particular type should be expected to have identical patterns or profiles. Allowing for some variation in nature, patients suffering from the same disorder can still be expected to be relatively similar in appearance. Empirical classification methods can be used to identify subgroups of highly similar patients, and by inference to define the number and nature of underlying disorders.

### GENERAL LOGIC OF CLASSIFICATION METHODS

The numerous alternative methods that have been proposed for use in grouping individuals or diseases according to similarities and differences on relevant indicators have two major features in common. Each requires a quantitative definition, or a measure, of the relative similarity between pairs of individuals or diseases. Given the quantitative indices of similarity, an algorithm is required for analysis of the similarity coefficients to detect homogeneous groups or subclasses. Thus, if one were to attempt to "classify" classification procedures, the method of defining multivariate similarity and the manner of analyzing the similarity coefficients would provide the critical distinctions. For any one method of defining multivariate similarity, a number of different algorithms exist for identifying classification groups. Conversely, a particular algorithm for classification grouping can usually be applied to any one of several different types of profile similarity indices.

Within this broad framework, somewhat different methods and conceptions are available for use with categorical data as opposed to quantitative measurement variables. It will not be possible, in the time available, to cover in detail all of the variants of classification methodology available for use with both categorical and quantitative measurements. In most of my discussion, I will concentrate on methods that have their primary utility in problems where the characteristics that are to be used as a basis for classification can be measured on quantitative scales of measurement. Methods such as "latent class analysis" which are especially appropriate for use with categorical attributes, will not be discussed in any detail. The reader should be alerted, however, to the existence of special methods that have been developed to deal with classification problems involving categorical or qualitative variables.

In the following section of this chapter, a variety of somewhat related multivariate profile similarity indices will be considered. The two major types of profile similarity indices are the *distance function* and the *vector product* indices. In spite of differences in the nature of calculations, both are variations on the same basic model. For each of the numerous special cases of the distance function index, a corresponding and equivalent vector product index can be defined. Certain logical and statistical bases for choice between alternative methods of defining multivariate similarity will be discussed.

Given matrices of multivariate similarity or difference coefficients, the next step is the analysis to identify subgroups of similar individuals or diseases. Once again, the logic of classification analysis is that individuals who are relatively similar on specified observable characteristics belong to the same family, suffer the same underlying disease process, or can for practical purposes be treated alike. The second section of this paper is concerned with the problem of arriving at a classification grouping or typology, once similarities among all pairs of individuals or diseases have been defined in objective terms. Somewhat different algorithms are required, depending on whether multivariate similarities have been represented in distance function or vector product coefficients. These methods are the subject of the second section of the present paper.

## INDICES OF MULTIVARIATE PROFILE SIMILARITY

The profile similarity indices that are currently in widest use for classification research are of two general types—distance function and vector product. The several variants of each can be

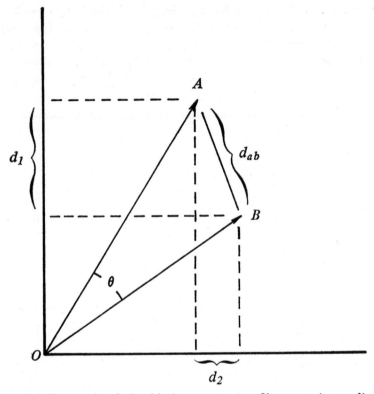

Figure 5–1. Geometric relationship between two profile vectors in two-dimensional space.

related in terms of a simple geometric model. The original multiple measurements, or linear functions of them, are taken as coordinate axes defining a Euclidean hyperspace. Individuals or diseases can be located as points, or vectors, in the hyperspace according to scores on the variables with which the coordinate axes are identified. This geometric model is represented in simplified form in Fig. 5–1 where only two orthogonal (right angle) measurement axes are displayed. The multivariate similarity of any two individuals can be defined, using a generalization of the familiar Pythagorean theorem, as a *distance* represented by the sum of squares of differences in projections on the coordinate axes $(d^2_{a\beta} = d_1{}^2 + d_2{}^2)$. Alternatively, in terms of the same geometric model, the similarity between two individuals can be defined in terms of the *angular disparity* (cosine) between their score vectors. Since the *distance* between profiles is measured along the "side opposite" to the *angle* between the profile vectors, it is obvious the two indices provide similar information.

## Selection of Measurements for Classification Research

A great deal has been said, by this author and by others, concerning desirable characteristics of measurements used in classification research. In general, the measurements should be relevant, reasonably independent, and comparable in metric. Obviously, if the units of measurement are quite different for different elements within the multivariate profiles, it may not be meaningful simply to add the squared differences to obtain a single composite index without taking the differences in metrics into account. Similarly, if two or more profile elements tend to measure the same thing, the influence of the redundantly represented source of variance will be increased in its effect on the value of a distance function or vector product similarity index. An obviously ideal solution is to choose for classification research variables that can be defined on a priori grounds as being independent and of comparable metric. As we shall see, one begins to run into problems when forced to use *statistical properties* of the multiple measurements in an attempt to transform original scores to achieve comparability of metrics and statistical independence; nevertheless, at times such transformations may be deemed necessary.

A first problem that one encounters in attempting to re-scale measurements for classification research is that it is really the *within class* or the error variance that is the relevant unit for classification and discrimination. According to the theory of types, individuals within categories or sub-types are conceived to be identical except for a multivariate distribution of errors. The difficulty encountered in attempting to re-scale measurements in terms of this error variability is that the classes are not known at the outset; hence the within-class variances and covariances are difficult to estimate in advance.

A second problem is conceptually even more vexing. We can either examine relationships between persons using measurements or functions of measurements as the coordinate axes, or we can examine relationships between measurements using persons as coordinate axes. The *variance* of a measurement variable can be derived geometrically as the squared length of the measurement vector, which in turn is a function of the sum of squares of projections on *orthogonal person axes*. The *covariance* between two measurement variables can be derived geometrically as the sum of products of projections on the same *orthogonal person axes*. These geometric derivations do not follow unless persons are accepted as representing orthogonal axes.

In a directly analogous manner, in the study of relationships between persons (or diseases), the lengths and angular separations between person vectors have their usual geometric meaning only with reference to *orthogonal measurement axes*. Thus, the *statistical* properties of measurement variables and person variables are each defined with reference to the other. With regard to the geometric model, one has to start by postulating or assuming an orthogonal reference frame. In the study of differential relationships among persons, it appears most logical to accept measurement variables as defining the orthogonal axes of the system. It appears both circular and inconsistent to use the assumption of independence among persons to define orthogonality of measurement vectors, and then to turn around and to rely on this definition of orthogonality to study differential relationships among persons. Somewhere one must begin by postulating something!

The view currently held by the present speaker is that we are on as firm ground, or more firm ground, in defining an orthogonal reference frame in terms of a *fixed* set of specified variables than we are in using randomly sampled individuals to define such a reference frame. The orthogonal reference frame is fixed and constant, and conclusions are reached within the context of the specified set of measurement variables. The same reference frame (measurements) can be applied in the same manner to other samples of individuals or diseases. Admittedly, this view is diametrically opposite that held by the present speaker a few years ago.[5] It has developed partly out of the frustrating attempt to reach a firmer conceptual bedrock and partly out of empirical research which has raised serious questions concerning the effects simple statistically based orthogonal transformations have on the reliability of similarity indices.[6] This is not to say that one should not give rational consideration to the problem of choosing measurements that represent reasonably distinct attributes and which have reasonably comparable metrics. If the original units of measurement are not at all comparable, re-scaling in terms of the expected *within class* standard deviations may be desirable.

## Distance Function Indices

The simplest and perhaps most generally useful index of multivariate similarity is the simple distance function. It is calculated as the sum of squares of differences between corresponding scores in two multivariate profiles. With reference to the geometric model illustrated in Fig. 5–1, the square of the distance between two profile points ($d_{ab}$) is equal to the sum of squares of differences in projections ($d_1$ and $d_2$) on the orthogonal reference axes. For simple distance function calculations, each original measurement variable is associated with a distinct orthogonal axis. Scores on these original measurements are then employed as Cartesian coordinates to locate each profile as a point, or vector, in the multidimensional hyperspace. Differences between *scores* for two individuals or diseases can thus be conceived as differences in *projections* on orthogonal reference axes. According to a generalization of the Pythagorean theorem ("The square on the hypotenuse is equal to the sum of squares on the other two sides."), the square of the distance between two profile points in p-dimensional space is equal to the sum of squares of differences in projections on p-orthogonal coordinate axes.

For simplicity, let $\underline{x}_i$ and $\underline{x}_j$ represent the score vectors for the i[th] and j[th] individuals regardless of any preliminary transformations that may have been effected on the data. The same calculations are required irrespective of prior transformations. The simple $d^2$ distance function index can be represented in vector notation as follows:

$$d_{ij}^2 = [\underline{x}_i - \underline{x}_j]' [\underline{x}_i - \underline{x}_j] = \underline{d}' \underline{d} \qquad (1)$$

If the scales of measurement for the several variables within the profiles are obviously quite different, it may be necessary to re-scale them to a common metric. The within-class standard deviation is an acceptable and meaningful metric; however, as previously mentioned, the classes are usually undefined at the beginning of classification research. The purpose of the research is to define the classes. Sometimes data are available, however, from external sources to provide estimates of variance within homogeneous groups of individuals. If the reliability coefficient is known for each measure within the profile, the *within-individual* variability can be derived as a meaningful scaling unit $[\sigma_\varepsilon^2 = \sigma_t^2 (1 - r_{tt})]$. If neither of these error variances can be estimated, one may have to resort to using as an initial approximation the standard deviations derived from a composite heterogeneous sample. In such event, it may be considered worthwhile to iterate the classification analysis using in a second analysis estimates of within-class standard deviations derived from an initial tentative classification. The adjustment for difference in units of measurement among the several profile components can be represented in matrix notation as follows:

$$d_{ij}^2 = [\underline{x}_i - \underline{x}_j]' V^{-1} [\underline{x}_i - \underline{x}_j] \tag{2}$$

where $V^{-1}$ is a diagonal matrix containing reciprocals of the within-class or the within-individual variance of the p profile elements.

If the several variables within the multiple-measurement profiles are substantially related, in the sense that they tend to reflect the same underlying classification dimensions, then some type of orthogonal transformation may be useful to insure a more equal consideration of all relevant dimensions. As previously stated, there seems to be little logic in requiring that profile elements be transformed to have precise statistical independence across all objects that are to be classified. An optimum approach is to define an orthogonal transformation that tends to maximize differences between classification categories, but, once again, it must be recognized that the classification categories are not available at the outset of a classification analysis. An expedient solution, but one which requires considerable computation, is to iterate the classification analysis starting with the simple $d^2$ of Equation 1, progressing to the variance corrected $d^2$ of Equation 2 and finally using as reference axes canonical variates obtained from discrimination among tentatively defined classes in the final step. The orthogonal transformation can be represented in matrix notation as follows:

$$d_{ij}^2 = [\underline{x_i} - \underline{x_j}]' W^{-1}[\underline{x_i} - \underline{x_j}] \qquad (3)$$

where $W^{-1}$ is the inverse of the *within-class* covariance matrix obtained by considering classification grouping from a previous iteration.

Where the number of elements within the profiles is large and the scores tend to be highly related, a canonical reduction to define a relatively small number of highly discriminating orthogonal dimensions will tend to provide more reliable and valid estimates of interprofile distance.

$$d_{ij}^2 = [\underline{x_i} - \underline{x_j}]' A \Lambda^{-1} A'[\underline{x_i} - \underline{x_j}] \qquad (4)$$

where A (p x r) is a matrix containing the first r solution vectors of the matrix equation $(B - \lambda_i W) a_i = 0$ and $\Lambda^{-1}$ is a diagonal matrix containing the reciprocals of the within-groups variances $\lambda_i$ of the linear functions defined by the normalized solution vectors.

The statistician will recognize this canonical reduction as a multiple discriminant analysis. The B and W matrices are between groups and within groups covariance matrices, and the vectors in matrix A define linear combinations of the original variables that have maximum potential for discriminating between members of different subclasses. Once again, Equation 4 cannot be used until a preliminary analysis has identified tentative classification groups. A logical progression involves use of Equation 1 to define profile similarity coefficients prior to any classification grouping. After classification grouping of the simple $d^2$ coefficients, Equation 2 can be used to obtain refined estimates of interprofile distances. Using a tentative grouping defined in the second iteration, a final set of interprofile distances can be computed using Equation 3 or 4. A final classification grouping can be obtained from the $d_{ij}^2$ values computed using the transformed variates.

## VECTOR PRODUCT INDICES OF PROFILE SIMILARITY

The Pythagorean distance function index of profile similarity has been represented as the squared length of one side of a triangle. It is thus dependent upon the angular disparity between the profile vectors and their respective lengths, as can be appreciated from the schematic diagram of Fig. 5–1. It is possible to define another statistic, which will be called a vector product index, that also depends upon angular disparity between profile vectors and their respective lengths. Expanding the distance function of Equation 1, we obtain

$$d_{ij}^2 = x_i' \, x_i + x_j' \, x_j - 2x_i' \, x_j \tag{5}$$

The first two terms represent sums of squares of total projections of the profile vectors on the orthogonal coordinate axes; thus, in terms of the geometric model, we conceive of them as the squared distances of the profile vector end-points from the origin, or the squares of the profile vector lengths. The cross-product term represents the cosine between the profile vectors multiplied by the product of the vector lengths.

$$d_{ij}^2 = l_i^2 + l_j^2 - 2l_i \, l_j \, \mathrm{Cos} \, \theta \tag{6}$$

The raw vector product index of profile similarity is simply the inner product of two score vectors. As described above, this raw vector product can be conceived as the cosine of angular separation between the two profile vectors multiplied by the product of their lengths.

$$v_{ij} = x_i' \, x_j = l_i \, l_j \, \mathrm{Cos} \, \theta_{ij} \tag{7}$$

It is obvious that the raw-score vector product index has one disadvantage as compared with the corresponding distance function. Whereas maximum possible similarity (identity) of two profiles results in $d^2 = 0.0$, the identity of two profiles results in a raw-score vector product equal to the square of the (common) vector length. Thus, the raw-score vector product index can have different values for different pairs of *identical* profiles. The vector length, or sum of squares of profile elements, can be large for one pair of identical profiles and smaller for another pair of identical profiles. For this reason, the vector product indices of profile similarity are almost universally computed using normalized profile vectors in which $\underline{x}_i' \, \underline{x}_i = \underline{x}_j' \, \underline{x}_j = 1.0$.

The simple $d^2$ index of profile similarity has the following expanded form when profile vectors have been normalized so that the sum of squares of elements in each is equal to unity.

$$d_{ij}^2 = 1.0 + 1.0 - 2\underline{x}_i'\underline{x}_j = 2(1 - \text{Cos } \theta). \tag{8}$$

Thus, 

$$d_{ij}^2 = 2 \, (1 - v_{ij}) \tag{9}$$

and 

$$v_{ij} = \underline{x}_i'\underline{x}_j = 1 - \frac{d_{ij}^2}{2} \tag{10}$$

The normalized vector product index has a maximum value of 1.0 corresponding to $d^2 = 0$, and the distance function index has a maximum value of $d^2 = 4.0$ corresponding to $\underline{x}_i'\underline{x}_j' = -1.0$. If the normalized profiles are not elevation-corrected and contain all positive scores, the maximum value for $d^2 = 2.0$ and the minimum vector product is $v = 0.0$.

For each transformed distance function index there is a corresponding transformed vector product index. In the face of incomparability of measurement units, a standard-score transformation may be required as follows:

$$d_{ij}^2 = [\underline{x}_i - \underline{x}_j]' \, V^{-1}[\underline{x}_i - \underline{x}_j]$$

so that 

$$d_{ij}^2 = \underline{x}_i' V^{-1}\underline{x}_i + \underline{x}_j' V^{-1} \underline{x}_j - 2\underline{x}_i'V^{-1}\underline{x}_j \tag{11}$$

where $V^{-1}$ is a diagonal matrix and contains the reciprocals of the within-class variances of the separate profile elements.

The associated vector product index is simply the following:

$$v_{ij} = \underline{x}_i' \, V^{-1} \, \underline{x}_j \tag{12}$$

In a similar manner, it may be considered on a priori or statistical grounds that some type of orthogonal transformation is required. Such transformation can be inserted into the vector product calculation in the same manner as it can be inserted into $d^2$ calculations.

$$v_{ij} = \underline{x}_i' \, W^{-1} \, \underline{x}_j \tag{13}$$

or 

$$v_{ij} = \underline{x}_i' \, A \, \Lambda^{-1}A'\underline{x}_j \tag{14}$$

It will be noted that these equations represent the third terms from expansion of Equations 3 and 4. The matrices $W^{-1}$ and $A\Lambda^{-1}A'$ are the orthogonal transformation matrices described with respect to the two related $d^2$ coefficients.

## CLASSIFICATION ANALYSIS BASED ON $d^2$ MATRIX

Numerous procedures are available for elucidating the subgroup configuration once indices of multivariate similarity have been computed. Most of these procedures are simple, logical decision sequences in which one starts with a "cluster" nucleus and adds to the cluster until no additional profile can be found that is similar enough to be included. At this point, a new cluster nucleus is identified and the search for additional group members begins again. The actual algorithms range from very simple to quite complex.

A computer program that can be used to group together similar individuals and to group into separate classes less similar individuals is presented in Appendix A. This program also appears in a textbook by Overall and Klett [8] in which a more detailed discussion of these and related methods can be found. The program actually consists of two sub-routines, one that results in calculation of a complete matrix of $d^2$ coefficients and another that operates on the $d^2$ matrix to accomplish homogeneous grouping. If $d^2$ coefficients are available from a prior analysis, the entry of raw data can be bypassed. The second sub-routine, which is of concern at this point, accomplishes cluster grouping as follows.

*Step 1:* The nucleus for the first cluster is sought. The ratio of the average distance of the two nearest profiles relative to the average distance to all other profiles is computed for each individual. The individual for whom this ratio is smallest is taken as a pivot point and together with the two individuals nearest to him forms the nucleus for the first cluster.

*Step 2:* Additional profiles are added to the first cluster according to the following decision procedure. The single individual having smallest average distance from individuals already in the cluster relative to the average distance from all other individuals is identified. If the average within-cluster versus extra-cluster ratio is smaller than a predefined critical value, say $B = .6$, the new individual is added. The process is continued until no new candidate is found to qualify for inclusion.

*Step 3:* A new cluster nucleus is sought following a procedure identical to that in Step 1, except that only individuals who are not already in a cluster are considered.

*Step 4:* Additional profiles are added to the new cluster following the procedure of Step 2, except that only individuals who are not already in a cluster are considered as potential candidates. This sequence is continued until all individuals are included in a cluster or until no further cluster nucleus can be identified.

The shortcomings and limitations of such a simple search-and-test procedure are obvious. The procedure is not subject to succinct mathematical description and the statistical sampling distributions for clusters identified in this fashion have not been worked out; thus, mathematicians and statisticians find little with which to work. A real problem with such a method is inherent in the possibility of chance factors operating to form a cluster nucleus. The starting point for any cluster depends on only three profiles. It is possible, by chance, to find three almost identical individuals who actually fall between two or more major clusters. This can distort the results, either by causing two or more distinct clusters to collapse around the off-center nucleus, or by defining an extra cluster which "pulls" away peripheral members from other larger clusters.

In spite of mathematical shortcomings and the possibility that unusual local densities will distort the results, the one thing that can be said for the simple cluster analysis procedure is that it usually works well, yields clinically meaningful results, and tends to produce rather stable results across replications with independent random samples. In view of the weakness of mathematical development and absence of statistical justification, a practical illustration may be of value at this point. The example should serve as an illustration of the potential utility of simple profile cluster analysis in defining underlying latent groups (disorders) in a mixed clinical population.

Psychiatric symptom descriptions available from a previous study of psychiatric diagnostic stereotypes, not real patients, were the data used. These data consisted of Brief Psychiatric Rating

Scale (BPRS) symptom rating profiles provided by a number of experts for "typical" cases of several different diagnostic types. Each "typical" patient was described by quantitative ratings of severity on 16 psychiatric sign and symptom constructs, such as "anxiety" and "motor retardation." For the present exercise, ten "typical" cases were selected *at random* to represent each of three major diagnostic groups: depressive, undifferentiated schizophrenic, and paranoid schizophrenic. The 30 profiles were randomly arranged and subjected to computer cluster analysis using the program listed in Appendix A. The classification procedure was repeated six times using six different independent random samples. The results are presented in Fig. 5–2. The symbols S, P and D indicate schizophrenic, paranoid and depressive diagnostic types and the numerals I, II and III represent empirically derived clusters.

It should be stressed that the computer was not provided with any information concerning actual group membership nor was the classification grouping based on any kind of a previously derived discriminant function technique. The computer program merely sorted each heterogeneous sample of 30 profiles into three homogenous groups. The fact that exactly three clusters were obtained in each analysis is interesting because the number was not fixed in advance. It will be noted that the classification resulting from the empirical similarity grouping agreed very well with the underlying or latent diagnostic classification in all six replications. Such demonstrations, if consistently successful in identifying a known class structure, provide an empirical basis for the expectation that the method can lead to identification of latent class structure in clinical areas where the number and nature of underlying disorders is not known.

## AN INTERNATIONAL CLASSIFICATION FOR PSYCHIATRIC DISORDERS

To illustrate potential utility of the simple cluster analysis program for the development of a classification of *diseases,* as contrasted with individuals, psychiatric diagnostic stereotype data obtained from investigators in France, Germany, Czechoslovakia and Italy will be used. In each of these countries, several dozen

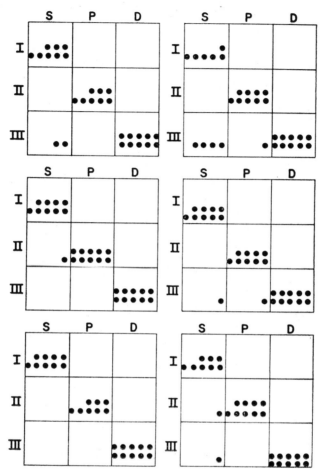

Figure 5–2. Cross-tabulation of cluster analysis results with clinical designation. (Six samples of 30 profiles.)

expert psychiatrists were asked to provide objective rating-scale descriptions of the psychiatric diagnostic types recognized by his countrymen. As a result, 65 to 125 independently derived rating profiles were obtained for each of 11 or 12 different diagnostic types in each of the four countries. Each profile consisted of the 16 symptom rating variables included in the Brief Psychiatric Rating Scale (BPRS).[7] This was a situation in which the specific disease groups (psychiatric diagnostic stereotypes) were previously specified so that it was possible to obtain multiple independent profiles representing each diagnostic type. The purpose of the analysis was not to discover underlying diagnostic types, but instead the objective was to examine relationships among the diagnostic concepts from different countries and to determine whether an empirically valid international classification of psychiatric disorders appears feasible.

The first step in the analysis was to compute a multiple discriminant analysis to define a reduced number of composite variables (canonical variates) that should have maximum utility in distinguishing between the several diagnostic types. In multiple discriminant analysis, the discriminant functions are computed in such manner that they are statistically independent and have unit variance across the several rating profiles *within* the original diagnostic groups. The method of multiple discriminant analysis is described by Rao [9] and the computations are illustrated in greater detail by Overall and Klett.[8] It is sufficient for the present purpose to recognize that the preliminary multiple discriminant analysis resulted in an orthogonal transformation of the original profile scores such that each new orthogonal variate was scaled to have unit variance within the diagnostic stereotype groups. Given an orthogonal transformation matrix (A) and a diagonal matrix $(\Lambda^{-1})$ containing the reciprocals of the within-groups variances of the orthogonal functions, as obtained from the characteristic roots and vectors of the matrix equation $(B - \lambda W)$ $\underline{a} = 0$, Equation 4 was used to compute distance function coefficients between *mean profiles* representing the international diagnostic stereotypes.

The matrix of $d^2$ coefficients was analyzed using the computer program listed in Appendix A. The cluster analysis method sorted the total of 47 mean profiles representing psychiatric diagnostic stereotypes from four European countries into four major classes. Examination of the cluster compositions shown in Table 5–I reveals that at least one diagnostic type from each country fell into each of the empirically derived classes. Thus, each of the empirically identified types is represented in the diagnostic nomenclature of each country. The American concepts of schizophrenia, paranoid syndrome, depression, and mania appear to correspond well to the four classification categories that were found to be represented consistently across four European countries.

Some interesting relationships are apparent in the cluster-groupings which can perhaps lead to better understanding of the

TABLE 5–I

SUMMARY OF D² CLUSTER ANALYSIS OF PSYCHIATRIC DIAGNOSTIC PROTOTYPES FROM FOUR EUROPEAN COUNTRIES

*Type I—Schizophrenia*

Schubförmige Katatone Schizophrenie (German)
Hebephrene Schizophrenie (German)
Schizophrenia Simplex (German)
Schizophrener Persönlichkeitswandel (German)
Schizophrenia Simplex (Czechoslovak)
Schizophrenia Hebefrenická (Czechoslovak)
Schizophrenia Katatonicka (Czechoslovak)
Schizophrenia Katatonicka Agiţovaná (Czechoslovak)
Chronicka Schizophrenia bez výraznějších příznakiu
    (without florid symptoms) (Czechoslovak)
Jiné Funkční Psychotické Stavy (Czechoslovak)
Schizophrénie Paranoide (French)
Etat Confusionnel (French)
Excitation Atypique (French)
Hébéphrénie (French)
Schizophrenia Ebefrenica (Italian)
Schizophrenia Catatonica (Italian)
Schizophrenia Simplex (Italian)
Stato Confusionale o Amenza (Italian)

*Type II—Paranoid States*

Schubförmige Paranoide Schizophrenie (German)
Schubförmige Paranoide—Halluzinatorische (German)
Paranoia (German)
Mischpsychose (German)
Schizophrenia Paranoidní (Czechoslovak)
Paranoidní Stavy (Czechoslovak)
Schizoafektivní Psychóza (Czechoslovak)
Chronická Schizophrenia s Floridními Príznaky
    (with florid symptoms) (Czechoslovak)
Psychose Paranoiaque (French)
Bouffée Délirante (French)
Psychose Hallucinatoire Chronique (French)
Paraphrénie (French)
Schizophrenia Paranoide (Italian)
Paranoia (Italian)
Paraphrenia (Italian)

TABLE 5–I (*Continued*)

*Type III—Depression*
Caenästhetische Schizophrenie (German)
Endogene Depression (German)
Endoreaktive Dysthymie (German)
Deprese Psychotická (Czechoslovak)
Dépression Réactionnelle (French)
Depression Atypique (French)
Mílancolie (French)
Melancolia (Italian)
Depressione Atipica (Italian)
Melancolia Involutiva (Italian)
*Type IV—Mania*
Manie (German)
Manie (Czechoslovak)
Manie (French)
Mania (Italian)

nature of particular European diagnostic concepts. For example, the French stereotype "Schizophrenie Paranoide" does not belong to the Paranoid class, but instead falls within the Schizophrenia class, while French "Boufee Delirante" and "Psychose Hallucinatoire Chronique" fall within the Paranoid classification. The French investigator who was responsible for the original study (Prof. Pichot) has confirmed that this grouping represents actual phenomenological similarities as distinct from transliteration of terminology. Thus, the example appears to confirm how classification analyses are capable of contributing to better understanding of diagnostic terminology used in different countries. The present analysis confirmed that, while terminology may not translate directly, the same four major types of psychiatric disorders are recognized in each of the different countries.

## A CRITERION OF ADEQUACY OF CLASSIFICATION RESULTS

The aim of classification analysis is to cluster individuals or diseases into homogeneous subgroups that are maximally discriminable. A good classification result is one in which individuals within groups are maximally similar relative to the differences between groups. A statistic that represents the ratio of multivariate variability within clusters to the multivariate variability across all clusters provides an index of the adequacy of the classification outcome. Alternative classification groupings can be compared for degree of cluster separation.

A multivariate analogy of the univariate "variance" is the determinant of the variance-covariance matrix. Anderson[1] calls such a determinant the "generalized variance." It should be noted that we are here concerned with the variances and covariances of the p-profile elements computed across individuals. The ratio of the generalized variance within classes to the generalized variance across all classes provides an index of the discriminability or relative separation of classes in the multivariate measurement space. In practice, the determinants of sums of products matrices, rather than covariance matrices are usually employed.

$$\Lambda = \frac{|\,W\,|}{|\,W + B\,|} = \frac{|\,W\,|}{|\,T\,|} \tag{15}$$

where $|\,W\,|$ is the determinant of the within-class sums of products matrix computed across all individuals within groups and $|\,T\,|$ is the determinant of the total sums of products matrix computed across all individuals disregarding groups.

The $\Lambda$ ratio is a well-known statistic that is employed in multivariate analysis to test the significance of differences between groups. It has a maximum value of 1.0 and a minimum value of zero. Small values of $\Lambda$ indicate that profiles for individuals within the clusters are relatively homogeneous as compared with the differences between clusters. Large values of $\Lambda$ indicate that the differences between classes are relatively small as compared with the variability of profiles within classes. Obviously, smaller values of $\Lambda$ are consistent with best classification results.

Although the $\Lambda$ statistic provides an excellent criterion for goodness of cluster configuration, methods that insure the obtaining of the absolute minimum value of $\Lambda$ are not available for most practical problems. Given unlimited computer resources, it would be possible to examine every possible cluster grouping of n objects or individuals and to choose the one that yields the minimum value of $\Lambda$. More practically, one can compare various feasible and likely solutions to choose the one that results in smallest $\Lambda$ value.

A procedure that the present speaker has employed has involved a preliminary cluster grouping using the methods described in the preceding section. A mean profile is computed for each tentative cluster, and the within-cluster covariance matrix is obtained. Individuals are then reassigned among the clusters using a maximum likelihood decision model based on the assumption of multivariate normal distributions of measurements within groups.[8] This will usually result in a change in cluster membership for some peripheral members of the previous tentative clusters. Within-cluster means and covariance matrix are recomputed using the new tentative grouping. At each stage, the $\Lambda$ index is computed and compared with that obtained from the previous tentative grouping. The procedure is terminated when $\Lambda$ fails to decrease in value between two iterations.

## ANALYSIS OF VECTOR PRODUCT MATRICES

Methods that are essentially identical to those described for cluster analysis of matrices of $d^2$ coefficients can be employed with vector product coefficients. The only real difference is that in dealing with vector product indices, larger coefficients indicate greater similarity rather than less similarity. The basic cluster analysis algorithm can easily be modified to key on larger rather than smaller coefficients, or alternatively vector product coefficients can be converted to $d^2$ coefficients using the relationship expressed in Equation 9. This conversion is strictly appropriate only if the profiles from which vector product coefficients are derived were normalized initially. As previously noted, vector product indices are usually computed from normalized profiles in order to eliminate the vector length in evaluating angular disparity (Fig. 5–1). Given a Q-type matrix of vector product coefficients computed from normalized profiles, or computed from raw-score profiles and subsequently scaled to unity in the principal diagonal, the associated matrix of $d^2$ coefficients can be obtained as specified previously.

$$d_{ij}^2 = 2\,(1\,-\,v_{ij})$$

The $d^2$ cluster analysis program presented in Appendix A can then be employed to identify homogeneous subgroups.

Although it is possible to cluster analyze vector product coefficients directly or to convert them to $d^2$ coefficients for subsequent analysis, more interesting and powerful methods are available for analysis of matrices of vector product coefficients. Cluster grouping is one of the potential outcomes of these methods; however, other valuable results include prototype profiles and weighting coefficients defining each individual as a linear composite of underlying pure types.

### Linear Typal Analysis

Linear typal analysis is essentially a factor analysis of a Q-type vector product matrix. Although mechanically much like factor analysis, the assumptions upon which the theoretical model rests and some details of the computation are quite different. To emphasize the distinctive theoretical model, the terminology of factor analysis will be avoided except with regard to a preliminary step in the actual computations.

Linear typal analysis is based on the theoretical conception that the multivariate score profile for an individual is a linear combination of *pure types* from which his characteristics are derived. A relatively few pure types underlie any heterogeneous population. Most individuals tend to be predominantly like one of the pure types, although some individuals are frank mixtures. A genetic analogy can be drawn in the case of several pure inbred strains into which a minor degree of cross-breeding has been introduced. After several generations, the foreign genes will tend to permeate the formerly pure strains in somewhat uniform fashion, although some individuals will manifest more and some less of the alien influence. Each individual can be conceived as a weighted average of the several pure types even though he will be predominantly like the prototype for one of the pure strains.

Within the medical domain, one can conceive of a heterogeneous group of patients manifesting somewhat variable symptom patterns. Most patients in the population will suffer predominantly from a single disorder; however, some individuals will in fact have two or more underlying disorders. In addition to the possibility that two or more disorders can be present in a single individual, certain chance factors, such as measurement or genetic errors, operate to produce a somewhat mixed appearance for most individuals. The multivariate score profile for each individual can be conceived as a weighted combination of prototype profiles representing the underlying pure disease states, plus a component of random error.

The typal model is thus a simple linear model in which the observed score vector for each individual (or disease) is represented as a weighted combination of pure-type profiles (or syndromes).

$$
\begin{bmatrix} x_1 \\ x_2 \\ x_3 \\ \cdot \\ \cdot \\ \cdot \\ \cdot \\ x_p \end{bmatrix} \approx b_1 \begin{bmatrix} Z_{11} \\ Z_{21} \\ Z_{31} \\ \cdot \\ \cdot \\ \cdot \\ \cdot \\ Z_{p1} \end{bmatrix} + b_2 \begin{bmatrix} Z_{12} \\ Z_{22} \\ Z_{32} \\ \cdot \\ \cdot \\ \cdot \\ \cdot \\ Z_{p2} \end{bmatrix} + \ldots + b_r \begin{bmatrix} Z_{1r} \\ Z_{2r} \\ Z_{3r} \\ \cdot \\ \cdot \\ \cdot \\ \cdot \\ Z_{pr} \end{bmatrix} \quad (16)
$$

The individual profile vector $\underline{x}$ will obviously resemble most closely the pure type vector $Z$ with the largest associated $b_1$ coefficient.

Since the observed score profiles for n individuals are conceived as weighted combinations of pure type profiles (except for a random error component), the prototype profiles representing the r underlying pure types can be approximated as weighted combinations of the individual profiles. In such a weighted combination, the individuals who are most like the pure type are given heaviest weight.

$$
\begin{bmatrix} Z_{1i} \\ Z_{2i} \\ Z_{3i} \\ \\ \\ \\ Z_{pi} \end{bmatrix} = a_1 \begin{bmatrix} x_{11} \\ x_{21} \\ x_{31} \\ \\ \\ \\ x_{p1} \end{bmatrix} + a_2 \begin{bmatrix} x_{12} \\ x_{22} \\ x_{32} \\ \\ \\ \\ x_{p2} \end{bmatrix} + \ldots + a_n \begin{bmatrix} x_{1n} \\ x_{2n} \\ x_{3n} \\ \\ \\ \\ x_{pn} \end{bmatrix} \quad (17)
$$

The objectives of linear typal analysis are to determine the nature and number of underlying pure types and to specify the weighting coefficients that define the pure-type composition of each individual. If a clear typal structure is defined in which most individuals relate primarily to one or another particular pure type, classification according to pure-type similarities will be simple and meaningful.

The matrix $Z(p \times r)$ contains prototype profiles for r pure types. It is obtained by applying a properly chosen transformation matrix $A(n \times r)$ to the original data matrix $X'(p \times n)$. The matrix A contains r columns of weighting coefficients, each including a different subset of nonzero elements. The non-zero elements in each column are asociated with a distinct subset of individuals. Thus, each pure type profile in Z is a weighted combination of several individual profiles recorded in the matrix X'.

$$
\begin{array}{ccc}
X & A & = & Z \\
nxp & pxr & & nxr
\end{array}
\tag{18}
$$

The problem, of course, is to specify an objective method for defining the matrix A in such manner that a good typal structure will result. This problem is solved by an oblique approach. (There are actually numerous ways that one can arrive at a good A matrix. The conventional factor analysis method is mentioned here to avoid the necessity of a lengthy discussion of alternative computational procedures). An orthogonal factor analysis of the matrix $Q = X X'$ is undertaken to define r independent factors. These factors are then rotated to obtain the best possible approximation to an orthogonal simple structure.[10] The matric of rotated factor loadings $F(nxr)$ is used as the basis for defining the matrix A.

Let $\hat{A}(nxr)$ be a matrix obtained by setting equal to zero all except the largest element in each of the n rows of F. The matrix $\hat{A}$ will thus contain r columns in which most elements are zero and in which the nonzero elements are associated with a distinct homogeneous subset of individuals. The matrix A, required in Equation 18, is obtained by scaling the columns of $\hat{A}$ using a diagonal matrix $D(rxr)$ that contains the reciprocals of the sums of the r columns of $\hat{A}$.

$$
X' \hat{A} D = X' A = Z
\tag{19}
$$

where $[\hat{A}D]$ is a matrix in which each
of the r columns sums to unity.

Since each column of $A = \hat{A}D$ sums to unity, the pure-type profile vectors in Z should be recognized to be weighted means of the original individual profiles.

The matrix B which contains n sets of weighting coefficients that define each of the original profiles (approximately) as functions of the r pure types (Equation 16) can be obtained as follows:

$$XX' \hat{A} D \Sigma^{-1} = B, \tag{20}$$

Where $\Sigma^{-1}$ is the inverse of
the matrix $\Sigma = D\hat{A}' XX' \hat{A}D$

The matrices Z and B satisfy the basic model equation:

$$\begin{matrix} X & = & B & Z \\ nxp & & nxr & rxp \end{matrix} \tag{21}$$

## CORRECTION TO A MEANINGFUL
## MULTIVARIATE ORIGIN

In the preceding discussion of linear typal analysis, no mention was made of preliminary transformations that may prove advantageous prior to calculation of $Q = XX'$ and the subsequent analysis. It is not infrequent that different variables within the score vectors will have arbitrary and quite different mean values. As a general procedure that can be employed safely without concern for metric properties, it is recommended that each of the p variables constituting the profile elements be standardized to unit variance and mean of $m = 0.5$. The present speaker also prefers to adjust individual (standard score) profiles to a mean of $m = 0.5$ to remove the average elevation effects in the study of pattern differences. This is tantamount to standardizing the p variates, subtracting out the individual profile means and adding the constant $m = 0.5$. In more general form, the elements of the double-corrected, constant-elevation profiles can be defined as follows:

$$x_{ij} = S_{ij} - \overline{S}_{i\cdot} - \overline{S}_{\cdot j} + \overline{S}.. + 0.5, \tag{22}$$

where $S_{ij}$ are the standardized scores. (Actually, standardizing of the p variables results in the column means $\overline{S}_{\cdot j} = 0$ and a grand mean of zero, but equation 22 is desireable as a general form.)

The question of a proper origin for use in multivariate profile analysis has been discussed by several authors. Gollob[3] has proposed that the raw data matrix should be double-centered so that both rows and columns sum to zero. Disregarding the problems created by differences in scales of measurement, this can be accomplished by adjusting each element in the data matrix as follows:

$$x_{ij} = X_{ij} - \overline{X}_{i\cdot} - \overline{X}_{\cdot j} + \overline{X}_{\cdot\cdot}$$

Subtraction of the variable mean from each score has the effect of moving the origin to the center of the person configuration and thus reducing the rank of $Q = XX'$ by one. Analysis of $Q = XX'$ will result in too few factors for proper representation of the cluster configuration unless the proper elevation factor is reintroduced.

Nunnally [4] and Tucker [11] have proposed the use of uncorrected raw scores in profile analysis, but this can produce problems also. The origins, and therefore the mean values, for most measurements in common use are essentially arbitrary and the scales of measurement may be quite different. If the arbitrary origin is too far from the center of the person space, the elements in $Q = XX'$ will be uniformly large and a single large general factor plus $r - 1$ "pattern" factors will emerge. Tucker [11] has suggested that the general factor should be extracted to remove the average of mean effects from the raw score matrix and that the remaining $r - 1$ factors should be used to study individual differences. As he points out, this is essentially equivalent to double-correcting the original score matrix and thus involves similar problems for linear typal analysis.

It is unfortunate that discussions of the proper placement of the origin in the multivariate measurement space have tended to polarize around two extremes. The original raw score origin is frequently arbitrary and too far from the center of the person configuration to yield simple results in linear typal analysis; however, the complete elimination of average profile elevation has an undesirable effect of eliminating a meaningful cluster dimension. The addition of $m = 0.5$ to the standardized scores places the origin at a uniform point at the low end of the score distributions. Although a small number of negative values will remain among the adjusted scores, this should pose no conceptual problem.

The addition of m = .5 to each score in the double-corrected matrix is an arbitrary approximation that has been found to be generally satisfactory. The optimum location of the origin in the multivariate measurement space actually depends on the number of underlying pure types represented in the data matrix, and this in turn depends on the true rank of the data matrix. If the number of pure types can be estimated in advance, even crudely, a good approximation to the optimum origin can be obtained by adding the constant $m = 1/\sqrt{r-1}$ to each score in the double-corrected data matrix, where r is the anticipated number of pure types.

If one desires to place the derived pure-type profiles back into raw score perspective, the following reverse transformation is suggested:

$$Z_{ij} = \sigma_j(z_{ij} - 0.5) + \overline{M}_j, \qquad (23)$$

where $\sigma_j$ is the original standard deviation and $\overline{M}_j$ is the original mean value for the $j^{th}$ profile element.

## SUMMARY

In this paper an attempt has been made to summarize a number of options and alternatives that are available in classification methodology. Multivariate classification methods tend to have two aspects in common. A measure or quantitative definition of multivariate similarities among individuals or diseases is required, and then an algorithm for identifying homogeneous sub-groups on the basis of the similarity indices must be specified. Multivariate similarity indices tend to be of two major types: distance function and vector product. Although the two types of indices are computationally quite different, they tend to be equivalent in the nature of information conveyed and in fact a direct translation from one to the other is usually possible. Various computational alternatives for both distance function and vector product indices include corrections for differences in metrics and dependencies among the profile elements.

Somewhat different algorithms are useful for homogeneous grouping based upon distance function as opposed to vector product coefficients. A simple d² cluster analysis program has been appended because it is difficult to describe in mathematical terms the simple logic of cluster analysis. In general, one starts with a cluster nucleus composed of highly similar profiles and adds to the cluster until no suitable candidate can be found. A new cluster nucleus is then identified and the process is repeated. The same cluster analysis algorithm can be employed in analysis of either distance function or vector product coefficients with only slight modification. The modification involves recognition of *largest* vector product coefficients as representing greatest similarity in contrast to *smallest* d² coefficients. Another possibility is to convert vector products to algebraically equivalent distance function indices and then to proceed with analysis using the d² cluster analysis method.

While cluster analysis provides a good basis for classification categorization, the theory and method of linear typal analysis may be even more useful. The general theoretical model for linear typal analysis assumes that each individual is a additive mixture of several underlying pure types. If the typal structure is reasonably simple, most individuals can be recognized as having characteristics that are predominantly those of a particular pure type. In addition to providing a basis for classification grouping, linear typal analysis results in definition of prototype profiles for the underlying pure types and weighting coefficients representing the pure type composition of each individual.

## ACKNOWLEDGMENTS

This work was supported in part by grant DHEW 5 RO 1 MH 14675–03 from the Psychopharmacology Research Branch, NIMH.

The author is indebted to the following European colleagues for data used in examples: Drs. Pichot (Paris), Hippius (Berlin), Engelsmann (Prague-Montreal) and Rossi (Genova).

## REFERENCES

1. Anderson, T. W.: *An Introduction to Multivariate Statistical Analysis.* New York, Wiley, 1958.
2. Frederickson, P. S., *et al.*: (NIH Group) A system of phenotyping hyperlipoproteinemias using L & H electrophoretic method. *Circulation, 31:*321, 1965.

3. Gollob, H. F.: Confounding of sources of variation in factor-analytic techniques. *Psychol Bull, 70:*330–344, 1968.
4. Nunnally, J.: The analysis of profile data. *Psychol Bull, 59:*311–319, 1962.
5. Overall, J. E.: Note concerning multivariate methods for profile analysis, *Psychol Bull, 61:*195–198, 1963.
6. Overall, J. E.: Investigation of reliability of different profile similarity indices. In Lorr and Lyerly (Eds.) : *Proceedings Conference on Cluster Analysis Methodology.* The Catholic University of America, Washington, D.C., 1967.
7. Overall, J. E. and Gorham, D. R.: The brief psychiatric rating scale. *Psychol Rep, 10:*799–812, 1962.
8. Overall, J. E. and Klett, C. J.: *Applied Multivariate Analysis.* New York, McGraw-Hill, 1972.
9. Rao, C. R.: *Advanced Statistical Methods in Biometric Research.* New York, Wiley, 1952.
10. Thurstone, L. L.: *Multiple Factor Analysis.* Chicago, University of Chicago Press, 1947.
11. Tucker, L. R.: Comments on "Confounding of sources of variation in factor-analytic techniques." *Psychol Bull, 70:*345–354, 1968.

## APPENDIX

```
C     PROGRAM FOR CLUSTER ANALYSIS OF INTER-
      PROFILE DISTANCE MATRIX
      DIMENSION A (60,60) ,X (60) ,Y (60) ,Z (60),R (60)
      DEFINE FILE 1 (60,120,U,L1) ,2 (30,120,U,L2)
    1 FORMAT (314)
    2 FORMAT (18F4.2)
    6 FORMAT (/20H PROFILES IN CLUSTER, I4)
    7 FORMAT (30F4.0)
    8 FORMAT (1X,16F5.2)
    9 FORMAT (/10X,24H MEAN VECTOR FOR CLUS-
      TER, I4)
   10 FORMAT (1X,10F6.1)
   11 FORMAT (/10X,38H DISTANCES WITHIN AND BE-
      TWEEN CLUSTERS)
      READ (2,1) NPRO,NVAR,NODAT
C     NODAT IS CODE ZERO IF RAW DATA CARDS ARE
      TO BE READ
C     NODAT IS CODE NON-ZERO IF DISTANCE FUNC-
      TION MATRIX IS TO BE READ
      FNPRO=NPRO
```

```
        T1=.6
        INDX=0
        L2=1
        DO 666 I=1,NPRO
666   Z (I) =0.0
        IF (NODAT) 554,555,554
554   DO 556 I=1,NPRO
        DO 556 J=I,NPRO
        IF (I-J) 553,556,553
553   READ (2,557) A (I,J)
556   CONTINUE
557   FORMAT (F6.3)
        DO 558 I=1,NPRO
        DO 559 J=I,NPRO
559   A (J,I) =A (I,J)
558   A (I,I) =0.0
        GO TO 65
555   DO 12 I=1,NPRO
        READ (2,2) (X (J) ,J=1,NVAR)
C     AT THIS POINT TRANSFORM PROFILE SCORES
        IF NECESSARY, ALSO
C     AT THIS POINT REMOVE PROFILE ELEVATION
        AND VARIABILITY IF DESIREABLE
12   WRITE (1' I) (X (J) ,J=1,NVAR)
C     BRING BACK PROFILE VECTORS AND COMPUTE
        D-SQR MATRIX
        DO 24 I=1,NPRO
        READ (1' I) (X (J) ,J=1,NVAR)
        DO 24 I2=I,NPRO
        READ (1'I2) (Y (J) ,J=1,NVAR)
        SSQ=0.0
        DO 23 J=1,NVAR
23   SSQ=SSQ+ (X (J) −Y (J) ) **2
        A (I,I2) =SSQ
24   A (I2,I) =SSQ
C     FIND   CLUSTER   NUCLEUS   CONSISTING   OF
        THREE PROFILES
```

```
65 NPR1 = -1+NPRO
   NPR2 = -2+NPRO
   XBAR = 0.0
   DO 66 J = 1,NPRO
   DO 66 J2 = J,NPRO
66 XBAR = XBAR+A (J,J2)
   XBAR = XBAR/ (NPRO*NPR1/2)
99 SML = 9999.
   DO 70 J = 1,NPRO
70 X (J) = 0.0
   DO 79 J1 = 1,NPR2
   IF (Z (J1) ) 79,71,79
71 J11 = J1+1
   DO 78 J2 = J11,NPR1
   IF (Z (J2) ) 78,72,78
72 J22 = J2+1
   DO 77 J3 = J22,NPRO
   IF (Z (J3) ) 77,73,77
73 DIST = A (J1,J2) +A (J1,J3) +A (J2,J3)
   IF (DIST-SML) 74,77,77
74 SML = DIST
   M1 = J1
   M2 = J2
   M3 = J3
77 CONTINUE
78 CONTINUE
79 CONTINUE
   RATIO = SML/ (3.0*XBAR)
   IF (RATIO-.5) 80,81,81
80 X (M1) = 1.0
   X (M2) = 1.0
   X (M3) = 1.0
   Z (M1) = 1.0
   Z (M2) = 1.0
   Z (M3) = 1.0
   XN = 3.0
   GO TO 88
```

```
C      FIND CLUSTER NUCLEUS CONSISTING OF TWO
          PROFILES
   81  SML=9999.
       DO 89 J1=1,NPR1
       IF (Z (J1) ) 89,82,89
   82  J11=J1+1
       DO 87 J2=J11,NPRO
       IF (Z (J2) ) 87,83,87
   83  IF (A (J1,J2) −SML) 84,87,87
   84  SML=A (J1,J2)
       M1=J1
       M2=J2
   87  CONTINUE
   89  CONTINUE
       RATIO=SML/XBAR
       IF (RATIO−.5) 90,900,900
   90  X (M1) =1.0
       X (M2) =1.0
       Z (M2) =1.0
       Z (M1) =1.0
       XN=2.0
C      COMPUTE RATIOS OF AVERAGE CLUSTER AND
          NON-CLUSTER DISTANCES
   88  DO 33 J=1,NPRO
       C2=0.0
       C3=0.0
       DO 34 I=1,NPRO
       IF (X (I) ) 35,36,35
   35  C2=C2+ A (I,J)
       GO TO 34
   36  C3=C3+A (I,J)
   34  CONTINUE
       C2=C2/XN
       C3=C3/ (FNPRO−XN−1)
   33  Y (J) =C2/C3
C      IDENTIFY PROFILE WITH SMALLEST CLUSTER
          RATIO
```

```
          MIN=1
          TEST  =9999.
          NN=0
          DO 37 J=1,NPRO
          IF (Z (J) ) 42,42,37
      42  NN=NN+1
          IF (Y (J) -  TEST) 38,37,37
      38  MIN=J
          TEST=  Y (J)
      37  CONTINUE
          IF (NN)  41,41,39
C         DETERMINE  ADEQUACY  OF  NEW  CLUSTER
              CANDIDATE
      39  IF (Y (MIN) -  T1) 40,40,41
      40  X (MIN) =1.0
          Z (MIN) =1.0
          XN=XN+1.0
          IF (XN-FNPRO-1) 88,41,41
C         PRINT  VECTOR  IDENTIFYING  PROFILES  IN
              CLUSTER
      41  INDX=INDX+1
          WRITE (3,6) INDX
          WRITE (3,7)  (X (J) ,J=1,NPRO)
C         STORE CLUSTER INDICATOR ON DISK
          WRITE (2'L2)  (X (J) ,J=1,NPRO)
          GO TO 99
     900  CONTINUE
          IF (NODAT)  560,561,560
C         COMPUTE MEAN VECTOR FOR EACH CLUSTER
     561  DO 201 J=1,INDX
          READ (2' J)  (X (I) ,I=1,NPRO)
          DO 200 I=1,NVAR
     200  Y (I) =0.0
          FNN=0
          DO 199 I=1,NPRO
          IF (X (I) ) 199,199,198
     198  FNN=FNN+1
```

```
      READ (1' I) (R (K) ,K=1,NVAR)
      DO 197  K=1,NVAR
  197 Y (K) =Y (K) +R (K)
  199 CONTINUE
      DO 195  K=1,NVAR
  195 Y (K) =Y (K) /FNN
      WRITE (3,9) J
  201 WRITE (3,   8) (Y (K) ,K=1,NVAR)
C     COMPUTE AVERAGE WITHIN AND BETWEEN
      CLUSTER DISTANCES
  560 WRITE (3,11)
      DO 302 J=1,INDX
      READ (2' J) (X (I) ,I=1,NPRO)
      DO 301 J2=1,INDX
      READ (2'J2) (Y (I) ,I=1,NPRO)
      SUM=0.0
      FN=0.0
      DO 300 I=1,NPRO
      DO 300 I2=1,NPRO
      IF (I−I2)  298,300,298
  298 XX=X (I) *Y (I2)
      IF (XX) 299,300,299
  299 SUM=SUM+A (I,I2)
      FN=FN+1.0
  300 CONTINUE
      IF (FN)  309,309,312
  309 R (J2) =0.0
      GO TO 301
  312 R (J2) =SUM/FN
  301 CONTINUE
  302 WRITE (3,10) (R (J2) ,J2=1,INDX)
      CALL EXIT
      END
```

## Chapter 6

# STATISTICAL CLASSIFICATION METHODS*

### JEROME CORNFIELD

CLASSIFICATION PROBLEMS ARISE in many different contexts and a variety of abstract formulations of the problem have been developed. No general theory of classification, of which each specific problem is a special case, exists, nor is it clear that any useful purpose would be served by seeking one. Medical diagnosis presents a special subset of classification problems which are by no means trivial, and I shall concentrate on some aspects of this subset. On the general principle that "when a man knows he is to be hanged in a fortnight, it concentrates his mind wonderfully," the aspects reviewed are largely those that have emerged as most relevant to the development of methods for computer diagnosis of the ECG.[1]

### GIVEN AND DERIVED CATEGORIES

A broad initial division is given by distinguishing between problems in which the diagnostic categories can be treated as *given* from those in which they are to be *derived*. No standard terminology exists to distinguish them. Kossack[2] suggests *discrimination* for the former and *identification* for the latter. Many recent discussions refer to the latter problem as that of *cluster* analysis.[3,4] Whatever the terminology, they are vastly different problems. It clearly makes a difference whether we know that "Every boy and every gal that's born into this world alive is either a little liberal or else a little conservative," or whether we must deduce the number and nature of political groupings from information available.

The key phrase here is "information available." In many prob-

* The preparation of this manuscript was supported by Research Grant GM–15004 of the National Institutes of Health.

lems of medical diagnosis it appears useful to consider what is
achievable with partial information; the ECG alone in the case of
pulmonary emphysema,[5] the x-ray alone for tuberculosis,[6] or clinical history alone for differential diagnosis of chest pain.[7] For such
problems the main question is the extent to which the partial information can discriminate between different diagnostic categories
"known" to be present on the basis of more complete information.
It is then useful to act as if the diagnostic categories are given and
to ask how the partial information can most nearly reproduce
them.

These known diagnostic categories must in turn have come
from something, however, and the more basic, and difficult, but
fortunately often less pressing problem, is how they should be derived. It is hard to see how a complete formulation of the derivation problem can proceed by empirical methods alone, no matter
how sophisticated mathematically, since biologically well-grounded
theoretical constructs will often be essential to the formulation of
diagnostic categories. Classes of infectious disease are more than
groupings of symptoms; they presuppose a germ theory. Similarly,
categories of congenital heart disease presuppose a theory of the
circulation, inborn errors of metabolism presuppose a theory of
inheritance, etc. Furthermore, unless categories developed from a
given information set can also predict similarities with respect to
new information, they will not survive advances in knowledge. In
what follows I shall restrict attention to the case in which diagnostic categories are given, deliberately overlooking the possibility
that with proper use of the information available these categories
might be improved.

We shall assume that these given categories are (a) mutually
exclusive, (b) exhaustive, and (c) that it is known without error
to which category each individual to be classified on the basis of
the partial information truly belongs. None of these assumptions
will in general be strictly true. New diagnostic categories presumably still remain to be discovered and the lack of exhaustiveness
must be taken care of by excluding some cases by various informal
means, such as significance tests, as suggested by Bailey.[4] (For an
interesting, but hypothetical, case study of the recognition of a
new diagnostic entity see Crichton.[8]) Furthermore, there is noth-

ing to prevent an individual from having two or more diseases and indeed in the experience of the outpatient departments of The New York Hospital almost half of them do.[9] This poses no problem in principle since diagnostic categories can be redefined to include all possible combinations of diseases, but since with m diseases this redefinition leads to $2^m$ mutually exclusive diagnostic categories, the practical complication can be considerable. That this complication can be more than theoretical is indicated by the observation of Warner *et al.*[10] that neither pulmonary stenosis nor atrial septal defect can by itself produce cyanosis, but that the two together will.

To determine the category to which an individual truly belongs some superior and, in principle, infallible, diagnostic method must be used—catheterization for congenital heart disease,[10] x-rays of the upper gastrointestinal tract for duodenal ulcers,[11] clinical, radiologic, and pulmonary function criteria for pulmonary emphysema,[5] etc. But clearly even such diagnosis may sometimes err. and a certain amount of contamination of the true diagnostic categories may be unavoidable. Even worse, it may not always be possible to assure that the "true" classification is entirely independent of the partial information set to be appraised. It is hard to be sure, for example, that all "true" cases of myocardial infarction are diagnosed without reference to the ECG, and in fact one category, the silent infarct, is defined solely with respect to electrocardiographic abnormalities. Whether such cases are treated as infarcts, normals, or excluded entirely, a certain amount of blurring appears inevitable.

## ASSIGNMENT, BAYES' PROCEDURES AND DECISION TREES
### The Error Matrix

Given mutually exclusive, exhaustive, and infallible diagnostic categories we can now review the formalism involved in evaluating a diagnostic procedure. We initially consider any such procedure as resulting in the assignment of an individual to a diagnostic category on the basis of the partial information available, without yet considering how this information is used to make that assignment. Someone who knows the true disease category for each individual can compute the proportion in each category that were correctly and incorrectly assigned, or more generally, the proportion in that category assigned to each of the other categories. It is thus useful to define for any assignment procedure as follows:

$$p_{ij} = \text{probability that an individual truly in the } i^{th} \\ \text{disease category is assigned to the } j^{th} \quad (2.1)$$

$p_{ii}$ is then the probability of correctly assigning an individual truly in the $i^{th}$ disease category to that category. If there are m categories in all, these probabilities provide a m x m error matrix.

Clearly $\sum_{j=1}^{m} p_{ij} = 1$ for every i; that is, for every true disease category. This matrix provides a description of the consequences of an assignment procedure and can be used to compare the merits of two or more such procedures. Thus if the probabilities of error of a second assignment procedure are denoted by $p_{ij}^{*}$ we should clearly regard the first as more diagnostic if

$$p_{ii} \geq p^{*}_{ii} \text{ for all } i \\ \text{and } p_{ij} \leq p^{*}_{ij} \text{ for all } j \neq i \text{ and all } i \quad (2.2)$$

with at least one of the inequalities strict.

### Bayes' Theorem

The situation described in Equation 2.2 would be an extreme one, but before considering less clear-cut cases it is useful to introduce a little more formal structure.

1. We assume that for each individual the partial information available consists of the values of each of k different variables: $x_1, x_2 \ldots x_k$ and that these same variables are available for each disease category. It is convenient to denote this k-dimensional variable by the single symbol x.

2. Given that an individual is truly in disease category i, the conditional probability that the vector x will be observed is denoted by $f(x \mid i)$.

3. In the patient material to which the error matrix 2.1 applied, each true disease category occurs with a certain frequency. Call the

relative frequency, or probability, of the $i^{th}$ disease category, $g_i$, with $\Sigma\, g_i = 1$.

4. Given that an individual has the vector value $\mathbf{x}$, the conditional probability that he falls in the $i^{th}$ disease category, $P(i \mid \mathbf{x})$ is by Bayes' theorem [12] given by the following:

$$P(i|\mathbf{x}) = \frac{f(\mathbf{x}|i)\, g_i}{\underset{j}{\Sigma}\, f(\mathbf{x}|j)\, g_j} \qquad (2.3)$$

Standard terminology refers to

 — $g_i$ as the prior probability of category i
 $P(i|\mathbf{x})$ as the posterior probability of category i and
 $\lambda f(\mathbf{x}|i)$ as the likelihood of i, where $\lambda$ is any quantity, possibly dependent on $\mathbf{x}$, but not on i.

Equally standard and perhaps more perspicuous for the problem of diagnosis would be to call the terminology as follows:

 $g_i$ the unconditional probability of category i
 $P(i|\mathbf{x})$ the conditional probability of category i, given $\mathbf{x}$
 $f(\mathbf{x}|i)$ the conditional probability of $\mathbf{x}$ given category i.

### Bayes Procedures

Some of the problems involved in giving empirical content to this conceptual structure are the subjects of later sections. Here we use it to review how information must be used for assignment. The more complete discussion by Birnbaum and Maxwell [13] is recommended. A: Suppose one sought an assignment procedure which maximized the overall probability of a correct classification, namely $\underset{i}{\Sigma}\, g_i\, p_{ii}$. It can be shown that the unique assignment procedure with this characteristic is the following: *Assign an individual with observational vector* $\mathbf{x}$ *to that disease category for which the posterior probability given by 2.3 is greatest.* B: Misclassifications need not all be equally serious, and a generalization of the criterion of maximizing the probability of a correct classification is to minimize the average cost of an incorrect one. Thus, if the unit cost of assigning an individual truly in category i to category j is $c_{ij}$ (with $c_{ij} \geq 0$ and $c_{ii} = 0$), the quantity to be minimized is $\underset{i}{\Sigma}\, g_i\, \underset{j}{\Sigma}\, p_{ij}\, c_{ij}$. It can be shown that the assignment procedure that minimizes this is the following: *For an individual with observational vector* **x** *compute the average cost of assignment to category* j, $\bar{c}_j$, *where*

$$\bar{c}_j = \sum_i c_{ij} P(i|\mathbf{x}) \qquad (2.4)$$

*and* $P(i \mid \mathbf{x})$ *is given by 2.3, and assign to that category for which* $c_j$ *is a minimum.* For $c_{ij} = 1$ for all $j \neq i$ and $= 0$ for $j = i$ this reduces to the procedure given in A. C: To one who finds unattractive the problems involved in quantifying prior probabilities and unit costs, a more modest objective than minimizing average cost might be appealing. Returning to 2.2 let us say that assignment procedure 1 *dominates* procedure 2. Call a procedure that is not dominated by any other procedure *admissible.* There may be more than one such procedure, but a more modest objective could be to avoid inadmissible procedures. It can be shown that for given $f(\mathbf{x} \mid i)$ the procedure described in B is admissible for any nonzero set of $g_i$ and $c_{ij}$ and that any other procedure that does not correspond to procedure B for some $g_i$ and $c_{ij}$ is inadmissible.

Call procedure B a *Bayes procedure* relative to given $f(\mathbf{x} \mid i)$, $g_i$ and $c_{ij}$. Then C tells us that we can reject out of hand any procedure that is not a Bayes procedure relative to some set of priors $(g_i)$, likelihood $\lambda f(\mathbf{x} \mid i)$, and unit costs $(c_{ij})$ and that from this formal point of view the empirical problems in diagnosis relate entirely to the determination of these quantities.

## Comparison with Decision Trees

Clearly any Bayes procedure can be cast into the form of a decision tree,[14,15] but the converse is false. Not all decision trees are Bayes procedures and hence not all decision trees are admissible. Some elaboration follows.

It is easy to see that a Bayes procedure can be cast into the form of a decision tree. For given **x** choose diagnostic category 1 in preference to category 2 if $\bar{c}_1 < \bar{c}_2$ (Equation 2.4) and category 2 otherwise. Compare whatever category is chosen in the first step with category 3 and choose category 3 if $\bar{c}_3 < \min (\bar{c}_1, \bar{c}_2)$, but the category chosen in the first step otherwise, and so on. This decision tree will obviously choose the category with the minimum average cost and hence is a Bayes procedure.

Second, consider a seemingly mild modification of the above tree which leads to a non-Bayes, and hence inadmissible, procedure. Since the first step involves only a choice between 1 and 2, $c_{13}$, $c_{23}$, $c_{14}$, $c_{24}$, etc. might be considered irrelevant since they involve diagnostic categories 3, 4, etc. One might at step 1 therefore use only the first two items of 2.4 and choose category 1 in the first step of the decision tree if

$$c_{11}\,P(1 \mid \mathbf{x}) + c_{12}\,P(2 \mid \mathbf{x}) < c_{21}\,P(1 \mid \mathbf{x}) + c_{22}\,P(2 \mid \mathbf{x}) \qquad (2.5)$$

and category 2 otherwise, with similar modifications for subsequent steps. It is easy to convince oneself that this need not lead to the choice of the category with minimum $\bar{c}_i$ and hence is not a Bayes procedure.

A variant of this non-Bayesian decision tree is sometimes seen. Equation 2.5 chooses category 1 if $f(\mathbf{x} \mid 1)/f(\mathbf{x} \mid 2) > c_{12}/c_{21}$ (since $c_{11} = c_{22} = 0$ and everything else in the posterior probabilities cancel). But since the choice depends only on the ratio of the likelihood of 1 to 2, it might seem plausible to use not all k variables, but only those that distinguish between categories 1 and 2, with a similar restriction at each other step in the decision tree. But this is not a Bayes' procedure—as will often be seen by the failure of the posterior probabilities for an individual to sum to unity when all pairwise likelihood ratios do not include the same variables.

That this use of different variables at different pairwise decision points in the tree is self-contradictory can also be seen without appeal to Bayes. Consider three variables and three diagnostic categories. Variable A is treated as distinguishing between categories 1 and 2, variable B between categories 1 and 3 and variable C between categories 2 and 3. But if variable B for an individual points towards category 1 rather than 3 while C considers categories 2 and 3 equally probable, then variables B and C together point towards category 1 rather than 2 and it is contradictory to treat only A as containing information bearing on this choice.

### Beyond Assignment

The assignment of each individual to one of m diagnostic categories provides a useful way of comparing different assignment procedures and of assessing the informational content of any partial information set. It is too simple, however, to serve as a complete model of diagnosis. A more general formulation would substitute decisions for assignments. On the basis of **x** one could decide, for example,

1. Admit the patient to an intensive care unit.
2. Keep for further observation.
3. Send him home with assurances of health, etc.

The cost of the $j^{th}$ decision $(j = 1,2 \ldots n$ and $n \neq m$ necessarily) when the true disease category is the $i^{th}$ is denoted by $c_{ij}$ and a *Bayes decision procedure* is to select the decision for which the average cost, $\bar{c}_j$, defined in 2.4, is a minimum. Various special cases are possible. Thus, the first m decisions could be to assign to one of the m diseases categories and the $m + 1^{th}$ to suspend judgment, with $c_{1(m+1)} < \min (c_{11} \ldots c_{1m})$.

Even when all the elements for a complete decision are known, the prior probabilities, the likelihood and a cost matrix, and computers are available for combining these elements, there are advantages to computing various intermediate results so that the humans involved in the system can control it. A particularly useful intermediate result, which is independent of the costs and only partially dependent on the prior probabilities has been variously termed the average likelihood ratio,[16] the Bayes factor,[17] and the rbo (for relative betting odds).[18] It comes from rewriting 2.3 as follows:

$$\frac{P(i \mid \mathbf{x})}{1 - P(i \mid \mathbf{x})} \bigg/ \frac{g_i}{1 - g_i} = \left[ \frac{1}{1 - g_i} \sum_{j \neq i} \frac{f(\mathbf{x} \mid j)}{f(\mathbf{x} \mid i)} g_i \right]^{-1} \tag{2.6}$$

The quantity $P(i \mid \mathbf{x})/[1-P(i \mid \mathbf{x})]$ is the posterior betting odds on category i, given **x**, the quantity $g_i/(1-g_i)$ the prior odds, and their ratio the relative betting odds. A particular value, e.g. 2, is interpreted to mean that whatever your prior odds on category i, knowledge of **x** has doubled them. The right-hand side of 2.6 shows that this quantity is the weighted harmonic mean of the individual likelihood ratios, the weights being the prior probabilities. Thus, the prior probabilities influence the results only as weights, and when there are only two disease categories are not involved at all.

## EMPIRICAL IMPLEMENTATION

The argument of the preceding section supplies the conceptual framework within which diagnostic decisions can take place. Detailed implementation raises a number of statistical problems, to which we now turn.

### Models for Estimating Conditional Probabilities

The formal counterpart of the data base required for diagnostic decisions is the conditional probability, $f(x \mid i)$ of Bayes' Theorem (Equation 2.3). This provides a description of the expected multivariate distribution by the variables $x_1, x_2 \ldots x_k$ of individuals, who are truly in disease category i. A formal and only mildly restrictive way of representing this distribution is in terms of a k-dimensional table showing the proportion of individuals in the $i^{th}$ disease category who have each particular combination of values of the variables. If each variable is dichotomized, the table has $2^k$ cells, or more generally, if the $\alpha^{th}$ variable is broken into $r_a$ disjoint categories, the table has $\prod_\alpha r_a$ cells. Denote for those in disease category i the probability of falling in the $j^{th}$ cell $(j = 1,2 \ldots \prod_\alpha r_a)$ by $p_j(i)$. Then $f(x \mid i) = p_j(i)$ and the statistical problem is to estimate this quantity from the data available.

The most straightforward estimate is to set each probability equal to the observed proportion falling in the cell. But even with only ten dichotomized variables the table will contain 1024 cells and unless the data base is very large indeed the probabilities will be poorly estimated. If the same body of data is used both to estimate the conditional probabilities in this fashion and to compute the error matrix, the poor quality of the estimates may not be obvious. But if the estimated probabilities are used to assign a new group of individuals and the error matrix is calculated for this new assignment, poor quality will manifest itself in a much higher misclassification rate.

An appropriate general response to this problem is to assume some structural model, such as independence, for the k-way table. The effect of using a model is to base the estimate of $p_j(i)$ on something more than the observed proportion in the $j^{th}$ cell and hence to reduce its variance. If the model is inappropriate, it will also lead to an increase in bias. The problem is to find models for which the increased bias is more than compensated for by decreased variance. The simplest model is that of independence and can lead to better estimates than are obtained with the complete k-way table, even when untrue. Although assignments based on this model have led to acceptably small misclassification errors, the associated posterior probabilities tend to be unrealistically close to unity.[19]

A class of models that will often be less restrictive can be obtained by assuming that the $p_j(i)$ are described by some multivariate distribution whose mathematical form is known, but whose parameter values must be estimated from the data. The only such distribution for which routine calculating methods are now available is the multivariate normal, although more general families leading to the same likelihood function have been suggested.[20] The k-variate normal probabliity density function for the $i^{th}$ category is as follows:

$$f(\mathbf{x} \mid i) = [(2\pi)^k \mid \Sigma_i \mid]^{-1/2} \exp\left[-\tfrac{1}{2}(\mathbf{x} - \mu_i)' \Sigma_i^{-1}(\mathbf{x} - \mu_i)\right] \quad (3.1)$$

where $\mu_i$ is the vector of means and $\Sigma_i$ is the variance-covariance matrix and a prime denotes a row vector. It is usually further assumed that $\Sigma_i$ is the same for all categories. With these assumptions the log of the likelihood ratio implicit in Equation 2.3 is given by

$$\log \frac{f(\mathbf{x} \mid j)}{f(\mathbf{x} \mid i)} = (\mathbf{x} - (\mu_i + \mu_j)/2)' \Sigma^{-1} (\mu_j - \mu_i) \quad (3.2)$$

and will be recognized as Fisher's linear discriminant function. In practice of course $\mu_i$, $\mu_j$ and $\Sigma$ are unknown and must be estimated. The next section considers some of the problems arising because of this.

It is a rare set of data that is even approximately multivariate normal and with equal variance-covariance matrices. It does not necessarily follow, however, that posterior probabilities computed assuming multivariate normality will be incorrect. Truett *et al.*[21] assumed multivariate normality in an analysis of seven possible risk factors in coronary heart disease. The departures from normality in this case were substantial, but it was nevertheless demonstrated that posterior probabilities estimated from discriminant functions were in good agreement with the empirically observed ones. An even more striking demonstration that the absence of multivariate normality is not necessarily fatal is provided by alternative analyses of six yes-no questions on chest pain used to discriminate between 376 patients with acute myocardial infarction and 383 patients having either an old myocardial infarction or angina pectoris. Using linear discriminant functions on these six dichotomous variables Pipberger *et al.* were able to classify 78 per cent of the patients correctly.[7] Using $2^6$ tables for each of the diagnostic categories and assigning a patient in the $j^{th}$ cell ($j=1,2 \ldots 2^6$) to that diagnostic category for which $p_j(i)$ was largest, thus achieving minimum misclassification error for the 759 patients under study, 80 per cent of the patients were correctly classified. The improvement is somewhat less than phenomenal, despite the obvious lack of multivariate normality.

For the posterior probabilities to agree with the empirically observed ones it is sufficient that the linear discriminant given by Equation 3.2 be univariate normal for both disease categories and with equal variances. But, because of the central limit theorem for dependent random variables, a linear function can be univariate normal even when the individual x's are not multivariate normal. Truett's Fig. 6–2 makes it clear that the distribution of her linear function was approximately normal even with only seven variables and that this was the reason for the accuracy of the posterior probabilities yielded by the model.

It does not necessarily follow, however, that the application of multivariate normal theory to non-normal data is without consequence. Although the posterior probabilities associated with each value of the linear function may be correctly estimated, the linear function itself need not be appropriate, as in the case, for example, in which combinations of variables are more diagnostic than their linear compound. For such cases the effect of an inappropriate assumption is an increased misclassification rate. Thus not all the information contained in the data need be extracted, even though what is extracted need not be misleading. This contrasts with the independence model which can lead to misleadingly high posterior probabilities in the presence of dependence.

As an introduction to the use of less restrictive models note that independence assumes the complete absence of interactions;* use of observed proportions in the complete k-way table assumes the presence of all interactions up to k-variable interactions, and multivariate normality assumes that the k-way table can be constructed knowing only the k one-way tables for each category and the $\binom{k}{2}$ two-way tables. It is not necessary to choose between these extreme assumptions, however, and methods now exist that allow one to assume the presence of only those interactions indicated by the data. These methods will in general lead to improved estimates as compared to either of the extremes. There are two somewhat different implementations of this idea, one due to Birch [22] and applied with great effectiveness in the National Halothane Study [23] and the other a straightforward application of Bayesian methods to this problem, due to Cornfield.[24] The application of Birch's procedure involves acting, on the basis of significance tests, as if some, but not necessarily all, of the interactions are zero. The Bayesian procedure has the effect of using all interactions but giving them decreased weight, the actual decrease being larger the less-well determined the interaction. Both methods are applicable to any estimation problem involving multidimensional tables, of which the problem of diagnosis is of course only one. Neither method appears to have been applied to diagnosis so that their contribution to this problem remains to be assessed. At a minimum, both provide ways of investigating the sensitivity of assignment procedures to departures from independence or multivariate normality and at a maximum improvement in these procedures when sensitivity to departures is large. Other alternatives to assuming independence or using the complete k-way table are discussed by Dickey [25] and Brunk and Lehr.[26]

---

* If $x_{ij}$ is the value in the $i^{th}$ row and $j^{th}$ column of a two-way table and $x_{ij}$ can be written as $K + c_i + r_j$ for all i and j we say that there is no interaction. Interaction is defined as any departure from this additive model. The magnitude, indeed presence, of interaction may depend on the scale in which the variables are expressed. In the discussion from Equation 3.4 below on, the scale assumed is log p.

**TABLE 6–I**

**OBSERVED FREQUENCIES IN A 2x2x2 TABLE**

| | | | Question 3 | | |
|---|---|---|---|---|---|
| | | | Y | N | *Total* |
| *Question 1* | Q2 | Y | $x_{111}$ | $x_{112}$ | $x_{11.}$ |
| Y | | N | $x_{121}$ | $x_{122}$ | $x_{12.}$ |
| | | Total | $x_{1.1}$ | $x_{1.2}$ | $x_{1..}$ |
| | Q2 | Y | $x_{211}$ | $x_{212}$ | $x_{21.}$ |
| N | | N | $x_{221}$ | $x_{222}$ | $x_{22.}$ |
| | | Total | $x_{2.1}$ | $x_{2.2}$ | $x_{2..}$ |
| | Grand Total | | $x_{..1}$ | $x_{..2}$ | $x_{...}(=n)$ |

Birch's approach will be illustrated by use of three dichotomized variables, which can be thought of as yes-no answers to each of three questions. (The correct analysis for this special case had been given earlier by Anderson and Bancroft.[26a]) The notation is summarized in Table 6–I. The observed number responding affirmatively to all three questions is $x_{111}$ and $Ex_{111} = p_{111}n$. Also $x_{111} + x_{112} = x_{11.}$; $x_{11.} + x_{12.} = x_{1..}$, etc. Thus, the number responding affirmatively to questions 1, 2 and 3 are respectively $x_{1..}$, $x_{.1.}$ and $x_{..1}$. Assuming independence, an estimate of $p_{111}$, say $\hat{p}_{111}$, is given by the following:

$$\hat{p}_{111} = x_{1..} \cdot x_{.1.} \cdot x_{..1}/n^3 \tag{3.3}$$

This assumes no interactions, i.e. the following:

$$\frac{p_{111}}{p_{121}} \frac{p_{122}}{p_{112}} = 1 \quad \text{for } i = 1,2 \tag{3.4}$$

This assumption can of course be tested. It might turn out that in fact this quantity is equal to $\theta$ for $i = 1,2$ and $\theta \neq 1$, i.e. that there are two factor interactions, but that, since $\theta$ is the same for a yes or no answer to question 1, that there are no three factor interactions. The estimates of $p_{ijk}$ with these assumptions are given by the following:

$$\hat{p}_{ijk} = \frac{x_{ijk} + \lambda}{n} \text{for all combinations of i, j, and k on the left hand side of equation 3.6}$$

$$= \frac{x_{ijk} - \lambda}{n} \text{for all combinations of i, j, and k on the right hand side of equation 3.6} \tag{3.5}$$

where $\lambda$ is uniquely defined (for $x_{ijk} \neq 0$ for all i, j, and k) by the following:

$$(x_{111} + \lambda)(x_{122} + \lambda)(x_{221} + \lambda)(x_{212} + \lambda) = \\ (x_{211} - \lambda)(x_{222} - \lambda)(x_{121} - \lambda)(x_{112} - \lambda) \qquad (3.6)$$

The generalization to more general contingency tables is straightforward.

## Effects of Estimating Unknown Parameters

A given assignment procedure will usually lead to a smaller error rate in the data from which the conditional probabilities have been derived than when applied to a new body of data.[27] This attenuation has a number of sources, of which the selection of the discriminating variables on the basis of the data on hand is an important but theoretically perplexing one, and will be discussed in the next section. Nevertheless a clear-cut theoretical model of a simpler situation, in which only the effect of estimating unknown parameters is considered, can lead to considerable insight for more complex cases.

We shall consider initially two-category discrimination when multivariate normality and equality of the variance-covariance matrices obtain, and the k discriminating variables are taken as given. The basic result is summarized in Table 6–II and discussed in the paragraphs after Equation 3.10. The same problem has been considered for k-dimensional tables by Cochran and Hopkins,[28] Hills,[29] and Dunn and Varady [29a] with broadly similar results. The argument leading to the result in Table 6–II follows.

TABLE 6–II

SAMPLE MISCLASSIFICATION RATE, $\Phi(-\sqrt{Ez^2}/2)$, BY RATIO OF NUMBER OF DISCRIMINATING VARIABLES TO NUMBER OF CASES AND TRUE MISCLASSIFICATION RATE FOR EQUAL-SIZED GROUPS
$(n_1 = n_2)$ and $n_1 >> 3)$

| Ratio of Number of Variables to Number of Cases $(k/(n_1+n_2))$ | True Misclassification Rate $(\Phi(-\zeta/2))$ | | | | |
|---|---|---|---|---|---|
| | .50 | .40 | .31 | .16 | .023 |
| | | Sample Misclassification Rate | | | |
| 3/4 | .00 | .00 | .00 | .00 | .000 |
| 1/2 | .16 | .14 | .11 | .04 | .001 |
| 1/5 | .31 | .28 | .23 | .11 | .010 |
| 1/10 | .37 | .34 | .27 | .14 | .016 |
| 1/20 | .41 | .37 | .29 | .15 | .019 |

When the parameters of the distributions are known, a linear compound $\zeta$ of the discriminating variables, given by 3.2, is defined for each individual in the two groups. The compound $\zeta$ will have a univariate normal distribution with means $\bar{\zeta}_1$ and $\bar{\zeta}_2$ in the two groups and common variance $\sigma^2$. A measure of the distance between the two groups obtained with the given discriminating variables is then

$$\zeta^2 = \frac{(\bar{\xi}_1 - \bar{\xi}_2)^2}{\sigma^2} = (\mu_1 - \mu_2)' \Sigma^{-1} (\mu_1 - \mu_2) \qquad (3.7)$$

If each individual is assigned to the group having the larger likelihood, given x, then a sketch of the relevant univariate distributions makes clear that the proportion misclassified in each of the two groups is $\Phi\left(-\zeta/2\right)$, i.e. the probability given by the standard normal integral from minus infinity to $-\zeta/2$.

When the parameters are unkown and estimates are made on the basis of observations on $n_1$ individuals in group 1 and $n_2$ in group 2 an estimated value, y, of the linear compound for observed vector x will be obtained, where, corresponding to 3.2 it is as follows:

$$y = (x - (\bar{x}_1 + \bar{x}_2)/2)' S^{-1} (\bar{x}_1 - \bar{x}_2) \qquad (3.8)$$

where $x_1$, $x_2$ and S are sample estimates of $\mu_1$, $\mu_2$ and $\Sigma$ respectively. Conditional on $x_1$, $x_2$ and S the compound y will have univariate normal distributions in the two groups with sample distance given by the following:

$$z^2 = \left(\frac{\bar{y}_1 - \bar{y}_2}{s^2}\right)^2 = (\bar{x}_1 - \bar{x}_2)' S^{-1} (\bar{x}_1 - \bar{x}_2) \qquad (3.9)$$

and misclassification rate given by $\Phi(-z/2)$, where $s^2$ is the pooled variance of the y.

The question then is what is the relation between $z^2$, the sample distance, and $\zeta^2$, the true distance? It has been independently observed by Cornfield [30] and Lachenbruch [31] that the expected value of $z^2$ over repeated samples of size $n_1$ and $n_2$, say $Ez^2$, is given by the following:

$$Ez^2 = \frac{n_1 + n_2 - 2}{n_1 + n_2 - k - 3} \left[ k \left( \frac{1}{n_1} + \frac{1}{n_2} \right) + \zeta^2 \right] \qquad (3.10)$$

where, k, as before, is the number of discriminating variables.

Clearly, the expected sample distance exceeds the true distance. The magnitude of the average excess may be surprising, however. Consider, for example, the case in which no discrimination whatsoever exists, i.e. $\zeta^2 = 0$, but with $n_1 = n_2 = k$, i.e. half as many discriminating variables as there are individuals. Then $Ez^2 = $

$\dfrac{n_1 + n_2 - 2}{n_1 + n_2 - k - 3} \left[ k \left( \dfrac{1}{n_1} + \dfrac{1}{n_2} \right) \right] > 4$ and the misclassification rate

corresponding to the expected value of the sample distance is $\Phi[-\sqrt{Ez^2}/2] < .16$, as compared with $\Phi(0) = .50$ for the true misclassification rate with variables totally lacking discriminatory power.

A comparison of $\Phi[-\sqrt{Ez^2}/2]$, which we refer to as the sample misclassification rate, for various true misclassification rates and ratio of number of variables to number of cases is shown in Table 6–II. Clearly, with this ratio equal to or greater than $\frac{1}{2}$ the sample rates can be grossly misleading, no matter how large $n_1$ and $n_2$ or the degrees of freedom, and only with ratios $1/20$ or less do the biases appear to become small. A less unreliable method of estimating misclassification rates would be to compute an unbiased estimate of $\zeta^2$, say $\hat{\zeta}^2$, where from 3.10 we receive the following:

$$\hat{\zeta}^2 = \frac{n_1 + n_2 - k - 3}{n_1 + n_2 - 2} z^2 - k \left( \frac{1}{n_1} + \frac{1}{n_2} \right) \qquad (3.11)$$

and to compute an adjusted misclassification rate as follows:

$$\phi[-\sqrt{\max(0, \hat{\zeta}^2)}/2] \qquad (3.12)$$

The results in Table 6–II also indicate that calculation of posterior probabilities by substitution of the sample estimates $x_1$, $x_2$ and $S$ for population parameters in 3.1 may lead to likelihood ratios whose departure from unity is exaggerated, a point to which attention has been called by Lachenbruch.[31] An argument of Geisser's [32] indicates that an appropriate way of allowing in the estimation of posterior probabilities for the fact that parameters are estimated is to use instead of 3.1 with sample estimates substituted for unknown parameters, the following expression for the probability density function:

$$f(\mathbf{x} \mid i) \propto \left(\frac{n_i}{n_i + 1}\right)^{(1/2)k} \frac{\{\Gamma(n - m + k)\}}{\{\Gamma(n - m)\}}$$

$$\left[1 + \frac{n_i(\mathbf{x} - \bar{\mathbf{x}}_i)' \, S^{-1}(\mathbf{x} - \bar{\mathbf{x}}_i)}{(n_i + 1)(n - m)}\right]^{-(1/2)(n - m + k)} \qquad (3.13)$$

where $n = \sum_{i=1}^{m} n_i$, and as before m is the number of diagnostic
groups and k is the number of discriminatory variables. This is
Geisser's case 8 with v set equal to 2. This result is obtained by
integrating the density 3.1 over the posterior distribution of the
unknown parameters and is an appropriate Bayesian way of allowing for the effects of estimation in the calculation of the posterior
probability of belonging to the i[th] category. As n-m increases for
fixed k, 3.13 (with proportionality constants included) approaches
3.1.

The adjusted misclassification rate yielded by 3.12 is still an
underestimate of the rate to be expected when the *sample* discriminant, 3.8, is applied to the population; it estimates only the
rate to be expected when the *true* discriminant based on these k
variables, 3.2 is so applied. On the basis of Cochran and Hopkins'
Table 4 this underestimate appears to be considerably smaller than
the difference between the true and sample misclassification rate.

### Selection of Variables

We shall assume that we are given a large but finite number
of variables on which information is available for all disease categories, and from which the discriminatory variables are to be
selected. (This contrasts with pattern recognition problems in
which even the initial finite set of variables is not given.) We
suspect however that some, and perhaps many, of the variables in
this initial set have little or no discriminatory power. The way one
proceeds from this point depends on whether this suspicion is
formally incorporated into the mathematical structure via appropriate prior probabilities, or simply motivates the search for an
algorithm which will identify most of the nondiscriminating vari-

ables without being formally incorporated into the algorithm. I shall concentrate on the latter approach only because of the present availability of systematic procedures for implementing it. Many consider, however, that as the former approach is investigated, it will prove to be the more penetrating.

In general one can start with the complete set of variables and eliminate one by one those which make no "significant" contribution to discrimination, or one can start with the single most discriminating variable and add additional ones as long as "significant" increases in discrimination are achieved. These step-down and step-up procedures need not lead to the same choice of variables nor need either set be an optimum one. Numerous computer routines are available for performing the selection, of which only the Biomed package will be mentioned.

No formal criteria are known for choosing between the two procedures, although intuitively it would appear to depend upon whether the nondiscriminating variables are a large or small proportion of the total. It has been a common experience that a point of diminishing returns is reached very rapidly as the number of discriminating variables is increased. This would seem to argue for step-up procedures.

A crude statistical model makes it clear why there does appear to be a point of diminishing returns. We consider only the case of independence, chiefly because of its simplicity, but also because step-up procedures may tend to select variables with low correlations and partly because departures from independence further slows down the already slow rate at which discrimination increases with increasing numbers of variables.

Consider the signed square-root of the distance between two disease categories obtained with any *one* variable (Equation 3.7) and assume that the distribution of distances for the k variables being considered is normal with mean 0 and variance V. Or, since the sign of the difference is irrelevant, assume that the distances themselves are distributed as $V\chi^2$ where $\chi^2$ is distributed as chi-square with one degree of freedom. Denote the $i^{th}$ order statistic from this distribution by $\chi_i^2$ ($\chi_1^2 \geq \chi_2^2 \geq \ldots \chi_k^2$). Then the distance between the two populations, using the j most discriminating variables is $V \sum\limits_{i=1}^{j} \chi_i^2$ and the percent misclassified, $P_j$, is the following:

$$P_j = \Phi \left[ -\frac{1}{2} \left( V \sum_{i=1}^{j} \chi_i^2 \right)^{1/2} \right] \qquad (3.14)$$

At the same level of crudity as the model itself we may eliminate V by noting the following:

$$P_1 = \Phi \left[ -\frac{1}{2} \sqrt{V\chi_1^2} \right], \qquad (3.15)$$

solving for V and substituting in 3.14 to obtain the following:

$$P_j = \Phi \left[ \frac{\Phi^{-1}(P_1)}{\chi_1} \left( \sum_{i=1}^{j} \chi_i^2 \right)^{1/2} \right] \qquad (3.16)$$

To illustrate, consider the six chest pain variables of Pipberger *et al.* previously discussed. The best single question resulted in 29.3 percent misclassified, so that

$$P_1 = .293$$

and from any standard normal (or probit) table

$$\Phi^{-1} (.293) = -.545.$$

The 1 degree of freedom chi-square order statistics as calculated from gamma order statistics given by Harter [33] are 3.03, 1.48, 0.81, 0.43, 0.19, 0.06, so that

$$P_6 = \Phi \left[ \frac{-.545}{\sqrt{3.03}} (3.03 + 1.48 + 0.81 + 0.43 + 0.19 + 0.06)^{1/2} \right]$$
$$= .222$$

Thus with this model the proportion misclassified with the best variable, .293, should decrease to .222 with the six best. It in fact decreased to .204.

An even more extreme case of the slow decrease in the percent misclassified with increasing numbers of questions is given by the data of Collen *et al.* on symptoms associated with asthma,[34] in which the best question (question 2) misclassified 27 out of 230 asthmatics and 23 out of 517 non-asthmatics, while the best six misclassified 24 of the former and 24 of the latter—for almost no improvement. The above model would have led to an expectation of a decrease from 8.1 percent misclassified with the best question (equal weighting of the two groups) to 2.5 percent with six, and the failure to achieve even this improvement may be due to non-independence between the questions.

At any point in a step-up procedure there are two groups of variables, those already selected and those yet to be investigated, say $k_1$ in the first group and $k_2$ in the second. Because of inter-correlations, the actual distances between two disease categories for any one of the variables in the second group may be "explained" by those in the first group. Adjusted differences for each variable can be obtained by standard covariance procedures. To decide whether any of these adjusted distances is of sufficient magnitude to warrant moving one or more of the variables from the second to the first group one might consider the combined distance statistic (Equation 3.9) on the adjusted variables in the second group, either via a significance test or an unbiased estimate of its magnitude (Equation 3.11). There is a difficulty in principle when the number of variables in the second group exceeds the number of individuals since S is then singular and cannot be inverted. This suggests that even when the inversion can be performed that the effects of a small number of discriminating variables may be swamped by a large number of useless ones. A compromise is to consider only the $l$ largest adjusted distances in the second group, where $l$ is some small integer. In many computer routines $l$ is set equal to unity, but this would seem to invite the kind of multiple comparison error that multivariate statistical procedures were originally designed to avoid. A compromise would involve setting $l = k_1 + 1$. If the distance statistic so obtained is considered large enough, the single variable with the largest adjusted distance is moved from the second to the first group and the process repeated. If not, the process terminates.

The major shortcoming of such procedures is not so much their failure necessarily to achieve an optimum choice of variables, as the inability to obtain any analytic indication, such as that given by Equation 3.10, of how well the variables obtained will work for a new body of data. Clearly the estimate given by 3.12 may still be too low. Traditionally this problem has been met by "validating" the variables selected on a new body of data, where this new body can consist of a portion of the original sample set aside for this purpose. This latter procedure has the disadvantage of basing the selection and estimation on only a portion of the information. When the number of variables is given, an ingenious adaptation of jackknife procedures by Lachenbruch [35] appears to handle this problem, but its suitability when the variables have been selected is not so clear. Experimentation with the performance of step-procedures in split samples might produce some empirical modification of Equation 3.10 appropriate for the variable selection case, but the best hope for a deeper theoretical understanding (and hence simpler procedures) appears to involve the Bayesian formulation. A first step in that direction is reported by Lindley.[36] This hope is strengthened when one considers that these are the problems with the mathematically tractable multivariate normal model and that choice of variables within the framework of the less restrictive models discussed in the section entitled "Models for Estimating Conditional Probabilities" will not be less difficult.

## REFERENCES

1. Pipberger, H. V.; Cornfield, J. and Dunn, R. A.: Diagnosis of the electrocardiogram, Chapter 18, this volume.
2. Kossack, C. F.: Discriminant analysis. In John A. Jacquez (Ed.) : *The Diagnostic Process.* Ann Arbor, Mallory Lithographing, 1964, pp. 69–77.
3. Gower, J. C.: A comparison of some methods of cluster analysis. *Biometrics, 23:*623–638, 1967.
4. Bailey, N. T. J.: *The Mathematical Approach to Biology and Medicine.* New York, Wiley, 1966.
5. Kerr, A.; Adicoff, A.; Klingeman, J. D. and Pipberger, H. V.: Computer analysis of the orthogonal electrocardiogram in pulmonary emphysema. *Am J Cardiol, 25:*34–45, 1970.
6. Yerushalmy, J.: Statistical problems in assessing methods of medical diagnosis with special reference to x-ray techniques. *Public Health Rep, 62:*1432–1439, 1947.
7. Pipberger, H. V.; Klingeman, J. D. and Cosma, J.: Computer evaluation of statistical properties of clinical information in the differential diagnosis of chest pain. *Methods Inf Med, 7:*79–92, 1968.
8. Crichton, M.: *Andromeda Strain.* New York, Dell, 1970.

9. Van Woerkom, A. J. and Brodman, K.: Statistics for a diagnostic model. *Biometrics, 17:*299–318, 1961.
10. Warner, H. R.; Toronton, A. F. and Veasey, L. G.: Experience with Bayes' theorem for computer diagnosis of congenital heart disease. *Ann N Y Acad Sci, 115:*558–567, 1964.
11. Rubin, L.; Collen, N. M. F. and Goldman, G. E.: Frequency decision theoretical approach to automated medical diagnosis. *Proceedings of the Fifth Berkeley Symposium on Mathematical Statistics and Probability, 4:*867–886, 1967.
12. Cornfield, J.: Bayes theorem. *Rev Inter Stat Inst, 35:*34–49, 1967.
13. Birnbaum, A. and Maxwell, A. E.: Classification procedures based on Bayes theorem. *Appl Stat, 9:*152–169, 1961.
14. Kemeny, J. G., Snell, J. L. and Thompson, G. L.: *Introduction to Finite Mathematics.* Englewood Cliffs, N.J., Prentice-Hall, 1957.
15. Lusted, L. B.: *Introduction to Medical Decision Making.* Springfield, Thomas, 1968.
16. Dickey, J. M.: Personal communication.
17. Good, I. J.: A Bayesian significance test for multinomial distributions. *J Roy Stat Soc,* (B) *29:*399–431, 1967.
18. Cornfield, J.: The Bayesian outlook and its application (with discussion). *Biometrics, 25:*617–657, 1969.
19. Lodwick, G. S.; Turner, A. H.; Lusted, L. B. and Templeton, A. W.: Computer-aided analysis of radiographic images. *J Chron Dis, 19:* 485–496, 1966.
20. Day, N. E. and Kerridge, D. F.: A general maximum likelihood discriminant. *Biometrics, 23:*313–323, 1967.
21. Truett, J.; Cornfield, J. and Kannel, W.: A multivariate analysis of the risk of coronary heart disease in Framingham. *J Chronic Dis, 20:*511–524, 1967.
22. Birch, M. W.: Maximum likelihood in three-way contingency tables. *J Roy Stat Soc,* (ser. B) *25:*220–233, 1963.
23. Bunker, J. P.; Forrest, W. H., Jr.; Mosteller, F. and Vandam, L. D. (Eds.) : *The National Halothane Study,* National Institutes of Health, National Institute of General Medical Sciences, U. S. Govt. Printing Office.
24. Cornfield, J.: Bayesian estimation for cross-classification, in press, 1970.
25. Dickey, J. M.: Estimation of disease probabilities conditioned on symptom variables. *Math Biosciences, 3:*249–265, 1968.
26. Brunk, H. D. and Lehr, J. L.: An improved Bayes' method for computer diagnosis. In *Proceedings of Conference on the Use of Computers in Radiology,* Univ. of Chicago Center for Continuing Education, to be published.
26a. Anderson, R. L. and Bancroft, T. A.: *Statistical Theory in Research.* New York, McGraw-Hill, 1952, pp. 144–47.

27. Armitage, P.: Recent developments in medical statistics. *Rev Inter Stat Inst, 34:*27–42, 1966.

28. Cochran, W. G. and Hopkins, C. E.: Some classification problems with multivariate qualitative data. *Biometrics, 17:*10–32, 1961.

29. Hills, M.: Allocation rules and their error rates (with discussion). *J Roy Stat Soc,* (B) *28:*1–31, 1966.

29a. Dunn, O. J. and Varady, P. D.: Probabilities of correct classification in discriminant analysis. *Biometrics, 22:*908–924, 1966.

30. Cornfield, J.: Discriminant functions. *Rev Inter Stat Inst, 35:*142–153, 1967.

31. Lachenbruch, P.: On expected probabilities of misclassification in discriminant analysis, necessary sample size, and a relation with the multiple correlation coefficient. *Biometrics, 24:*823–834, 1968.

32. Geisser, S.: Posterior odds for multivariate normal classifications. *J Roy Stat Soc,* (B) *26:*69–76, 1964.

33. Harter, H. L.: *Order Statistics and their Use in Testing and Estimation, vol. 2, Estimates Based on Order Statistics of Samples from Various Populations,* U.S. Govt. Printing Office, Washington, 1969.

34. Collew, M. F.; Rubin, L.; Heyman, J., et al.: Automated multiphasic screening and diagnosis. *Am J Public Health, 54:*741–50, 1964.

35. Lachenbruch, P. A.: An almost unbiased method of obtaining confidence intervals for the probability of misclassification in discriminant analysis. *Biometrics, 23:*639–646, 1967.

36. Lindley, D. V.: Bayesian analysis in regression problems. In D. L. Meyer and R. O. Collier, Jr. (Eds.): *Bayesian Statistics.* Itasca, Ill., F. E. Peacock Publishers, Inc., 1970.

## Chapter 7

# DIAGNOSIS AND THE BAYESIAN VIEWPOINT*

### Leonard J. Savage

I OWE THE PRIVILEGE of being here to those of you who are already interested in implications of the Bayesian viewpoint for diagnosis and who know my enthusiasm for that viewpoint in the related field of statistics. Perhaps it will be to our advantage that most of my applied statistical experience has been with medical problems but somewhat to our disadvantage that this experience has never been with problems of diagnosis, except in the diffuse sense that would see all problems of statistics as problems of diagnosis. I can therefore talk to you only in terms of general principles, and not necessarily realistic examples, with the hope of stimulating more substantive discussion and perhaps of paving the way for succeeding speakers and usefully underlining some of the points raised by preceding ones.

Even to such half-opened eyes as mine, diagnosis is suggestive of a great many themes, so this talk is confined to a few aspects of diagnosis where I best discern promise for the Bayesian viewpoint. This excludes many tantalizing and important topics such as the discovery of valid new diagnoses and of classification systems, effective nomenclature, and ills that ought not to be regarded as subject to diagnosis or classification in the usual sense but as points on a continuum of one or several dimensions. For focus, then, let us confine ourselves to reflections on diagnostic propositions that can reasonably be regarded as simply true or false, though we may not know which, such as, this child has measles and poison ivy, but not chicken pox; this man has homologous serum jaundice or obstructive jaundice, but not both.

* This research was supported in part by the Army, Navy, Air Force, and NASA under a contract administered by the Office of Naval Research. Reproduction in whole or in part is permitted for any purpose of the United States Government.
NOTE: Professor Savage died on November 1, 1971.

Prognosis under treatment seems to me so intellectually similar to recognizing a disease that it can be included without complication. For example, this patient will survive the proposed operation, and he will not survive without it. The inclusion of such alternative prognoses in the concept of diagnosis is vital for the attitude that stresses diagnosis as a facet of the process of patient management, or treatment tactics, which is ably stressed in later chapters; see especially Chap. 12 and Chap. 13.

A possible misunderstanding should be nipped in the bud; for if I seem to regard diagnosis as the making of unqualified pronouncements, you will not hear me out. My real thought is that the diagnostician says implicitly, if not explicitly, not that this or that is true but that it is probably true, almost certainly true, possibly true, or an eight to five bet, as he may see it. In fact, according to the Bayesian viewpoint it is not only worthwhile to make these probabilistic qualifications explicit but to make them much more quantitative than is yet customary.

Fortunately, many of you come here already well informed about the Bayesian viewpoint and the rest have had some, and will have more, opportunity to absorb it from other speakers; for the idea cannot be properly conveyed in the few moments allowed for its introduction in any one talk. To begin my own too succinct explanation, the Bayesian viewpoint—more strictly, the personalistic Bayesian viewpoint—takes the theory of probability as a model of disciplined, but subjective, personal opinion. Opinion, in this context, is ultimately given an economic interpretation in a broad sense. For example, I will bet five dollars to one that this little boy has only a green-apple bellyache; or, of these two dangerous operations, this one is most likely to succeed.

Along with the personal probability of events, or propositions, there goes the utility of consequences. Suppose, as an overly simple example, that a physician could schematize a particular medical problem thusly: The patient is almost surely in one of the three mutually exclusive states A, B, or C with probabilities $P(A)$, $P(B)$ and $P(C)$, perhaps .01, .09, and .9, respectively; if I do not perform an emergency operation now, he will die in case of A, recover very badly in case of B, and be fine tomorrow in case of C; if I do operate, he will recover but rather uncomfortably and be out of pocket half a year's salary. According to the theory of utility, any tenable decision of this physician can be represented by attaching numbers $U_1$, $U_2$, $U_3$, and $U_4$ to the four possible consequences, death, nonpostoperative recovery with its costs, speedy recovery, and postoperative recovery with its costs—all without regard for the probabilities of A, B, and C—in such a way that the operation is preferred if and only if

$$U_4 > U_1P(A) + U_2P(B) + U_3P(C).$$

Certain traditions oppose weighing a patient's life against hours or days of pain or against money, or even weighing pain against money, and some people might conclude that if the Bayesian view requires such callous calculations it is not suitable for medical decision. But to make a medical decision at all, we Bayesians contend, is implicitly to make appraisals of utility and probability, and it seems in accordance with the best traditions of the evolution of medical thinking that these appraisals of values and of chances should come to be made openly and explicitly, as exemplified later in this volume (see Chap. 13).

But no less open and explicit should be the recognition that numbers purporting to measure value and opinion will vary greatly from one valuer and opinioner to another and more often than not will be only crudely determined even for one individual. When a decision is hard to make because we vacillate in our judgment of the values or of the chances, we are in a quandary. Further reflection or fresh data sometimes clarify the situation, but the existence of quandaries remains a bitter fact of life not to be altogether dissipated by the adoption or the rejection of any particular theory or discipline. The explicit and numerical analysis recommended by the Bayesian viewpoint makes the presence of quandary painfully clear, and that is often seen as a reason to abandon such analysis for unanalyzed judgment. We Bayesians believe that to do so is to sweep under the rug indecision that ought to be recognized and bracketed.

An important and subtle feature of medical decisions is that while the probabilities to be used in the judgment should ordinarily be those of the responsible physician, the pertinent values are far more accurately described as those of the patient than of the physician. Even this is only an approximation; for of course the patient is often conspicuously in no position to make important value judgments, if only because he is ill. Also, it is by no means widely accepted that the patient should, for example, be allowed to choose death in preference to amputation or blindness. I was particularly pleased to hear the bold and radical defense of the thesis that medical values should be those of the patient made by Dr. Slack (see Chap. 1). His thesis was hotly debated, but even those who resisted his particularly thoroughgoing position should be able to acknowledge the elements of truth and importance in it. The topic is subtle and complicated, and informal discussion on a later occasion reminded us that public interest as well as that of the patient plays a part in some medical decisions. The allocation of extremely scarce medical resources was mentioned as one example, and of course many questions of public health such as quarantine and vaccination provide others.

From the Bayesian point of view, the activity of diagnosis is one of generating probabilities. The practical importance of probabilities is that, together with utilities—which do not derive from diagnosis—they provide a basis for decision. A typical misuse of probabilities, and one actually proposed in print (Herman and Dollinger, 1966), would be to take the possibility that has the highest probability as "the diagnosis." No one thinking in terms of decision would propose such a degradation of probabilities; appendicitis need not be the most probable diagnosis before an appendectomy, even with its attendant dangers and other costs, is indicated.

How are diagnostic probabilities to be generated? Many partial answers must be given. Whenever a person applies his judgment and skill to digest observations whether formal, casual, or sub-liminal, he is arriving at personal probabilities or reasonable facsimiles thereof. In many areas, humans have wonderful abilities to make such informal diagnoses, for which there is sometimes no formal substitute yet available—as when we recognize an odor or a face. Much of the fascinating new indoor sport of pattern recognition consists in trying to analyze those tasks of recognition and judgment that people perform so easily but mysteriously. These skills play an important part in medical diagnosis and presumably always will. They must be admired, emulated, and taught. But there are grave dangers in being overawed by the intuitive approach, which certainly ought not lead us to deride the keeping of, and of course no less the studying of, records. And it seems to be among the objectives of these conferences not to accept good intuitive diagnosis as an unanalyzable marvel but rather to scrutinize it empirically in various ingenious ways, studying how and where it goes systematically astray and could be helped by formal methods and how it may be better taught.

One important possibility for the improvement of intuitive diagnosis is that real, though not necessarily very mathematical, knowledge of probabilistic concepts might help experts in arriving at their opinions, even in contexts where they could not properly make very formal use of the theory. Moreover, merely learning to express ultimate diagnoses in probabilistic terms—which of course must not be uttered as mere jargon but with trained and practiced understanding—promises to be useful in communication between physicians and between physician and patient, and even in those situations in which the diagnostician and the physician responsible for treatment are the same. It seems especially important that when the two are not the same, the diagnosticians learn to speak meaningfully in terms of probability and that those to whom they report be trained to understand them. For though probability refers to personal opinion, it is a definite and well-defined kind of expression of opinion. Even one who knows and understands this notion can look inward to report his personal probabilities only imperfectly at best, but much better with suitable training and practice than without.

Diagnosis, the formation of probabilities, is an ongoing process; with the accumulation of data, our opinions are revised. Problems of what data to gather next in the light of the current costs and promised worths of the alternatives are among the most important, and frequently among the most difficult, as was emphasized later in the conference (see for example Chaps. 12 and 13). The simple formula according to which probabilities are updated in the light of new evidence is called Bayes' Theorem after Thomas Bayes, and it lies behind such expressions as "the Bayesian viewpoint." Numerous formal applications of Bayes' Theorem are under exploration by physicians and medical teams, and practice in the use of Bayes' Theorem is one of the aspects of probabilistic training that might be of value even in those diagnostic roles that tend to resist formalization.

Diagnosis often involves judgments by more than one person, and there is much room for invention and experimentation about how these persons can fruitfully communicate with one another, presumably in probabilistic terms. What, for example, should an internist ask of a radiologist in connection with a chest x-ray? (What is actually done I scarcely know but suppose it varies greatly.)

One conceivable, and intellectually tempting, solution would be for the internist to brief the radiologist as fully as possible about the case and then invite the radiologist to make a diagnosis of the chest, though not necessarily of the patient. This is very expensive in physicians' time at best and seems to be on the wrong track because it minimizes the diagnostic talents of the internist and puts great extra-radiological diagnostic demands on the radiologist. Further, as was brought out in discussion, the radiologist's specific contribution can easily be lost by his overreaction to clinical information.

Consider now another extreme, and perhaps equally unrealistic, possibility. The radiologist is shown the film but told nothing. At first glance, or at least at second glance, the radiologist can communicate no useful probabilities at all under such circumstances. Suppose, for example, he were to say I would lay three to one that these lungs are without any "radiographic" lesions at all. What could he really mean? And what might you as an internist do with his opinion? The radiologist must be making his assertion on the basis of some background hypothesis such as some population of films, perhaps those that are ordinarily sent to him. But you, the internist, have little interest in the population of films ordinarily sent to that radiologist and, worse, you have at best very vague ideas of what that population is. Extreme examples make your lack clear. If the radiologist is almost never consulted except in cases where there is serious suspicion of lung lesions, his judgment could justifiably be taken as great reassurance. If, however, he normally deals mainly with routine checks on astronauts, his attribution of probability $1/4$ to the possibility of a pathological shadow should be taken by you as very grave information about your sandblasting patient. But from the debacle there emerges an idea that, if not already in use, may ultimately be implemented in forms of practical value for radiology, pathology, and other such specialties. Suppose the radiologist and the internist can agree that the radiologist will report probabilities as though he were referring to a specified, if perhaps artificial, standard population of patients known both to himself and the internist and also let him report a rather full list of hypothetical probabilities such as probabilities of tuberculosis, histoplasmosis, silicosis, etc., each in several grades, including of course the condition of no shadow. With this data, it is in principle possible for the internist to say, "If the radiologist sees one chance in 50 that this patient has silicosis on the hypothesis that the patient comes from the standard hypothetical population in which only one in 5000 has it, then I, with my knowledge of this sandblaster's occupational hazard, must multiply the odds in favor of silicosis about 15-fold to conclude that the probability is about $1/3$ that he has radiological shadows due to silicosis." Of course, if the internist himself sees still other signs pointing in that direction, he will through further application of Bayes' Theorem arrive at still higher odds.

This rough scenario may sound quixotic and impractical, but experience in other areas suggests that with experience and resourcefulness something valuable can be made of it. Technically, and stripped to essentials, the idea is to have the radiologist report likelihoods—which are ratios of probabilities of the film for various diagnostic states—and not to attempt to form probabilities of diagnostic states themselves, since he cannot be expected to have either the data or the experience to do that. This separation of function is commonplace when what is consulted is not an expert but merely a laboratory procedure. When a physician obtains a quantitative reading from a laboratory and recognizes that the reading is afflicted with laboratory error, with day-to-day fluctuation in his patient, and with variation from patient to patient in the same basic state of health, he in effect reduces it to likelihood ratios in favor of various hypothesis, and these then contribute to his ultimate formation of the probabilities of the hypotheses.

Specifically in the area of chest radiology, it has been found that even the most skilled readers frequently differ from one another in diagnosis, and on reading the same plates on different occasions each reader differs from himself. Under such circumstances, it might be expected, and has been verified, that various ways of pooling judgments result in a composite judgment more reliable than any single one. One way to effect such pooling is to average the probabilities of two or more individuals—conceivably weighting the more skilled more than the less skilled. Some more subtle combination of several sets of probabilities might be appropriate in those situations where secondary opinion is sought only in case the primary opinion expresses particular doubt.

As was brought out in Dr. Lusted's discussion (see Chap. 3), a mechanism that has tended to exaggerate the apparent discrepancies among film readers is this. If, in accordance with the pre-Bayesian traditions of ordinary language, the film reader is asked to say merely whether there is or is not a lesion, he must in effect ask himself how large the likelihood ratio in favor of the presence of a lesion must be for him to report it. This of course depends on the relative costs of false positives and false negatives and on the general health of the population, and diverging opinions about the utilities and public-health statistics involved here have inadvertently been confounded with divergences of opinion about the significance of the film. Once more, conscious separation of function promises to lead to much better communication.

I have said very little that is new to people who are thinking professionally about diagnosis. Two ideas, whether new for you or not, that I would leave with you are these: The Bayesian viewpoint forms a good framework in which to discuss diagnosis; and with suitable effort it may lead to the development of language in which diagnoses and diagnostic information are much more sensitively transmitted than in the very crude language of "maybe" and "surely."

### REFERENCES

Herman, Louis M., and Michael B. Dollinger, "Predicting effectiveness of Bayesian Classification systems," Psychometrika, 31, 1966, 341–349.

## Chapter 8

# N = 1: DIAGNOSIS IN UNIQUE CASES

### Ward Edwards

IN A SENSE, every diagnostic problem is unique, just as every event is unique. In another, more important sense, every event and every diagnostic problem has intellectual linkages to the diagnostician's past experience—linkages that he must exploit in order to make a diagnosis.

Yet the statistical Bayesians seem to me to overestimate the availability and usefulness of one kind of non-uniqueness. They seem to feel that the only approach to Bayesian techniques in diagnosis is to use past experience with the symptoms and the diseases with which they may be linked to form a mathematical model (typically multinomial) of the data-generating process, and then use that model to produce inputs to Bayes' Theorem, and then use Bayes' Theorem to produce posterior probabilities of the various possible diagnoses. It is the first step in this chain that bothers me. For one thing, my friends who are expert about medical records tell me that to attempt to dig out from even the most sophisticated hospital's records the frequency of association between any particular symptom and any particular diagnosis is next to impossible—and when I raise the question of complexes of symptoms, they stop speaking to me. For another thing, doctors keep telling me that diseases change, that this year's flu is different from last year's flu, and so that symptom-disease records extending back over time are of very limited usefulness. Moreover, the observation of symptoms is well-supplied with error, and the diagnosis of diseases is even more so; both kinds of errors will ordinarily be frozen permanently into symptom-disease statistics. Finally, even if diseases didn't change, doctors would. The usefulness of disease categories is so much a function of available treatments that these categories themselves change as treatments change—a fact hard to incorporate into symptom-disease statistics.

All these arguments against symptom-disease statistics as a basis for diagnosis are perhaps somewhat overstated. Where such statistics can be obtained and believed, obviously they should be used. But I argue that usually they cannot be obtained, and even in those instances in which they have been obtained, they may not deserve belief. What then? That set of circumstances defines what I call the N = 1 problem.

A frequently encountered answer is that when you are stuck with the N = 1 problem, you have no choice but to depend on human intuition. I agree. The answerer usually goes on to express relief that in this world of computers, arithmetic, and the de-humanization of everything, there are still secure roles for men; this is one of them. Again I agree. He then goes on to express the pious (and often insincere) hope that 100 years from now, Bayesian arithmetic will have something to offer the diagnostician, but in the meantime . . . And at that point, I violently disagree.

I pointed out that three steps are required to apply a typical statistical Bayesian approach to diagnosis: formation of a model of the data generating process; use of that model to produce inputs to Bayes' Theorem; and use of Bayes' Theorem to produce outputs in the form of probabilities of various diagnoses. All the criticisms that followed were directed to only one step, the first. We often cannot form a meaningful model of the data generating process. That does not mean, however, that we cannot obtain inputs to Bayes' Theorem, or that we cannot use Bayes' Theorem to obtain probabilities of various diagnoses. In fact, there is by now considerable evidence that Bayesian procedures are extremely useful in the total absence of a model of the data-generating process, when dealing with really unique diagnostic problems. That is what this paper is about.

The crux of my argument is this. There are actually two intellectual steps in diagnosis after data collection is complete. One is the judgment of the meaning of each individual symptom; the other is the aggregation of the symptoms in order to reach a diagnosis. The first, I argue, is often inevitably a task for human expertise, either because this particular symptom or set of symptoms is essentially unique (N = 1) or because, though it is not unique, information about its association with diseases is unavailable. But the second step, aggregation, is readily mechanized by means of Bayes' Theorem, and such mechanization has great advantages over more intuitive, less formal methods of doing the same intellectual work.

Let me start with an example of what can go wrong with intuitive aggregation of evidence. Here's an imaginary bookbag full of poker chips. In my desk I keep two such imaginary bookbags, one containing 70 red and 30 blue chips and the other containing 70 blue and 30 red. I flipped an imaginary fair coin to determine which one to bring with me, and this is it. Now, on the basis of the story so far, what is the probability that this is the predominantly red bag? Since I picked one of two bags by flipping a fair coin, I hope you agree with me that that probability is 0.5. Next, let's consider some data. I'll reach in, stir up the poker chips, sample one randomly, look at it, put it back, stir them up again, sample again, and so on 12 times. In 12 such random samples with replacement after each sample I get eight red and four blue chips. Now, on the basis of all the evidence you have, what is the probability that this is the predominantly red bag? (Reader: please write down a guess in the margin before going on to the next paragraph or reading the footnote. The example is much more illuminating if you can compare your own unaided intuition with the formal arithmetic.)

The Bayesian arithmetic for this example is easy to do. When I do it * the probability that this is the predominantly red bag turns out to be 0.97.

---

* One way of writing Bayes's theorem is as follows:

$$\frac{P(H_1|D)}{P(H_2|D)} = \frac{P(D|H_1)}{P(D|H_2)} \cdot \frac{P(H_1)}{P(H_2)}$$

The first term is known as the posterior odds, the second is the likelihood ratio, and the third is the prior odds. The prior odds in this example are of course 1:1, or 1, so the posterior odds are equal to the likelihood ratio. A simple derivation shows that in such symmetric binomial examples (not, however, in asymmetric ones) the likelihood ratio can be written $(P/Q)^{s-f}$, where P and Q are the probability of a red and a blue chip in a single draw from, say, the red bag (in this example, therefore, $P/Q = .7/.3 = 7/3$) and s-f is the difference between the number of successes (red chips) and failures (blue chips) in the sample—in this case 4. So the posterior odds are $(7/3)^4 = 29.64$, to four decimal places. A little arithmetic translates those odds into 0.97 probability.

The point of this example was to illustrate a fact that by now is well-known, though perhaps not to physicians: Men, even highly trained men, are conservative information processors, unable to extract from evidence anything like the degree of certainty that the data justify. (Note: in the verbal presentation of this talk I tried the example with the audience of physicians, medical students, and other professionals; they were all conservative—typical estimates were in the 0.70–0.80 region.) This finding is by no means confined to casual demonstrations in conferences; it can be reproduced and made quantitative in carefully controlled experimental settings, using either naive or expert subjects.[2,5,6]

Why are men conservative? Our first idea was that asking people to estimate probabilities might make them conservative, but experiments in which we asked them to estimate odds [3,6] soon proved that idea wrong. So we then focused on two main theories of conservatism. One, the misperception theory, says that people perceive the diagnostic content of each datum as less than it in fact is, but combine data properly according to Bayes' Theorem. The other, the misaggregation theory, says that people perceive the diagnostic content of each datum correctly, but fail to aggregate data the way Bayes's Theorem specifies. (Obviously, both could be true; evidence presented below indicates that that is not the case.) For a discussion of these hypotheses see Edwards.[1]

Gloria Wheeler and I set out to do an experiment on the misaggregation-misperception argument. Bookbags and poker chips are poor tools for such an experiment, because they offer only a very small set of likelihood ratios to estimate. So we ended up using two normal distributions differing only in mean, the kind of task made so famous by signal detectability theory.[7] I should remind you that the separation between means of the distributions, measured in units of their common standard deviation, is called $d'$. In this first experiment, $d'$ was fixed at 1.6, which means that the likelihood ratio at the mean is 3.60.

When people think of experimenting on diagnosis using normal distributions, they sometimes think of numbers as stimuli and of pretty bell-shaped curves as displays of what the stimuli mean. Both ideas disturb me. Numbers as stimuli invite subjects to hunt for simple transformation rules that will change numerical stimuli into numerical responses. And pretty bell-shaped curves are misleading. When you sample from a normal distribution and lay the successive samples out in the order in which you obtained them, you will never see a bell-shaped curve. Instead, you will see a random histogram. To capture this fact about sampling from normal distributions, we exhibited the two distributions to subjects as shown in Fig. 8–1. Each bar in Fig. 8–1 is intended to represent a 7-inch-long child's pick-up stick, painted partly blue and partly yellow (since blue and yellow are the University of Michigan colors). The samples presented are not in fact random; instead, they are carefully chosen to be representative of their respective populations. Thus each half of the display is of one population, more or less as the subject might expect to see it.

In this experiment we had four groups. Two groups aggregated; two did not. Two groups estimated likelihood ratios; two did not. The members of the aggregated posterior odds group performed the standard Bayesian task. Starting from 50–50 prior odds, they revised their odds after seeing each of eight sticks by making

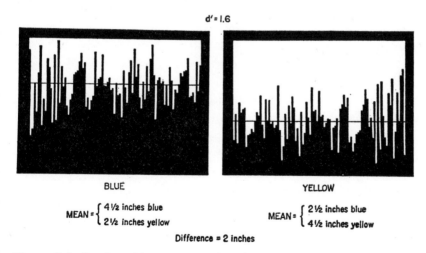

Figure 8–1. Random histograms representing two populations of pick-up sticks. Population A has a mean length of blue (represented by black in the figure) of 4½ inches. Population B has a mean length of blue of 2½ inches. d' is 1.6.

marks on odds scales logarithmically spaced, running from 1:1 to 1,000,000:1. (Space was provided if the subject wished to insert higher odds—and some did.) The members of the nonaggregated likelihood ratio group, seeing the same sequences of sticks, were asked after each stick "Is this stick more likely to have come from the predominantly blue or from the predominantly yellow population, and, in a ratio sense, how much more likely?" The members of the aggregated likelihood ratio group, again seeing the same sticks, were asked "Consider all these sticks. Are they collectively more likely to have come from the predominantly blue or the predominantly yellow population, and in a ratio sense, how much more likely?" The members of the nonaggregated odds group were asked to estimate posterior odds after each stick, but between each stick and the next the population was reselected and so the odds were reset to 50–50 (by a bit of trickery, they saw the same sticks as did the other three groups).

What would the two theories predict for this experiment? Misperception would of course predict that all groups would be conservative, since all four would equally perceive the data as less diagnostic than they actually were. The misaggregation hypothesis, on the other hand, would predict that the two aggregation groups would be conservative, while the two nonaggregation groups would be Bayesian. Fig. 8–2 shows what happened. Clearly, the nonaggregation groups were Bayesian, which should dispose of the misperception hypothesis. Thus we conclude in favor of misaggregation—a conclusion with great practical importance for medical diagnosis, as I will explain later.

But some of our colleagues came up with a disquieting objection. They complained that the aggregation groups were estimating ridiculous numbers like 100,000:1, while the nonaggregation groups were estimating almost no numbers outside the 10:1 to 1:10 ranger. What subject understands the meaning of 100,000:1? This argument, somewhat more elaborately put, has come to be known as the response bias hypothesis.

Gloria Wheeler decided to dispose of the response bias hypothesis for her Ph.D thesis. Again she did a pick-up stick experiment, but this time she used three different values of $d'$ (1.0, 1.6, and

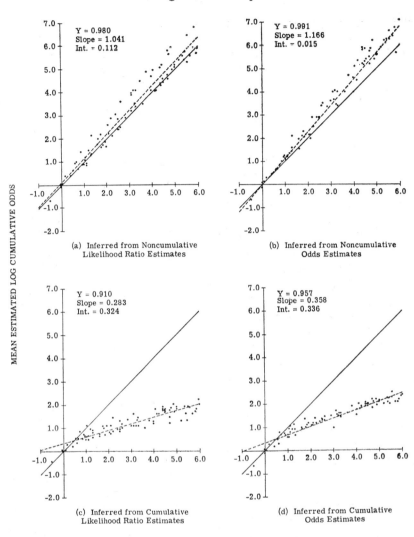

MEAN ESTIMATED LOG CUMULATIVE ODDS

(a) Inferred from Noncumulative
Likelihood Ratio Estimates

Y = 0.980
Slope = 1.041
Int. = 0.112

(b) Inferred from Noncumulative
Odds Estimates

Y = 0.991
Slope = 1.166
Int. = 0.015

(c) Inferred from Cumulative
Likelihood Ratio Estimates

Y = 0.910
Slope = 0.283
Int. = 0.324

(d) Inferred from Cumulative
Odds Estimates

Y = 0.957
Slope = 0.358
Int. = 0.336

LOG BAYESIAN ODDS

Figure 8–2. Results of the Wheeler-Edwards experiment. The two upper figures represent nonaggregated odds and nonaggregated likelihood ratio estimation groups. The two lower figures represent aggregated odds and likelihood ratio groups. The upper right-hand group uses the procedure called PIP in the text.

2.2) and a large number of very carefully gimmicked sequences of sticks. The most important ones for the current purpose were those in which the diagnosticities (likelihood ratios) of the sticks were carefully controlled so that posterior odds never got outside the 10:1 range. Still, subjects were conservative when they had to aggregate, and Bayesian when they did not. We feel that this effectively disposes of the response bias hypothesis—though I doubt if all of my colleagues would agree. Incidentally, the data from this experiment were fully as elegant as those from the previous experiment presented in Fig. 8–2. Subjects behave in a very orderly way in such experiments—at least on the average.

What does the fact that people (perhaps including doctors) are conservative aggregators of information mean for medical diagnosis? Taken at face value, it can mean one or the other or both of two things. A conservative information aggregator wastes information. If he is like our laboratory subjects, for typical situations he will waste from 50 percent to 80 percent of the information he gets. Thus, for a fixed amount of information input, he will be considerably less certain of the meaning of that input than he could be. This does not in itself do harm, though it may make the diagnostician unnecessarily uncomfortable; so long as he treats the patient appropriately, it makes little difference how certain he is of the appropriateness of that treatment. Of course, one could imagine scenarios in which conservatism would lead to misdiagnosis of rare diseases. But even if such scenarios are real, by definition they must be rare.

A more serious consequence of conservatism arises when the amount of information input is not fixed. Information costs money. A diagnostician who wastes information may well require more information than is necessary or (ideally) appropriate before proceeding with treatment. Moreover, in most medical situations, the information obtained early is relatively cheap, while information obtained later is considerably more expensive. Reduction in the use of expensive laboratory procedures might occur if conservatism in medical diagnosis exists and could be cured— and that might be an important ingredient in reducing the total cost of medical care.

I have never been able to study human conservatism in medical diagnosis, so I am unable to make anything but guesses about whether the speculations of the previous paragraphs are in fact

correct or not. I invite you, both doctors and patients, to examine
your own past experiences and make your own guesses.

Can conservatism be cured? One easy thought is to train people
to be less conservative in making inferences. In an unpublished
study, Manley did just that. He found that so long as the data came
from the same source and were of the same general nature in the
post-training test situation as had been used in training, training
would indeed cure conservatism. But as soon as he made even
fairly minor modifications of the data-generating process, conservatism was back as strong as ever. In other words, in his experiment the training did not generalize from one situation to another.
That finding, incidentally, agrees with my own experience. I have
known about human conservatism in general, and my own in
particular, for at least ten years. I now can estimate fairly nonconservative posterior odds, by the simple but inelegant procedure
of saying to myself "It feels like about 70–30, so I'll say 90–10."
In short, after ten years of working in the field, my intuition is
as conservative as ever.

But it makes little sense to try to cure conservatism by training
people anyhow. Bayes' Theorem is a nonconservative, optimal
rule for information aggregation. Why not use it?

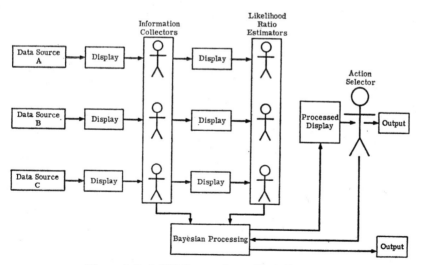

Figure 8–3. A PIP for use in medical diagnosis.

Fig. 8–3 presents a block diagram of a combination of men and machines that I call a Probabilistic Information Processing system, or PIP. The men on the left-hand side of the diagram are collectors of information, whether doctors or medical technicians or others. The information they gather, having been purged of irrelevancy and put into standard format, is displayed to the man or men whom I call Likelihood Ratio Estimators—in a medical context these would be doctors, or perhaps one doctor. The likelihood ratios they estimate, one for each symptom for each pair of diseases being considered, is passed on to the block called Bayesian Processor, which simply does Bayes' Theorem. The resulting posterior probabilities or odds of the various diseases are displayed to the decision-maker, who chooses the appropriate course of action. (In later, more sophisticated systems, the Bayesian Processor might suggest courses of action; that is why I have included the possibility of an output from it other than posterior probabilities of diseases. To do so, it would have to know the relevant costs and payoffs—a very difficult kind of knowledge to obtain.)

Does PIP work? We have done a number of laboratory experiments, from very abstract to as realistic as we could get in the laboratory, that indicate that it does. For one, see Reference 2. In our more realistic experiments we worked with vague, verbal, qualitative data and vague, verbal qualitative hypotheses—the epitome of the $N = 1$ problem. Here, just as with the pick-up sticks, the PIP procedure squeezes much more certainty out of the same amount of evidence than any other procedure. Data that would lead PIP to give 99:1 odds in favor of a hypothesis would lead its next-best competitor to give less than 3:1 odds.

Perhaps more important by now is the growing body of evidence that real-world applications of the PIP idea also work. PIP has been applied to the problem of information processing in the intelligence community (see Chap. 11). PIP has by now been applied in several medical contexts (see Chap. 15). We are now trying to apply the PIP idea to weather forecasting, but it is too soon to say anything firm about results.

I would be misleading you, though, if I failed to mention some of the intellectual difficulties in real-world applications of PIP. Perhaps the first one to occur to many is the problem of nonindependence. We all know that everything is correlated with everything else, and the simple form of Bayes' Theorem used in this talk and in the PIP experiments assumes a certain kind of independence.

The first step toward dealing with this problem is to recognize that there are two different kinds of independence: independence and conditional independence. The fact that everything is related to everything else, and in particular that symptoms correlate with one another, far from being a hindrance to the application of Bayes' Theorem, is the sole reason why Bayes' Theorem works. The most important reason why two symptoms correlate with each other is because they are both symptoms of the same disease— and it is that fact that the simple, independent form of Bayes' Theorem works with. Thus, nonindependence, far from being a problem, is what we must hope for if we are going to have any success at diagnosis at all.

Violations of conditional independence are a different and less happy story. Supposing that, within a population of patients all of whom have the same disease, two symptoms that are sometimes present and sometimes absent correlate with each other. More technically, suppose that if you know that the patient has the disease *and* that he exhibits symptom 1, this changes his probability of exhibiting symptom 2. That constitutes a violation of conditional independence, which is assumed in the simplest form of Bayes' Theorem. The difference between this and the preceding kind of nonindependence is that in this one we consider only patients having the disease, while in the previous one we considered all patients.

At least three procedures for coping with violations of conditional independence exist. One, often highly appropriate if the violation is not too severe, is simply to ignore it and calculate as though the symptoms were conditionally independent. The amount of error introduced may well be small compared with other sources of error.

A second, estimation of conditional likelihood ratios, may turn out to be the best of all, but no research has been done on it as yet, so I will not describe it. The third technique is the one now most commonly used. It is simply to combine conditionally nonindependent symptoms into one grand symptom, and obtain likelihood ratio estimates for that larger, more complex symptom. Dave Gustafson and others have clearly shown that this technique will work; no one yet knows whether some other technique might be better.

Closely related to conditional nonindependence is the problem of multistage inference. In a medical context, this is presumably a frequent event—as it is in the intelligence context also. Several symptoms may indicate the malfunctioning of some body system; in turn the fact that that body system is malfunctioning may imply some disease, not necessarily a disease only of that body system. Formal rules for such multistage inferences exist; they are more complex mathematically than Bayes' Theorem, but conceptually quite similar to it. For a discussion of the formal rules, see Gettys and Willke.[4] Some experimental data seem to indicate that in such multistage inference problems, men are radical, not conservative, perhaps because they tend to behave as though the middle-level hypothesis most favored by the datum is guaranteed true, whereas of course it is not.

I don't really care whether men are conservative or radical when they must perform diagnostic information processing in their heads. The obvious solution to either problem is to use the correct processing rule: Bayes' Theorem. Since men are good at estimating likelihood ratios and related quantities and poorer at aggregating evidence, a natural division of labor is to let them do the former and let Bayes' Theorem do the latter.

## REFERENCES

1. Edwards, W.: Conservatism in human information processing. In B. Kleinmuntz (Ed.): *Formal Representation of Human Judgment.* New York, Wiley, 1968, pp. 17–52.

2. Edwards, W.; Phillips, L. D.; Hays, W. L. and Goodman, B. C.: Probabilistic information processing systems: Design and evaluation. *IEEE Transactions on Systems Science and Cybernetics,* SSC–4:248–265, No. 3, 1968.

3. Fujii, T.: Conservatism and discriminability in probability estimation as a function of response model. *Jap Psychol Res, 9:*42–47, 1967.

4. Gettys, C. F. and Willke, T. A.: The application of Bayes' Theorem

when the true data state is uncertain. *Org Behav Human Performance, 4:*125–141, 1969.

5. Phillips, L. D.: Some components of probabilistic inference. Human Performance Center Technical Report No. 1, University of Michigan, 1966.

6. Phillips, L. D. and Edwards, W.: Conservatism in a simple probability inference task. *J Exp Psychol, 72:*346–354, 1966.

7. Swets, J. A. and Green, D. M.: *Signal Detection Theory and Psychophysics.* New York, John Wiley & Sons, Inc., 1966.

Chapter 9

# SYNTAX-DIRECTED CONCEPT ANALYSIS IN THE REASONING FOUNDATIONS OF MEDICAL DIAGNOSIS*

ROBERT S. LEDLEY

## INTRODUCTION: USE OF LOGIC

$T$HE REASONING FOUNDATIONS of medical diagnosis involve logical combinations of symptoms. In previous work, Dr. Lee B. Lusted and I have outlined the logical formulation of the diagnostic process. The concept of the "symptom complex" was introduced as a "positive-negative combination" of all the symptoms under consideration. Thus for three symptoms $S_1$, $S_2$, and $S_3$, a symptom complex could be $S_1 \cdot \bar{S}_2 \cdot S_3$, meaning $S_1$ positive, $S_2$ negative, and $S_3$ positive. For our illustration of three symptoms, there are $2^3 = 8$ conceivable symptom complexes (including $\bar{S}_1 \cdot \bar{S}_2 \cdot \bar{S}_3$). Similarly, if $n$ symptoms are under consideration, $2^n$ symptom complexes are conceivable. The number of conceivable symptom complexes could be very large; e.g. if we are considering 20 symptoms, there are $2^{20} = 1,048,576$ conceivable symptom complexes.

Medical knowledge enters the picture by telling us that not all conceivable symptom complexes are *possible*. Hence only a few of all the $2^n$ symptom complexes actually occur. For example, suppose that medical knowledge told us that $S_1$ and $S_3$ are related so that if a patient has $S_1$ he must have $S_3$ (but not necessarily the converse). Then the conceivable symptom complexes $S_1 \cdot S_2 \cdot \bar{S}_3$, and $S_1 \cdot \bar{S}_2 \cdot \bar{S}_3$ cannot occur. Hence upon taking into account

* The research in this paper has been supported by U. S. Public Health Service Grant RR–05681 from the National Institutes of Health to the National Biomedical Research Foundation.

152

medical knowledge, the number of possible symptom complexes is greatly reduced. However, the number may still be large; e.g. for 20 symptoms, even half of $2^{20}$ is 524,288.

Hence the question arises, how do physicians handle medical diagnosis, since they obviously do not remember all possible symptom complexes associated with a disease? Of course, physicians do not make a diagnosis with "mathematical rigor"—this is only required for computer aids to the diagnostic process. However, if our logical formulation is indeed a mathematical rationale for medical diagnosis, then the physician must somehow, even in a qualitative sense, take into account logical relationships when making a medical diagnosis.

The purpose of this paper is to explore one possible mathematical formalism that might serve in some sense to simulate the implicit reasoning processes utilized by a physician in handling the problem of the multitude of symptom complexes. This formalism can itself be used to program a computer to more easily process symptom complexes as an aid to medical diagnosis.

## TECHNICAL LANGUAGE AND HIERARCHICAL STRUCTURES

Technical language expresses concepts and relationships and is used as an aid to the reasoning processes associated with technical scientific topics in general, and with medical diagnosis in particular. Hence an analysis of some aspects of technical language will be useful in our consideration of the reasoning foundations of medical diagnosis. Such an analysis has been more highly developed in computer science than in most other sciences. This is because the computer scientist is so frequently faced with the problem of explicitly and precisely describing reasoning processes and therefore is also faced with the problem of formulating the *language* in terms of which these processes are described. Thus we will appeal to the computer scientist's analysis of his technical languages as a guide to our analysis of the medical diagnostic reasoning process and to the development of a formalism to aid in this reasoning process.

The fundamental idea used by computer scientists is that of the hierarchical structure of concepts in their relationship to each other. The meaning of this idea is best explained by means of an illustration.

The so-called "simple arithmetic expression" (sae) is most frequently used in computer science. We have all learned how to recognize an sae in elementary school, and so we hardly think about it anymore. For example, it is obvious to us that the following:

$$A + B * (C + D)/E$$

is an sae but that

$$A + - B */C + D +$$

is not a proper sae. (In computer science, "*" is multiplication and "/" is division.) But how do we tell the computer this? The answer to this question is that we must formulate a set of rules, such as the following:

Rule 0. A *variable* is a letter.

Rule 1. A *term* is a *variable,* or an sae enclosed in parentheses.

Rule 2. A *factor* is a *term,* or a *factor* followed by "*" followed by a *term,* or a *factor* followed by "/" followed by a *term.*

Rule 3. An sae is a *factor,* or + *factor,* or − *factor,* or sae + *factor* or sae − *factor.*

Then we can "diagram" an expression that is a candidate for an sae to determine if indeed it is an sae. The diagram for the following:

$$A + B * (C + D)/E$$

is shown in Fig. 9–1.

In this illustration we are applying the rules in order, and on the arithmetic symbols from left to right. We first build A up to an sae (steps 1, 2, and 3). But an sae followed by + could be a more encompassing sae if a factor followed the + (by Rule 3). So we build B up to a factor (steps 4 and 5). But a factor followed by * could be more expansive if the * is followed by a term, and so we place our attention on C, and so forth.

Note that we are making use of a hierarchical structure involving progressive generalizations. Thus an sae is at the top, encompassing factors, which themselves encompass terms. Also, we

A + B * ( C + D ) / E

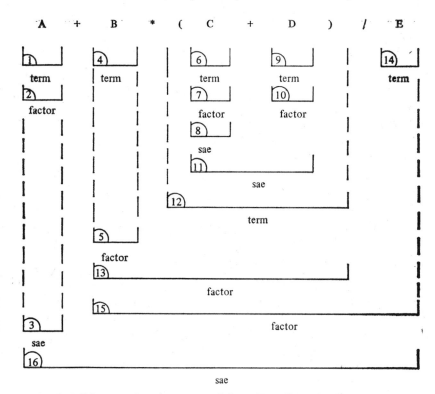

Figure 9–1. Diagramming the syntax of A + B * (C + D) /E. The numbers in the quarter circles are the "step numbers."

attempt to make the larger factors and sae's as the diagramming progresses. We are in fact diagramming the *syntax* of a simple arithmetic expression, just as school children used to diagram the syntax of English sentences.

It should be remarked that our second example, namely A + − B */C + D + will not result in an sae according to our rules, because the rules make no provision for the combination + −, or */, or for a term followed only by a + with nothing following the +.

Let us now summarize the results of our discussion on technical language and hierarchical structures. Our four relatively simple rules identified in a specific manner the concept of a simple arithmetic expression. There are of course a (countably) infinite number of actual arithmetic expressions that can be written, but by applying the rules any one of them can be identified.

What has this to do with medical diagnosis? We are faced with the problem that for many diseases the number of symptom complexes that may be presented by the patient can be very large. Perhaps we can learn by analogy with the methods of the computer scientist how to formulate a relatively few rules that would contain the "concept" of a particular disease, where an instance of the actual symptoms presented by the patient is analogous to an actual simple arithmetic expression.

### SOME SIMPLE SYMBOLISM

It is customary in computer science to use a symbolic notation for writing the syntax rules. Four symbols are used, namely "<," ">," "|," and "::=". A name enclosed in the angular brackets means it is a generic name, the vertical line means "or," and the four-dots-equals means "is defined as being." Hence our rules for a sae become the following:

Rule 0. <variable> ::= A|B|C|D|E|F|G|H|I|J|K|L|M|N|O|P |Q|R|S|T|U|V|W|X|Y|Z

Rule 1. <term> ::= <variable>|(<sae>)

Rule 2. <factor> ::= <term>|<factor>*<term>|<factor>/<term>

Rule 3. <sae> ::= <factor>|+<factor>|−<factor>|<sae>+<factor>|<sae>−<factor>

The correspondence with the word statement of the rules should be clear.

### CONCEPT RECOGNITION

Let us utilize another illustration to show how "recognition" can be obtained by these means. We will use pictures for the example, and we will write syntax rules for recognizing and distinguishing between a house and a church. To do this we must first introduce symbols that describe spatial relations; these are shown in Fig. 9–2. Using these relations we can symbolize a picture as shown in Fig. 9–3.

| Symbol | Meaning | Spatial Relation Correspondence |
|---|---|---|
| ⊥ | on top of | 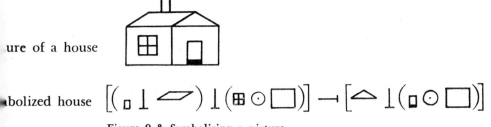 |
| ⊣ | adjacent to | |
| ⊙ | inside of | |

Figure 9–2. Spatial-relation symbols.

...ure of a house

...bolized house  $\left[ \left( \square \perp \diagup \right) \perp \left( \boxplus \odot \square \right) \right] \dashv \left[ \triangle \perp \left( \square \odot \square \right) \right]$

Figure 9–3. Symbolizing a picture.

Now let us consider the concept of a house. A four-year-old boy, if asked to draw a house, will most likely draw the following:

But if we show the boy a real house, with chimneys, roof shingles, gutters, bricks, screen doors, picture windows, carports, etc., he will still call it a house. Hence the question arises: How does the boy relate the real house to his simple concept of a house? Rather facetiously we answer: He uses syntax rules, as shown in Fig. 9–4.

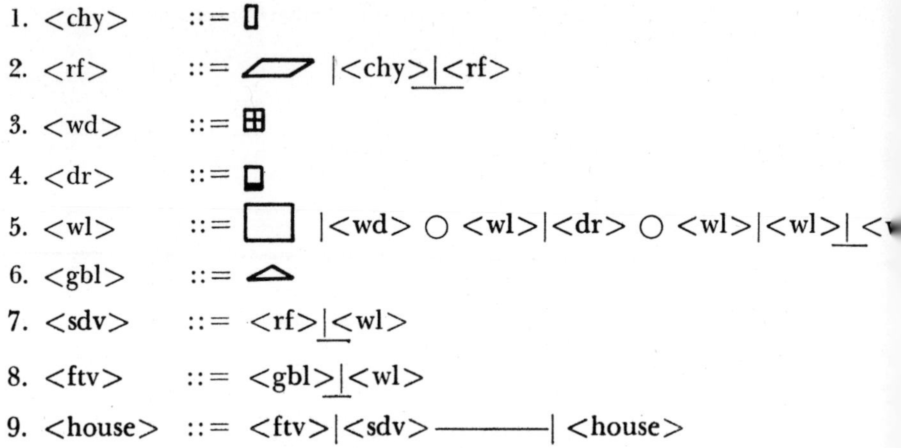

1. \<chy\>     ::= ▯

2. \<rf\>     ::= ▱ |\<chy>|\<rf\>

3. \<wd\>     ::= ⊞

4. \<dr\>     ::= ▯

5. \<wl\>     ::= ☐ |\<wd\> ○ \<wl>|\<dr\> ○ \<wl>|\<wl\>| \<w

6. \<gbl\>    ::= △

7. \<sdv\>    ::= \<rf>|\<wl\>

8. \<ftv\>    ::= \<gbl>|\<wl\>

9. \<house\>  ::= \<ftv>|\<sdv\>————| \<house\>

Figure 9–4. Syntax rules for a house.

By the method used above for an sae, we can diagram the recognition process for determining that our more complicated house is
really the same as the four-year-old boy's concept of a house, as
shown in Fig. 9–5.

What was really done was to recognize a roof with or without a
chimney, a wall with or without windows or doors, a side view as

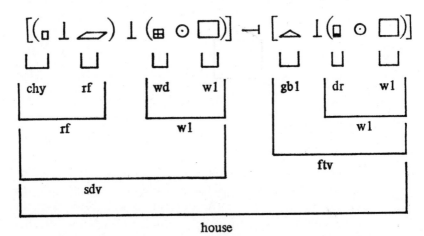

Figure 9–5. Diagram of recognition process for a house.

a wall with a roof, a front view as a gable on a wall, and a house as a front view (the four-year-old boy's concept) with or without a side view.

If we wish to distinguish between a house or a church, we need merely add three more syntax rules, namely

Rule 6′. <stpl>　　　::= △
Rule 8′. <cfv>　　　::= <stpl>|<wl>
Rule 9′. <church>　::= <cfv>|<sdv>————| <church>
after rules 6, 8, and 9, respectively. In this case, all of the forms shown in Fig. 9–6 represent pictures that could be correctly identified as houses or churches.

What has all this to do with medical diagnosis? The relation to medical diagnosis is threefold. First, by giving two widely differing examples using the same methods, I hope to impress the reader with the generality of the method, leading him into its application to medical diagnosis. Second, note that the procedure really has nothing to do with the context of the subject field of the application. Like any mathematical technique, it will work if the interpretation of the model is correct. For instance, the definitions of the sae can be stated in terms of numbers as follows:

Rule 0. = A|B|C|D|E|F|G|H|I|J|K|L|M|N| . . .
Rule 1. = 0.|(3.)
Rule 2. = 1.|2.*1.|2./1.
Rule 3. = 2.|+2.|−2.|3.+2.|3.−2.

HOUSES　　　　　　　　　　　　CHURCHES

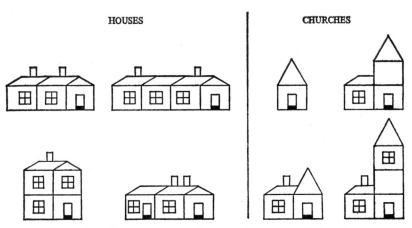

Figure 9–6. Representative pictures of houses and churches.

Hence it can be programmed for a computer to process in a straightforward manner, and hence also, by relating the method to aspects of medical theory, the computer can serve as an aid to diagnosis. Third, the examples have served to give insight into how the syntax lines are written in the first place. These examples indicate that in order to make use of the syntax-directed methods, the field of medical diagnosis should be first analyzed in terms of hierarchical relationships.

## HIERARCHY IN MEDICAL DIAGNOSIS

Before we proceed with a discussion of the hierarchical relationships that occur in medical diagnosis, let us first delineate that aspect of the reasoning foundations of medical diagnosis which is under consideration here. We are concerned with only the nonprobabilistic, logical aspects, the goal of which is to eliminate from consideration all possibilities not consistent with the presenting symptoms or, in other words, to determine the disease or diseases that the patient could possibly have.

The hierarchical aspect of our discussion has to do with the fact that many specific findings and symptoms can be categorized in terms of more general concepts, and in fact it is only these more general concepts that are involved in the disease-diagnosis decision. For example, in the case of oral diseases, it is necessary to know whether or not the patient has malaise, where by "malaise" we mean fever, aching, etc.—i.e. those symptoms brought about by a general systemic infection. The specific form of the malaise is not really important; we only wish to know if the oral disease is an aspect of a more generalized infection, or only a local oral problem. Similarly, the exact location of an oral lesion is often not as important in making an oral diagnosis as knowing whether the lesion is diffusely scattered throughout the oral mucosa or is located in only one portion of the mouth.

In Table 9–I we illustrate a possible syntax for defining and distinguishing between four oral diseases. The illustration was not constructed to be exemplary of the context, but was composed to give the reader a more specific idea of how syntax-directed concept analysis can be utilized in medical diagnosis. The purpose of the illustration is to identify certain aspects of such a syntax

TABLE 9–I
SYNTAX FOR FOUR ORAL DISEASES

*Location*

1. $<$tongue$>$    $::=$ lateral edges | top of | posterior of
of tongue | tongue | tongue

2. $<$cheek$>$    $::=$ buccal | $<$cheek$>$ anterior | $<$cheek$>$ posterior

3. $<$gum$>$    $::=$ gingival | $<$gum$>$ lingual | $<$gum$>$ buccal

4. $<$diffuse$>$    $::=$ $<$tongue$>$$<$cheek$>$$<$gum$>$

5. $<$localized$>$    $::=$ $<$tongue$>$ | $<$cheek$>$

*Type of Lesion*

6. $<$bullae$>$    $::=$ round small diameter

7. $<$glossy$>$    $::=$ smooth surface

8. $<$leukoplacia$>$    $::=$ white | $<$leukoplacia$>$ leathery | $<$leukoplacia$>$ patches

*Character of Oral Symptoms*

9. $<$inflamed$>$    $::=$ hyperaemic | red tender

10. $<$necrotic$>$    $::=$ sloughing | $<$necrotic$>$ bleeding | $<$necrotic$>$ inflamed

11. $<$pain$>$    $::=$ gum pain | cheek pain | tongue pain

*Other General Symptoms*

12. $<$systemic$>$    $::=$ skin lesions

13. $<$malaise$>$    $::=$ fever | aching bones | sweating | $<$malaise$>$ $<$malaise$>$

*Disease Definitions*

14. $<$lichen planus$>$    $::=$ $<$localized$>$$<$glossy$>$ $<$leukoplacia$>$

15. $<$cancerous$>$    $::=$ $<$localized$>$$<$leukoplacia$>$ | $<$gum$>$$<$leuko-
placia$>$ | $<$localized$>$$<$necrotic$>$ | $<$gum$>$
$<$necrotic$>$ | $<$cancerous$>$$<$pain$>$

16. $<$Vincent's
infection$>$    $::=$ $<$gum$>$$<$necrotic$>$$<$pain$>$ | $<$Vincent's$>$ $<$malaise$>$

17. $<$erythema
multiformus$>$    $::=$ $<$diffuse$>$$<$bullae$>$$<$pain$>$$<$systemic$>$

analysis, and to point out certain characteristics that syntax-directed concept analysis has when applied to medical diagnosis.

The illustration distinguishes four oral diseases: lichen planus; a general cancerous or precancerous conditions (normally a carcinoma) ; Vincent's infection; and erythema multiformus. Another "disease," known as leukoplacia, is interpreted as a syndrome characteristic of either a precancerous lesion or lichen planus, depending on other symptoms. Note that the symptoms are categorized as identifying (a) location in the mouth, (b) type of lesion insofar as appearance is concerned, (c) character of the lesion insofar as inflammation, necrosis, and pain are concerned, and (d) any other more generalized symptoms that may also occur. The definitions have, of course, been severely limited in order to make the illustration short: for example, "systemic" is used to indicate only that there are other lesions elsewhere on the skin in addition to the oral lesions.

With these limitations in mind, we can now proceed to discuss the illustration from the point of view of the methodology involved. Note that in lines 1, 2, and 3 we reduce the exact location of the lesions to only three general areas. If the lesions occur all over the mouth at the same time, then they are called <diffuse>. We also assume that the adjectives "anterior," "posterior," "buccal," and "lingual" will be given after the major area is indicated, namely <tongue>, <buccal>, and <gingival>. Thus the term "buccal" is used in a dual sense, as the location on the gingiva, and as <cheek>. The syntax itself takes care of the intended meaning; for example, "buccal anterior" becomes "<cheek> anterior," which in turn becomes just "<cheek>," but "gingival buccal" becomes "<gum> buccal" which becomes just "<gum>." Similarly we could have written definition 1 as

<tongue>  ::=|<tongue> lateral edges|<tongue>
top|<tongue> posterior

On comparison of this with definition 1, it is clearly seen how to write syntax lines to include relationships involving the concept "part of."

Note that the definition of <localized> involves only the tongue and cheek. This is because Vincent's infection occurs only on the gums, while lichen planus occurs only on either the tongue or the cheek. Hence we can use the word <localized> in the definition of lichen planus and <gum> in the definition of Vincent's infection.

Finally, note that some words are enclosed in the brackets, <   > while others are not. The distinction is as follows: The words in the brackets are "derived words," being defined only by the lines of the syntax. The other words, not enclosed in brackets, are the "basic words," the meaning of which is outside the syntax and is assumed as being known. This dichotomy also existed for our other illustrations. For the simple arithmetic expression, the basic "words" were the following:

A, B, C, D, . . . . , X, Y, Z; *, /, +, −, (,)

and the derived words were the following:

<variable>, <term>, <factor>, <sae>

For the house-church example, the basic "words" were as follows:

□, ▢, ▱, ⊞, ⊙, △, ▮, ⊥, ⊣, △

and the derived words were the following:

<chy>, <rf>, <wd>, <dr>, <wl>, <gbl>,
<sdv>, <ftv>, <house>, <stpl>, <cfv>, <church>

A similar list of basic and derived words can be made for the syntax of our oral-diagnosis example. Note that there is one syntax line for each *derived word,* and that the left-hand term of each line gives a different derived word.

One of the main reasons for appealing to syntax was stated to be economy of notation in describing or stating symptom complexes. Unfortunately, this is difficult to illustrate in a simple example. The reason for that is that any technical language must be introduced with a plethora of specific terms descriptive of the nature of the subject matter. For instance, when starting gross anatomy the student must learn a whole list of terms, such as saggital, frontal, distal, mesial, anterior, posterior, dorsal, and so forth. However, these terms are actually used because of their economy in describing the subject matter. The number of such technical terms is quite small in comparison with the quantity of subject matter in a gross-anatomy book; but in describing just one anatomic item, the true economy of the terms does not become apparent.

## SYNTAX-DIRECTED MEDICAL DIAGNOSIS

Let us now utilize our syntax to make a medical diagnosis, or at least to distinguish between the four oral diseases. Consider a patient who presents inflamed buccal gingiva with sloughing and

burning, and also is running a fever. For the "symptom string" we
have the following:

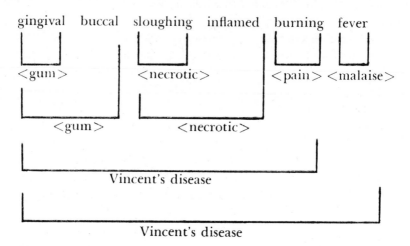

As another example, consider a patient who presents sloughing
and bleeding on the posterior buccal mucosa with pain. The
symptom string is as follows:

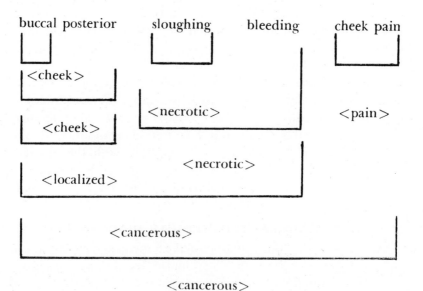

Next consider a patient with a white leathery lesion on the anterior buccal mucosa, with pain, fever, and sweating. The symptom string becomes as follows:

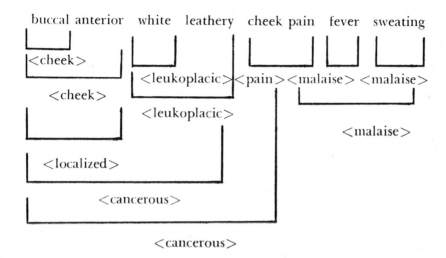

Here we have no combination in our syntax for <cancerous> followed by <malaise>. Hence the diagnosis is *not* within the purview of this syntax.

The above examples have indicated how the syntax can be used in constructing a diagnosis from the patient's symptom profile or symptom string. The exact computer program that can perform such a computation is described in previous publications by the author,* and an even more comprehensive computer program for performing such syntax analysis has been prepared for the IBM 360/44 computer. Since the details of these programs are beyond the scope of the present paper, we shall not dwell further on them at this time.

## SUMMARY AND CONCLUSIONS

Table 9–II summarizes the status of four types of mathematical approaches to the logical aspects of the reasoning foundations of medical diagnosis. The Boolean-algebraic approach (i.e. the use

---

* See for example, Reference 5.

## TABLE 9–II

| The Status of Various Approaches to the Logical Aspects of Medical Diagnosis | Capability Lacking | Status Feasibility Problems | Progress to Date |
|---|---|---|---|
| Logic (Boolean Algebra) | none | too many combinations | lots |
| Tree structure | recursive logic | complete set of symptoms required | lots |
| Finite state automaton | relational variety | no provision for relational logic | none |
| Syntax directed analysis | none | construction of syntax lines? | none |

*Type of Mathematical Approach* (row label spanning the four approaches)

of mathematical logic) presents all the necessary capabilities; however, it does have a feasibility problem in that there can be too many possible symptom profiles to record, as mentioned at the beginning of this article. Much progress has been made to circumvent this difficulty. The tree-structure or branching approach has the appeal that it does not necessitate any extensive mathematical knowledge as a prerequisite to its use. But it requires a complete symptom set, or else one may come to a node or branch point that requires a symptom result that is not available, in which case the method breaks down. Also, recursive logic is not incorporated into a tree-structure approach.* In cases where complete sets of symptoms are available though, tree structures have been utilized in medical diagnosis. The finite-state-automaton approach has not been tried in medical diagnosis. It is usually based on a single binary relation, and it is difficult to incorporate a variety of relations (in the mathematical sense) into the method.

Finally consider the syntax-directed-analysis approach. It has all required capabilities. It overcomes the feasibility problems of the Boolean-algebra, the tree-structure, and the finite-state-automaton approaches. However, it may have a potential problem:

---

* For instance, we could not apply a tree structure to the definition of a simple arithmetic expression because we cannot have ($<$sae$>$) become a $<$term$>$ without looping the tree; a tree with a loop is not a tree!

Can adequate syntax lines be constructed for the realistic application of the method? We believe that it is possible to feasibly construct such syntax lines in realistic situations, such as in medical specialties. The problem is that the individual who is constructing the syntax must be knowledgeable in the syntax-directed method *and* must be expert in the medical specialty under consideration. Formulating the syntax perhaps requires even more precision in thought and expression than writing a textbook on the subject matter. The required knowledge is in a good textbook, but the writing of syntax lines requires more precise thinking and terminology and greater consistency than many experts are prepared for. Of course, this statement can be made about almost any type of computer application—what you get out of a computer is no better than what you put in. Similarly, the syntax lines can tell one no more about a medical specialty than the originator of these syntax lines.

## REFERENCES

1. Ledley, R. S. and Lusted, L. B.: Reasoning foundations of medical diagnosis. *Science, 130:*9–21, July 3, 1959.
2. Ledley, R. S. and Lusted, L. B.: Medical diagnosis and modern decision making. *Proc Appl Math Symp, 14:*117–158, March 1961.
3. Ledley, R. S.: Local aid to systematic medical diagnosis (and operational simulation in medicine). *J Operations Res Soc Am, 4:*392, August 1956.
4. Ledley, R. S. and Lusted, L. B.: The role of computers in medical diagnosis. *Med Dokumentation, 5:*70–78, July 1961.
5. Ledley, R. S.: *Programming and Utilizing Digital Computers.* New York, McGraw-Hill, 1962.
6. Ledley, R. S.: *Use of Computers in Biology and Medicine.* New York, McGraw-Hill, 1965.
7. Ledley, R. S.: Computer aids to clinical treatment evaluation. *Operations Res, 15:*694–705, July–August 1967.
8. Ledley, R. S.: Computer aids to medical diagnosis. *JAMA, 196:*933–943, June 13, 1966.
9. Ledley, R. S. and Lusted, L. B.: The use of electronic computers in medical data processing. *Trans Med Electron, 7:*31–47, January 1960.
10. Ledley, R. S.: High speed automatic analysis of biomedical pictures. *Science, 146:*216–223, October 9, 1964.

11. Ledley, R. S. *et al.*: FIDAC: Film input to digital automatic computer and associated syntax-directed pattern-recognition programming system. In Tippett, J. A., *et al.* (Eds.): *Optical and Electro-Optical Information Processing.* Cambridge, Mass., MIT Press, 1965, pp. 591–614.

12. Additional references can be found at the end of Lee B. Lusted: *Introduction to Medical Diagnosis Making.* Springfield, Thomas, 1968.

Chapter 10

# DIAGNOSIS AND PREDICTION IN METEOROLOGY

Edward S. Epstein

I THINK THIS DISCUSSION is included in this volume in recognition of certain analogies between problems of meteorological prediction and of medical diagnosis. Certainly the analogies exist, and I will allude to them. However, it seems to me to be proper that I not try to identify or dwell on analogies at this time, but rather expound on things that I presumably know something about—the problems of meteorological prediction. I trust that many of the analogies will be apparent.

The atmosphere is a large, thermodynamically active, irreversible system. It consists (mostly) of a mixture of gases which fortunately are chemically inactive (mostly) and very nearly ideal (again mostly).* Some of the less abundant components of this gaseous mixture happen to have significant radiative properties, and one component in particular (water) has the nasty characteristic of changing state to both liquid and solid phases at temperatures and pressures frequently encountered.

The earth's surface forms the lower boundary of the atmosphere. It is not only an irregular terrain, but many of its significant properties vary in the course of time. Sometimes this lower boundary undergoes changes, in response to atmospheric influences, that markedly affect its characteristics. There are exchanges of momentum, heat, and even mass at this air-planet interface. A further complication is that the planet, to which the at-

---

* Meteorologists, by and large, have not paid sufficient heed to the chemically active gaseous components of the atmosphere, nor to the nongaseous components, or aerosols. Like everyone else, we'd like pollution just to go away. It further complicates an already complicated situation.

mosphere is attached by gravitational forces, rotates, which means that the natural system of coordinates for following the behavior of the atmosphere is itself an accelerating frame of reference.

The physical problem is formidable enough. There is the further complicating factor, however, that even if we understood the physics and the relevant mathematics perfectly, it would still be a practical impossibility to make a perfect forecast. This is because the equations are so complex that they must be handled numerically, and with any computer one can still do only a finite amount of arithmetic in a finite period of time. Time is a factor because weather forecasts, like medical diagnoses, are perishable commodities. Anything one does to solve the problem by doing a finite amount of arithmetic must introduce some errors.

A final complication that the meteorologist faces is that in order to predict tomorrow's weather he must first know the state of today's weather. Here we are limited by a much smaller finite number of observations, each of which is subject to error. On the average we have less than two observations of the winds, temperatures, and pressures at the important levels of the middle atmosphere for every one million square miles (about 300 observations over 200 million square miles of the earth's surface). Some large regions of the earth, including most of the southern hemisphere but many regions in the northern hemisphere as well, are almost wholly unobserved. Satellites are correcting the problem of inadequate coverage. This leaves only the problems of observational error, inadequately understood physics, and more arithmetic to do than any conceivable computer could handle.

With these limitations and difficulties in mind, the meteorologist tries to bring to the public, each day, forecasts of the weather one, two, even as many as five days in advance. The reputable meteorologist never doubts that there is uncertainty in his forecasts, and he sometimes is able to make specific reference to these uncertainties in his forecast.

Meteorologists—or better the weather services—maintain careful records to verify or substantiate predictions. When a forecast does not turn out very well he can then ask the question, "Was the error due to faulty initial data, a poor method of forecasting, or was it an error in the data by which I verified the forecast?"

In general, he has a great deal of difficulty distinguishing among those three sources of error. Yet he has been able to determine that there are some methods of prediction that work better for him than other methods.

The two classes of prediction methods available to meteorologists are methods based upon his knowledge of the physics of atmospheric behavior, and those based upon his knowledge of how the atmosphere has behaved in the past. The former is usually referred to as either "physical weather prediction" or "numerical weather prediction." (The latter is the more common term although clearly subject to misinterpretation.) The alternative approach is that of empirical or statistical prediction. There is also room for combinations of these two approaches, and such combinations are used in routine practice, but even then they tend to be clearly separable steps in the prediction methodology.

We have learned from experience that when it comes to extrapolating the behavior of the atmosphere over periods of 12 hours or more, none of the statistical methods known to us can compete with physical weather prediction. The reasons for this are summarized in two words: nonlinear and unstable.

By unstable I mean that two states of the atmosphere which are quite similar to each other initially will eventually develop to grossly dissimilar conditions. This instability apparently extends to pairs of initial conditions that are arbitarily close to one another. Since observations could never distinguish between such arbitarily similar initial conditions, this implies an upper limit to the range over which we could ever predict the state of the atmosphere, and also the presence of error in even short range predictions.

As long as the difference between any pair of initial states of the atmosphere remain small, the rate at which they become more dissimilar tends to be linearly related to the relevant parameters. Once this separation becomes larger though, the nonlinearities implicit in all atmospheric developments begin to dominate. Only by methods of physical prediction can we adequately deal with the nonlinear aspects of atmospheric evolution.

Certainly there exist statistical methods which can treat nonlinear processes, but the more complex the methods or the more complex the system being represented, the greater is the requirement for developmental data. Those methods which have had the greatest success in application to meteorological problems have been linear or almost linear in their general attributes. To give you some idea of the data that would be necessary to develop statistical methods of sufficient complexity and nonlinearity to adequately handle the problem of a general 12-hour prediction of the global wind and pressure pattern in the middle atmosphere, let me relate the following finding. E. N. Lorenz [3] went through five years of twice daily sets of values of the pressure patterns at three levels in the northern hemisphere searching for analogs, i.e. pairs of situations close enough to one another that they would subsequently follow similar patterns of change. He found none. By extrapolating some of his results he estimated that in order for him to be likely to find a single good analog pair he would have to increase the length of his data sample to include 140 years of data (i.e. 140 years $\times$ 365 days/year $\times$ 2 sets of observations/day $\cong 10^5$ sets of observations). Observations of the type he examined exist in relatively complete form for only the last 25 years or so. It is difficult to identify unknown interactions (nonlinearities) without any replications.

Even though statistical methods are of limited use for forecasting over periods of 12 hours or greater, they have seen considerable use in meteorological prediction of very specific weather elements for short periods of time. In a few cases, statistical methods have been used for extrapolations of 12 or more hours, but in these cases it has been the lack of suitable physical models, rather than the adequacy of the statistical methods that has led to this result. One example is the prediction of the positions of hurricanes. Only in the last few years have meteorologists begun to learn enough about tropical meteorology to develop suitable physical models of these storms. Some of the most successful predictions of the behavior of tropical storms have been by statistical means. These predictions, which would not be considered good according to the standards of our ability to forecast the positions of large extratropical storms, have been based primarily on methods of multiple regression, with the predictors having been chosen by appropriate screening techniques. Multiple regression with screening is also being widely used in meteorology to specify specific local conditions in the light of values of some of the larger scale meteorological factors that are predicted by physical models. For example, effective procedures for forecasting maximum and minimum temperatures make use of multiple regression equations involving such parameters as the maximum and minimum temperatures of the preceding period and forecast values of the temperatures and pressures at various levels in the atmosphere at selected locations.[2] Similar methods are used to forecast precipitation.[1]

I should interrupt this discussion here to say a little about the actual procedures followed by the Weather Bureau in bringing forecasts to the public. A great deal of calculations are made at the National Meteorological Center just outside of Washington and many of the immediate results of these calculations are sent via facsimile to local weather stations. In addition, experienced meteorologists at the National Meteorological Center analyze the results of these calculations in the light of all their experience and all the other data that may be at their disposal and these analyses are also transmitted to the local weather stations. The local forecasting office also receives a great deal of more recent and local data that may not have been incorporated into the products emanating from the NMC. The calculated statistical predictions referred to above are among the information which is available to the local forecaster. He has the opportunity to examine these forecasts and to either accept them at their face value or to modify them according to his personal judgment. Because there are very careful records kept comparing his forecasts, the advisory forecasts that he receives, and the subsequent weather, he soon learns that extent to which he is able and ought to modify his advisory material. *None of the automated procedures that have been developed have ever reached the point where some improvement is not possible if done carefully and imaginatively by an experienced meteorologist.*

There are two statistical techniques that have been found particularly effective for short range prediction of specific meteorological elements. Both of these techniques have been developed primarily for the short range (up to seven hours) prediction of airport ceiling and visibility. These methods are multiple discriminant analysis (MDA) and the regression estimation of event probabilities (REEP). Both methods provide probabilities that each of a set of mutually exclusive, operationally significant categories will occur. These methods were developed in this context by R. Miller and J. Bryan at the Travelers Research Corporation. For both procedures, it was found useful to express all the possible predictors in terms of dummy variables, i.e. binary digits which indicate whether or not a specific precursive event occurred. For example the relative humidity, a continuous variable, may be subdivided into four or five categories (e.g. 0–50%, 50–75%, 75–90%, 90–95%, 95–100%), each of which represents a separate binary predictor. The use of dummy variables in this way introduces an element of nonlinearity into otherwise linear methods. It also simplifies certain machine computations.

In multiple discriminant analysis a subset of the possible predictors is selected by a screening procedure and these predictors are then used to define a set of linear discriminant functions.[4] In the space (discriminant space) defined by these functions, the separation between the different categories of that which is predicted is maximized in comparison to the spread within the categories. One obtains from MDA conditional probabilities of the several categories, given particular values of the predictors, by finding the point in discriminant space represented by the values of the predictors, and evaluating the relative frequency of the various groups among previous observations in the immediate vicinity of that point in discriminant space. This procedure proved to be an effective forecast tool, but it had the disadvantage of requiring not only a considerable amount of calculations to derive the appropriate discriminant functions, but also it requires a considerable amount of calculations each time one wishes to determine a probability. If there are four discriminate functions (the maximum number of such functions is one less than the number of categories being discriminated) and several thousand previous observations, then for each application it is necessary to determine distances in four-dimensional space between the new point and all previous points to find which are nearest. This requires a computer with considerable speed and storage capacity.

The REEP method uses the same dummy variables as predictors, but one simply develops five simultaneous linear regression equations between the predictors and the five dummy variables representing the predicted groups. Since for each observation, one and only one of the predicted groups can be observed, the sum of the values calculated from the five regression equations will always be unity. It is reasonable to think of the outputs of the five regression equations as being probabilities of the individual events. It is possible for values greater than one or less than zero to be indicated by these equations, but such occurrences are very rare and it is not difficult to devise procedures to accommodate such occurrences.

REEP equations are very easy to apply in practice. It is only necessary to sum algebraically the coefficients corresponding to the particular dummy variables that occur. REEP procedures are now being introduced to give forecasts of visibility and ceiling at a large number of airports throughout the United States. The forecasts thus produced represent significant improvements over both climatology and persistance. (It is very difficult to do better than a persistance forecast over short periods of time. It is difficult to do better than a climatological prediction for extended time periods.) Here, too, there is some indication that the skilled forecaster could do as well as these statistical techniques, but no skilled forecaster could produce as many forecasts so quickly for such a large range of stations; and there is not a very large number of skilled forecasters.

Let me now return to the subject of the analogies between the diagnostic problem in medicine and the prediction problem in meteorology. We are both trying to deal with extremely complex systems, systems which we understand partially at best. In both cases our concern is considerably more than idle curiosity, for there are vital decisions that must be made in the light of the information that we can provide. In general, either because of limitations of our data, or because of limited knowledge and understanding, our analyses are imperfect. From the point of view of the decisions that must be made, the best information that we can give is our subjective probabilities that certain situations are, or will be, the case. I say subjective probabilities because it is manifestly impossible to observe, and quite difficult even to conceive of the necessary replications of particular situations to be able to talk meaningfully of relative frequencies.

While on the subject of probabilities I should introduce also the very important question of scoring rules for probability assessments. This is a subject which is of particular concern to meteorologists who are always comparing different forecasters and different forecast methods. A scoring rule is a function of the forecast and the observed event. Let $R = (r_1, r_2, \ldots r_k)$ be the forecast probabilities of k possible events (with the obvious condition that $\sum\limits_{i=1}^{k} r_i = 1$ and $0 \leqslant r_i \leqslant 1$ for all i). Also, let $O = (o_1, o_2, \ldots o_k)$ be the observation made subsequent to the event, and defined such that $o_i = 1$ if and only if the $i^{th}$ event occurred. A scoring rule S(R,O) assigns a number to each forecast after the fact of the observation. There is no limit to the different kinds of scoring rules that can be invented, but there are certain attributes that scoring rules should have. In particular, the scoring rule should be *proper*,[5] i.e. the forecaster should achieve his best score only if his forecast is consistent with what he really believes. The principal reason for this criterion is that subjective probabilities, in order to make sense, must be believed. The person who issues the forecast should not be encouraged to say something other than his belief.

As an example of this let me use a situation in which there are only two possible events, as in the meteorological case of rain or no rain. I will define three possible scoring systems.

$$S_1 = r_1\, o_1 + r_2\, o_2$$
$$S_2 = 1 - o_1\, (1\text{-}r_1)^2 - o_2\, (1\text{-}r_2)^2 = 1 - o_1\, r_2^2 - o_2\, r_1^2$$
$$S_3 = \log\, (r_1\, o_1 + r_2\, o_2)$$

The first scoring system $(S_1)$ assigns a score equal to the probability given for the event that occurs. The best score of 1.0 is earned if the event that occurs had been predicted with certainty. The second scoring system also gives a score of 1.0 for a perfect forecast, but extracts a penalty proportional to the square of the amount by which the probability assigned to the subsequently observed event departs from 1.0. The third system assigns a score of the logarithm of the probability assigned to the event that occurs. Here the score for a perfect forecast is 0.0.

Now let us consider the forecaster who *believes* that the probabilities of the two events are $p_1 = 0.1$ and $p_2 = 0.9$. It is reasonable that he should make the forecast $(r_1, r_2)$ that would maximize his expected score:

$$E(S) = p_1 S(r_1, r_2 \mid o_1 = 1) + p_2 S(r_1, r_2 \mid o_2 = 1)$$

$S(r_1, r_2 \mid o_1 = 1)$ means the score he would get for the forecast if the event i occurs. Table 10–I gives the expected scores for several possible forecasts.

TABLE 10–I

| Forecast | | $E(S_1)$ (Linear Scoring Rule) | $E(S_2)$ (Quadratic Scoring Rule) | $E(S_3)$ (Logarithmic Scoring Rule) |
|---|---|---|---|---|
| $r_1$ | $r_2$ | | | |
| .3 | .7 | .1 (.3) + .9 ( .7) = .66 | .1 (.51) + .9 (.91) = .87 | .1 (−.523) + .9 (−.155) = −.192 |
| .2 | .8 | .1 (.2) + .9 ( .8) = .74 | .1 (.36) + .9 (.96) = .90 | .1 (−.699) + .9 (−.097) = −.157 |
| .1 | .9 | .1 (.1) + .9 ( .9) = .82 | .1 (.19) + .9 (.99) = .91 | .1 (−1.0) + .9 (−.046) = −.141 |
| 0 | 1.0 | .1 (0.) + .9 (1.0) = .90 | .1 (0) + .9 (1.00) = .90 | .1 (−∞) + .9 (0) = −∞ |

The forecaster being scored by the linear scoring rule $(S_1)$, believing $p_1 = .1$, would forecast $r_1 = 0$, because this would give him an expected score of 0.90, significantly better than the score he would expect forecasting $r_1 = .1$. Put another way, the forecaster (or forecast method) achieving the best score would likely not be the one that gives the best, most honest, forecast. Thus *the linear scoring rule is not proper.* On the other hand the quadratic rule $(S_2)$ and the logarithmic rule $(S_3)$ both give the best scores when the forecast $(r_1, r_2)$ and the belief $(p_1, p_2)$ are identical. They are proper scoring rules.

In meteorology, the quadratic scoring rule (or one almost identical to it) is used most frequently. Scores achieved depend not only on the skill of the forecaster but also on the difficulty of the forecast problem. For example the score for precipitation probability forecasts * will vary from place to place and from season to

---

* Precipitation probability forecast should be interpreted as the probability of more than a trace (>.005 inches) of precipitation in a particular period (normally 7 AM–7 PM or 7 PM–7 AM) at any particular point in the forecast area.

season. Recent average values of $S_2$ for a 12-hour forecast in Detroit in winter have been near 0.91 and in summer about 0.87. The winter figure indicates considerably more skill than the summer figure because the higher frequency of precipitation in winter would otherwise tend to give rise to lower scores.

I must add that not all meteorologists agree with me that the output of a meteorological forecast system should be the probabilities of subsequent events. Even I must admit that I find it difficult to imagine the format in which one could inform the public at large, concisely and coherently, of the assessed probabilities of all possible subsequent weather events. The mere fact that we are doing it for the occurrence or nonoccurrence of precipitation over particular periods of time represents a certain amount of progress, but subsequent steps may prove more difficult. Note that one of the differences between the problem of medical diagnosis and that of weather prediction is that we regularly offer our judgments to the public, who are then in a perfect position to judge us right or wrong. Remember what Mark Antony said about Caesar. How fortunate you are that your diagnoses need not always be announced to the public, and that even if they were, the public need not always know whether they were right or wrong. On the other hand your diagnoses are directed to a more sophisticated and highly selected group of individuals who can more readily be made aware of the proper interpretation of probability statements.

In what I've said thus far it has been apparent that meteorology generally deals with prognosis while you are first concerned with diagnosis. Diagnosis is important whenever a possible treatment can affect the prognosis and one must make a decision as to which if any treatment to use. Recently meteorologists are learning about diagnosis in the area of weather modification. We now believe that the seeding of certain cloud systems with silver iodide (or certain other agents) can enhance precipitation. Seeding other clouds, though, may suppress precipitation. In the past much cloud seeding has been done rather indiscriminantly and with conflicting results. We are learning the necessity of diagnosing the clouds before prescribing a treatment. Of course, somewhere in the decision-making processes one also has to make explicit judgment as to whether more or less rain is desirable. That may prove the most troublesome question of all.

Every diagnosis, or every prediction, represents a subjective judgment. The use of automation can be a very significant adjunct to the diagnostic or predictive procedure. Yet the use of such a procedure does not necessarily imply that no diagnostician or forecaster, left to his own devices, could do as well. It is the meteorological experience that in most situations there exist particularly skilled people who can do as well as the automated empirical methods. In general, however, there are too few of these very skilled individuals. It is a much more satisfactory procedure, in view of the very many decisions and judgments that must be made, to train people to recognize when the automated procedures produce reliable results, and when those results should be given less credence. In any case, by having the best possible automated procedures and combining them with highly trained, imaginative interpreters, we are in general in a far better position to provide the best of services in the largest number of cases.

I wish us both lots of luck.

## REFERENCES

1. Klein, W. H.: The forecast research program of the techniques development laboratory. *Bull Am Meteor Soc, 51:*133–142, 1969.
2. Klein, W. H. and F. Lewis: Computer forecasts of minimum temperatures. *J Appl Meteor, 9:*350–359, 1970.
3. Lorenz, E. N.: Atmospheric predictibility as revealed by naturally occurring analogs. *J Atmos Sci, 26:*636–646, 1969.
4. Miller, R. G.: Statistical prediction by discriminant analysis. *Meteor Monogr* (No. 25). Boston, American Meteorological Society, 1964.
5. Murphy, A. H. and Epstein, E. S.: A note on probability forecast and "hedging." *J Appl Meteor, 6:*1002–1004, 1967.

## Chapter 11

# BAYES' THEOREM FOR INTELLIGENCE ANALYSIS

### Jack Zlotnick

THE INTELLIGENCE INTEREST in probability theory stems from the probabilistic character of customary intelligence judgment. Intelligence analysis must usually be undertaken on the basis of incomplete evidence. Intelligence conclusions are therefore characteristically hedged by such words and phrases as "very likely," "possibly," "may," "better than even chance," and other qualifiers.

This manner of allowing for more than one possibility leaves intelligence open to the charge of acting as the oracle whose prophecies seek to cover all contingencies. The apt reply to this charge is that intelligence would do poor service by overstating its knowledge. The very best that intelligence can do is to make the most of the evidence without making more of the evidence than it deserves. The best recourse is often to address the probabilities.

The professional focus on probabilities has led to some in-house research on possible intelligence applications of Bayes' Theorem. At the time of my participation in this research, I was an analyst in the Central Intelligence Agency, which sponsored the scholarship but took no position of its own on the issues under study. My personal views on these issues, as elaborated in the following pages, have no official character.

## THE BAYESIAN APPROACH

Bayes' Theorem in its odds-likelihood form served participants in our test program as their diagnostic rule for appraising new evidence. The odds-likelihood formulation of Bayes' Theorem is the following equation:

$$R = PL$$

R is the revised estimate of the odds favoring one hypothesis over another—the estimate of the odds after consideration of the latest item of evidence. P is the prior estimate of the odds—the odds before consideration of the latest item of evidence. There is no escaping some starting estimate of P. However, after the starting estimate was in hand, the participating analysts offered no judgments about P. It was a value carried forward in machine memory from previous analysis. R, the result of the mathematical processing, was what went back into machine memory to become the value of P used in consideration of the next item of evidence. The participating analysts offered judgments only about L, the likelihood ratio.

The likelihood ratio was the analyst's evaluation of the diagnosticity of an item of evidence. Evidence is diagnostic when the chances of its appearing are different if one hypothesis is true than if another hypothesis is true. Suppose intelligence is asked to estimate the comparative merits of two hypotheses—one of imminent war, the other of no imminent war. The estimate is to be expressed in terms of the odds favoring or disfavoring the war hypothesis. The latest evidence is deployment of foreign troops to a border area. Is the deployment deemed to be say two times more likely if the war hypothesis is true than if the no-war hypothesis is true? Then the evidence is certainly diagnostic. The value of L, a judgment of the analyst communicated to the machine processor, would in this case be the fraction $2/1$.

Three principal features of the Bayesian method distinguish it from conventional intelligence analysis. The first is that the intelligence analyst is required to quantify judgments which he does not ordinarily express in numerical terms. This requirement to quantify probabilistic judgment is the feature that perhaps draws most of the critical fire against the Bayesian approach in intelligence analysis. A debating point of the critics is that analysts are bound to disagree in their opinions of the exact figure that should represent the diagnostic value of an item of evidence. The Bayesian rebuttal is that disagreement among analysts is just as much a characteristic of traditional method and is no less serious for being implicit rather than explicit in the analysis. The critic returns to the debate by observing that the typical analyst, being a verbal and not a mathematical man, finds it inordinately difficult to express his degree of belief to the precision implied by a numerical value. The partisan of Bayes, for his part, takes the position that people have been quantifying probabilistic judgments since the beginning of time—whenever they offered or accepted betting odds on the outcome of any doubtful issue.

The second distinguishing feature of Bayesian method is that the analyst does not draw from the available evidence his conclusions about the relative merits of opposing hypotheses. He rather postulates, by turns, the truth of each hypothesis, addressing himself only to the likelihood that each item of evidence would appear, first under the assumption that one hypothesis is true and then under the assumption that another hypothesis is true. The analyst is under no ego-supporting need to hold to positions previously taken on the merits of the respective hypotheses; he does not feel called upon to reinforce his self-esteem by reaffirmation of opinions previously put on the record.

The third distinctive feature of Bayesian method is that the analyst makes his judgments about the bits and pieces of evidence. He does not sum up the evidence as he would have to do if he had to judge its meaning for final conclusions. The mathematics does the summing up, telling the analyst in effect: "If these are your readings of the individual items of evidence, then this is the conclusion that follows." The research findings of some Bayesian psychologists seem to show that people are generally better at appraising a single item of evidence than at drawing inferences from the body of evidence considered in the aggregate. If these are valid findings, then the Bayesian approach calls for the intelligence analyst to do what he can do best and to leave all the rest to the incorruptible logic of a dispassionate mathematics.

The Bayesian approach was not studied with any idea of its replacing other approaches in intelligence analysis. The responsibility of intelligence is to depict, as best it can, the current and prospective state of international affairs. The intelligence estimate is a closely reasoned analysis of such important matters of interest as the top political leadership of a foreign country, evolving popular attitudes in that country, changing force structures in its military establishment, its levels of scientific achievement, and the hard choices it is making in allocation of resources to the guns and butter sectors of the economy. The intelligence estimate is sketched in all the lights and shadows of descriptive, narrative, and interpretative commentary. This task is not reducible to terse statement of the odds favoring one particular hypothesis over another.

There are, however, areas of intelligence analysis where Bayes' Theorem might well complement other approaches. One crucially important area is that of strategic warning—the analysis directed to uncovering any pattern of activity by a foreign power suggestive of a major and imminent threat to U.S. security interests. The patterns of events leading to Pearl Harbor in 1941 and to the Communist invasion of South Korea in 1950 are cases in point. Strategic warning analysis focuses primarily on just the problem that Bayes' Theorem addresses—the odds favoring one hypothesis (say imminent attack) over another hypothesis (no imminent attack).

## THE RESEARCH TASK

One way to test the usefulness of Bayes' Theorem for intelligence analysis is to replay intelligence history. This means going back to international crises of years past. It means assembly of the evidence which was available before the outcomes of the crises were known. It means reading the old intelligence estimates and other studies in order to find out how the analysts of the day interpreted the evidence. It means assignment of L values—likelihood ratios—that honestly reflect these analyst's evaluations of the evidence at the time and not our present hindsight knowledge.

Another way to test Bayes' Theorem is on current inflows of evidence. The advantage of this kind of testing is that hindsight knowledge does not intrude; Bayes' Theorem is pitted fairly and squarely against the conventional modes of analysis. Offsetting this advantage for honest research, however, is a disabling disadvantage.

The disadvantage derives from the very nature of the hypotheses at interest in strategic warning. The alternative hypotheses are commonly of two types. One stipulates continuation of the status quo. The other stipulates sudden change from the status quo. Usually the situation today is pretty much what it is going to be a week from today. The status quo hypothesis, in other words, usually turns out to be the true one in strategic warning analysis. But the main test of strategic warning effectiveness is the capability to give forewarning of the sudden changes that occasionally do occur in the status quo. The intelligence interest in Bayes' Theorem is primarily in how well the Bayesian approach to strategic warning would meet this main test of performance in situations of general surprise, without chronic resort to cry-wolf false alarms. Unfortunately, intelligence research cannot be speeded up by focus on the particular current issues which will turn into occasions of intelligence surprise. If intelligence could pick out in advance the issues on which it was going to be surprised, it would by definition never be surprised, and it would have no interest in the possible contributions of Bayes' Theorem to improved analysis.

The outlook, then, is that many tests of Bayes' Theorem on current inflows of evidence will be needed to get the few interesting occasions that show Bayesian performance in circumstances of general intelligence surprise. And just a few interesting examples are not enough to make the case for or against the Bayesian approach, which may do better than conventional method sometimes and not as well other times. A large enough sample of interesting examples is needed to justify confident findings of comparative performance on the average.

The results of the testing so far have been interesting enough to make a good case for further testing of Bayes' Theorem in intelligence analysis. Among the interesting results has been an uncovering of problem areas that flank the path of intelligence analysis and that are not very easily outflanked.

### The Life-Span of Evidence

One such problem area has been called nonstationarity. In situations of nonstationarity, that is, when hypotheses are being effectively altered by the passage of time, evidence will have a limited life-span. An intelligence hypothesis about current Soviet policy is not exactly the same hypothesis on January 15 that it is on February 15. The date has changed, so the hypothesis is to a degree different; and evidence back in January which had a certain bearing on the hypothesis of what was then current Soviet policy does not have the same bearing on the hypothesis of what is current Soviet policy a month later.

Consider, for example, some evidence which was available to intelligence and to the public at large in the summer of 1962, before photographic confirmation was received of missiles in Cuba that could reach targets deep in the United States. Soviet leaders gave public assurances during this period that the expanding military aid to Cuba was for defensive purposes only. Now an analyst's appraisal of this kind of assurance will depend partly on how honorable or dishonorable he believes Communists to be. But whatever his views about the honor of Communists, he would certainly not consider any government's assurances to constitute a commitment for all eternity. Governments do make new decisions and reconsider old ones. This amounts to saying that the diagnostic value of evidence bearing on hypotheses about current government policy tends to erode over time. A mathematical logic for strategic warning analysis has to be attentive to this erosion. Perhaps the analyst can specify the expected rate of erosion when he first encounters an item of evidence. If he cannot or prefers not to, the Bayesian approach does not quite attain the mechanistic ideal that would require of the analyst only his one-time attention to each item of incoming evidence. The analyst instead finds himself looking back from time to time at his whole body of past evidence to consider whether its diagnostic value, as recorded in machine memory, is still valid and not outdated.

## Causal Evidence

Another problem area spotlighted in the testing is the occasional reversal in cause and effect relationship between hypotheses and data. The disease generates the symptoms of the disease, and so the physician can infer the disease from the symptoms. Similarly in his surveillance of the Soviet scene, the intelligence analyst in Washington can infer from Soviet actions a good deal about Soviet policy. But the analyst also has his eye cocked for relevant data other than Soviet actions, data which have less a derivative than a causal relationship to Soviet policy. I draw again on the Cuban missile crisis of 1962 for my historical example.

On several occasions that year, President Kennedy publicly warned that the United States would take a grave view of strategic missile emplacements in Cuba. How would a Bayesian analyst evaluate President Kennedy's warnings for their relevance to opposing hypotheses about Soviet missile shipments to Cuba? If the analyst were a mechanical, uncritical Bayesian, he would say to himself: "President Kennedy is more likely to issue these statements if the hypothesis of imminent Soviet missile shipments to Cuba is true than if the hypothesis of no such missile shipments to Cuba is true. My L in the Bayesian equation $R = PL$ is greater than 1/1, and so my mathematics works out to an increase in the odds favoring the missile hypothesis."

Well, the analyst in this case is surely not reasoning as President Kennedy reasoned. The President no doubt felt that the clear communication of American concern would either have no effect on Moscow or, hopefully, would dissuade the Soviet leadership from shipping strategic missiles to Cuba. He thought, in other words, that his statements would tend to reduce, not increase, the odds favoring the missile hypothesis.

The complication for the Bayesian analyst is the causal character of President Kennedy's statements. Soviet actions are direct derivatives of Soviet policy. President Kennedy's statements were not. They were important primarily for the chance that they would affect, not reflect, Soviet policy.

It can be shown that, in principle, Bayes' Theorem is as applicable to causal evidence as to derivative evidence. In practice, Bayes' Theorem often offers slippery ground to the analyst appraising causal evidence. In practice, the analyst does better by putting a little sand in his tracks. He gets better mental traction in this case by making a direct judgment about the impact of the causal evidence on the comparative merits of his hypotheses. He says to himself: "If the odds were even-money in favor of the missile hypothesis before receipt of the causal evidence, what would the odds be now after receipt of this evidence?" When the prior odds are even-money (that is, 1/1), the revised odds equate to the likelihood ratio, according to the Bayesian equation R = PL. So, by making a direct judgment of revised odds following a stipulation of even-money prior odds, the analyst obtains an effective likelihood ratio to give the computer.

This is an approach which respects the mathematics of Bayes but does violence to the spirit of Bayes. One of the attractive features about Bayesian method in its pristine purity is that the analyst need address himself to the merits of the hypotheses only at the very beginning of his analysis. In principle, he does not thereafter reaffirm his first opinion, admit to a change in opinion, or criticize anybody else's opinion on the subject. He is supposed to make a judgment, instead, of quite another sort, a judgment about the evidence which postulates the truth of each hypothesis in turn, a judgment which does not involve him again in debate about the merits of each hypothesis. His encounters with causal evidence, however, often do not allow him to quite keep this detachment from the hypotheses. He finds himself addressing R, not L.

### Catch-All Hypotheses

Another problem area encountered in our research has been examined in Bayesian literature as the nonindependence issue. Nonindependence enters into analysis as a complicating feature when the likelihood ratio—the L value of an item of evidence—is affected by the previous pattern of evidence.

Nonindependence is an arcane subject to analysts who are new to probability mathematics, mainly perhaps because items of evidence which are independent if one hypothesis is assumed true can be nonindependent if another hypothesis is taken as true. Analysis is easier when items of evidence are independent (or to put it more properly, conditionally independent) —that is to say, when the likelihoods of their being received do depend on which hypothesis is assumed true but when these conditional likelihoods hold regardless of the previous pattern of evidence. Intelligence analysts have their way of reaching for conditional independence, whether or not they have ever heard of the nonindependence issue. They reach for a new hypothesis to do service for some hypothesis that no longer seems suitable as originally worded.

Such an unsuitable hypothesis could be the one postulating continuation of the status quo in the strategic warning problem. This catchall hypothesis can be divided into two or more subhypotheses (and it can be divided different ways into different sets of subhypotheses). For an illustrative example, take any case in history of a big power threatening its much smaller neighbor and finally invading the little country when threats alone did not avail.

Suppose the invasion is preceded by reports that the big power is moving its troops toward the border. Considered later in time from the vantage point of hindsight, the troop movements certainly would seem to be strong evidence, which ought to have tipped the odds substantially in favor of the invasion hypothesis. But the analyst of the day would probably find himself reflecting on at least two relevant subhypotheses of the no-invasion hypothesis. Subhypothesis A might be that the big power will not invade the little country but will apply very strong pressures—psychological, political, and other—just short of military invasion. Subhypothesis B might be that the big power will neither invade nor apply other extremes of pressure against the little country.

Now the analyst using Bayes' Theorem introduces an initial opinion about the hypotheses when he begins his analysis. He must similarly introduce an opinion about the subhypotheses if he comes to make them explicit elements in his analysis. By the time he receives the reports of troop movements, the previous evidence will have inclined him to the opinion that subhypothesis A—strong pressures against the little country—is the only reasonable interpretation of the no-invasion hypothesis. The events leading up to the troop movements (the grim warnings, the shrill propaganda, the military alerts) will constitute such virtual contradiction of subhypothesis B—no extremes of pressure—as to give it a near-zero probability. If this is the analyst's view, then the troop movements toward the border must seem almost as likely under the no-invasion hypothesis as under the invasion hypothesis. His L is just about $1/1$. His Bayesian approach has done virtually nothing to change his current odds.

This undiagnostic character of incoming evidence near the climax of international crises may seem novel to novices; it is familiar enough to experienced intelligence analysts. The more experienced they are, the more rueful they are likely to be in their recollections of evidence that was ambiguous to contemporaneous vision but became telling in retrospective inquiries.

## False Evidence

Perhaps the most difficult problem area is the suspect character of some evidence. The intelligence analyst gets his information in accounts from sources of varying reliability. He does not know for sure which accounts to believe and which to disbelieve. So he has to appraise his evidence, not only for its bearing on the hypotheses, but also for its probability of being accurate. The estimated probability of accuracy will enter into the analysis and will affect final results.

Unfortunately, an analyst's opinion about a report's probable accuracy or inaccuracy will be influenced by his current opinion about the hypotheses. Does he find it hard to give credence to reports from Cuban refugees who claim to have seen objects resembling medium-range missiles near Havana? If he is skeptical, it may well be because he finds it hard to give credence to the hypothesis that the USSR will do anything so foolish as to ship such missiles to Cuba. So once again, we have a case of information not doing the work which critics later, in all the wisdom of hindsight, will say it should have done.

## THE RESEARCH PROMISE

My exposition of these problem areas is not meant to imply that they muddle only the Bayesian approach; they plague with fine impartiality all types of intelligence analysis—traditional method as well as Bayesian method, verbal logic as well as mathematical logic. Traditional method also must cope with the eroding diagnostic value of past evidence as it recedes into history. Traditional method also finds it harder to draw probabilistic conclusions about the state of the world from causal evidence than from derivative evidence. Traditional method also sometimes explains away evidence that can be explained away by a favored subhypothesis of a catchall hypothesis. Traditional method also has to contend with the implausibility of evidence that is not in character with the climate of prevailing opinion.

My purpose in expanding on the problem areas is to show that much of the difficulty in intelligence analysis is not the difficulty to which the Bayesian approach is addressed. The Bayesian approach seeks to insulate analysis from frailties of logic in aggregating the evidence. The working world of intelligence, however, is concerned not only about possible inconsistency in everyday thinking between the conclusion drawn from the body of evidence considered as a whole and the conclusion that should logically follow from judgments about the evidence considered item by item. Intelligence looks with concern also at the possibilities of mistaken judgments about individual items of evidence. The intelligence pragmatist is wistful about evidence which almost speaks for itself, evidence to which most people will attribute much the same probability values because the values can be documented by, say, actuarial statistics or other such extrinsic authority. The pragmatist feels that an increase in the amount of this kind of evidence would do more to help men reach sound conclusions than could any formal logic—Bayesian or other—for reasoning from uncertain propositions about the evidence.

Conceding this point, the Bayesian responds that intelligence must still do the best it can with what it has. In a world of fallible judgments about evidence, the Bayesian approach is not a path to perfection; it can be at best only a path to improvement. The promise of the research on Bayesian method is a mathematical logic to which intelligence can have recourse for substantiating or contradicting the verbalizations of the traditional analysis. When the different approaches lead to discrepant conclusions, intelligence should perhaps undertake to rethink, recalculate, and if possible reconcile. The research interest at this time should be to find out whether such a Bayesian cross-check on other reasoning would significantly improve the quality of analysis.

Chapter 12

# THE TESTING OF CLINICAL JUDGMENT—AN EXPERIMENTAL COMPUTER BASED MEASUREMENT OF SEQUENTIAL PROBLEM-SOLVING ABILITY*

G. Octo Barnett
John B. Baillieul
Barbara B. Farquhar

A SIGNIFICANT PART OF the educational experience in the last two years of medical school and in internship/residency consists of an apprenticeship program aimed at helping the embryonic physician learn the skills of clinical judgment. This term "clinical judgment" has been used to describe a variety of cognitive processes and there is often disagreement as to both the definition of the term and the processes involved. Excellent and stimulating discussions of aspects of this problem are given by Feinstein[1] and Weed.[2] The classical definition of clinical judgment usually has a major component relating to the skills in diagnosis. In this sense clinical judgment is evaluated in terms of a skill in taxonomy, e.g. given a patient with a certain set of symptoms, signs, and laboratory data, classify this patient with a term which relates the particular patient to other patients with similar attributes. In reality this classification decision is only the terminal decision of the physician's problem-solving activity. Of equal importance is the selection of strategy used by the physician in his collection of information about the patient. Obviously it is neither feasible nor desirable to collect all possible historical information, to do all conceivable physical examinations, or to carry out all available laboratory tests. Because of circumstances of avail-

* This investigation was supported in part by grant HS–00240 from the National Center for Health Services Research and Development.

able time, possible hazard or inconvenience to the patient, and financial cost, the physician must select only the most appropriate subset of information to collect. Furthermore, this selection process is not a static decision, but a dynamic activity where each new item of information modifies the current hypothesis and therefore influences the judgment of what additional information would be most useful. This model of the diagnostic process has been developed in detail by Gorry [3] and has been shown to have practical applicability in certain areas of computer-assisted diagnosis.[4,5]

The typical medical school curriculum gives little emphasis to the teaching of any formal model of clinical problem-solving, and the testing of a student's ability is usually by subjective evaluation by his preceptor. As schematically illustrated in Fig. 12–1, this problem-solving task can be considered to have two components. The first is the ability to make the correct classification given the available information; one classification is the decision that more information is required to clarify the differential diagnosis. The second component of clinical judgment can be considered to be the ability to choose the most appropriate information item to seek; an information item may be a particular historical datum, a physical examination, or a particular laboratory test.

The testing of clinical ability can thus be defined as the measurement of the student's judgment in these two tasks. Clearly, such a measurement is limited in that many other aspects of clinical ability are ignored, e.g. it includes no recognition of the nonverbal communication aspects of history collection; it does not evaluate the manipulative features of the physical exam; it does not recognize the importance of the emotional commitment every good physician must have. Nevertheless, the cognitive aspects of clinical problem-solving are important in the educational process, and the apprenticeship philosophy of most clinical teaching has sufficient weaknesses that supplementation with a more formal technique may have some use.

It is the purpose of this chapter to describe one such technique which is based on a model of Bayesian sequential diagnosis. This technique allows not only the evaluation of a student's ability to

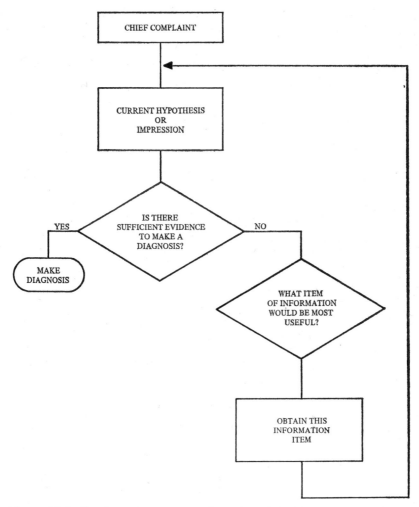

Figure 12–1. A schematic representation of an idealized clinical problem-solving activity. The student begins with the chief complaint and then collects information in an interactive fashion until he has sufficient data to justify making a diagnosis. In the computer-based examination, measurement of the examinee's performance is done at the two decision points indicated by the diamond-shaped boxes.

classify, but also of the student's ability to select the most appropriate strategy of information collection.

## METHODS

The testing of clinical judgment was carried out by having the user attempt to diagnose a "patient" through an interactive dialogue with a computer system. This interaction takes place at a typewriter-like device connected to an on-line, real-time computer.[6] The "patient" actually consists of a set of test results which are stored in the computer in numerical form. (Here we use the word "test" to include not only laboratory tests but also such things as questions asked in taking a history and physical examination findings. Results of tests are called *attributes*.) The student is told that the patient represents an individual who comes to an ambulatory clinic complaining of chest pain. For each case, the computer first presents the age, sex, and primary location of the pain. The student is given a vocabulary of tests that can be re-

```
THIS IS A 61 YEAR OLD MALE
WHO ENTERS WITH THE CHIEF COMPLAINT OF
CHEST PAIN LOCATED ON THE LEFT SIDE OF THE CHEST



SYM # = 7   PAINS FIRST STARTED : GREATER THAN 2 MONTHS AGO
SYM # = 5   NATURE OF THE PAIN : SQUEEZING
SYM # = 4   PAIN RADIATES : NO RADIATION

GIVEN THE DATA YOU HAVE THIS FAR, WHAT IS YOUR TENTATIVE
 IMPRESSION? WHAT DO YOU THINK IS THE MOST LIKELY
DIAGNOSIS #= 5 ANGINA

 OUTSTANDING,  JOHN



YOU MAY NOW COLLECT MORE INFORMATION IF YOU CHOOSE TO DO SO

SYM # = 21  RELATION OF PAIN TO EXERCISE : STARTS SOON AFTER BEGINNING
SYM # = 13  RELIEF OF PAIN BY NITROGLYCERIN : COMPLETELY
SYM # = DIAGNOSIS
DIAGNOSIS #= 5 ANGINA VERY GOOD

YOUR SCORE WAS 98
```

Figure 12–2. The examination is carried out through an interactive dialogue between the student and the computer, wherein the student selects a test (e.g. the presence of a particular symptom) by entering a vocabulary code. The computer immediately gives back the information for the patient under consideration. The student may make the diagnosis at any time by entering a "D." For purposes of illustration, the student's entries are underlined.

quested, and a list of diseases. He is told that the patient must have one and no more than one of these diseases.

As illustrated in Fig. 12–2, the student asks for one test item at a time by entering the appropriate code for the information item. The result for that patient is immediately retrieved from storage and reported by the computer. When the student feels that he has sufficient information to make a diagnosis, he enters a "D" and the computer requests the diagnosis number.

For purposes of evaluation of this technique, the computer program was used by 19 Harvard medical students who were on the medical service rotation in the summer of 1970 and by 11 members of the MGH medical house staff. Each examinee was given the same three cases of simulated patients with chest pain. The score that was assigned the examinee was a function of the "value" of each test selected and the correctness of each diagnosis. The purpose of the experiment was to determine whether this method of computer-based evaluation of clinical judgment could be demonstrated to have educational validity.

In order for the computer program to evaluate clinical judgment in quantitative terms, it is necessary to incorporate in the computer program an idealized analytical model of clinical problem solving. As previously indicated, any such model must have two components—a component which is a model of classification and a component which is a model of information gathering. These models will be intimately linked in the problem-solving situation. The classification model must always provide a *current view* (e.g. the differential diagnosis or "impression") of the patient under consideration based on the information the information gathering model has acquired. This current view will in turn be used by the information gathering component to decide what is the most useful item of information to acquire next.

For a given model of classification it is possible to have a number of different information gathering models. All such models will operate in essentially the same way, in that they will all attempt to "improve" the current view held by the classification model. A further degree of flexibility comes in the number of possible ways of defining what we mean by "improving" the current view. For example, one reasonable information gathering model is one which would attempt to confirm the diagnosis currently held most likely in the patient. Another form of an information gathering model would be one that attempted to "rule-out" the diagnosis which is currently held to be the second most likely.

Each examinee's "clinical judgment" was evaluated in terms of the closeness of match between his behavior in test selection and classification and the computer's behavior given the same clinical situation. The computer's behavior is determined by an idealized model of classification and idealized model of information gathering (or test selection).

The model of classification which we have chosen is a simple Bayesian one, the essence of which is the representation of the current view by a probability distribution:

$$p(D_1), P(D_2), \ldots \ldots, p(D_n)$$

where $p(D_j)$ is the probability of the patient having disease $D_j$. For example, a current view might be the impression that the diagnosis of angina is likely but not certain (expressed as odds, this could be stated that there is a four out of five chance that the patient has angina; expressed as a probability, this would be stated that the probability of angina is 0.8). In addition, one might believe that muscular-skeletal pain was still a fair possibility (expressed as odds, this could be stated as a one out of five chance; expressed as a probability statement, the probability of muscular-skeletal disease is 0.2). The current view expressed as a probability distribution is thus a listing of the diseases under consideration and their associated probabilities at each stage of the interaction.

As each new test is performed, there is new information, and these probabilities are changed in accordance with Bayes' Theorem. The Bayesian model was chosen because it has been widely used in computer-based medical diagnostic problems, and because it has a simple mathematical formulation and can be easily implemented in a computer program. We recognize the limitations of this technique (particularly the errors introduced by the assumption of independence of symptoms, the requirement that all diseases be represented and that the probability of each of the symptoms in each disease be known). However, these limitations do not appear to invalidate the use of the model in a teaching and testing program, particularly since no other model seems to be significantly superior and as easy to implement.

The choosing of a computer model for determining appropriate test selection behavior is more complicated. The purpose of the model is to allow the evaluation in quantitative terms of the student's information gathering activities. The computer must be able, at each point of the interaction, to assign a score or value to each possible test that could be asked (the value of test T may be represented as $V_T$). The critical issue is to choose the test selection model which assigns the most appropriate $V_T$. In order to make this selection it is necessary to decide what is the appropriate value for a given test at each point in the interaction. Different models may give different values for a test at a particular point in the interaction. The selection of the appropriate model requires clear-cut criteria as to what is desirable test selection behavior. We were unable to find any reference material on clinical judgment which would suggest that one model was superior; indeed the relative dearth of quantitative or even explicit discussion of clinical judgment make this type of education research very difficult. We have examined a number of different models for test selection. The particular model and the scoring procedure which we used are described briefly in the Appendix. In this model the examinee's score is a function of the strategy used in selection of tests; in addition the score is influenced by the student's performance in selecting the correct diagnosis as soon as sufficient information is accumulated.

We made the assumption that if a valid model were used in the computer program, then "good" clinicians would score higher than "bad" clinicians in a test situation. Although this form of circular reasoning seems quite acceptable in educational research, it requires that there be some absolute standard to discriminate "good" from "bad." Obviously there is no such absolute standard in medical education. We choose to use as a standard the ability of the test to discriminate between the medical student population and the medical house staff population. We made the assumption that the medical house staff had better "clinical judgment" since they had more years of training and experience. In these terms the ability of the computer-based examination to measure clinical ability was marginally significant. Three different test cases were given—one of angina, one of chest pain secondary to gastrointestinal disease, and one of chest pain due to muscular-skeletal disease. In all three cases the average score of the residents was higher than that for the students, but in only two of the cases was this difference significant at the p value of .1 (one tailed t-test significance).

## SUMMARY AND CONCLUSION

This technique of attempting to measure clinical judgment in an objective and uniform fashion seems to offer a promising approach. The usual method of evaluation of a student is to have his preceptor observe his performance in a clinical situation. The limitations of this preceptor evaluation are many; the most important being there is no precise definition of what is "good" clinical judgment and the fact that the subjective biases of the evaluator always enter in. The model we have described can be rigorously defined as to what is being measured and our means of measurement. Thus the act of measurement can be objective and reproducible.

The computer-based examination also has weaknesses. Of these, the most fundamental are the artificiality of the test situation and the attempt to isolate one part of the cognitive activity from all other aspects of clinical judgment. It will have to be demonstrated that a student's performance on such an examination adequately reflects his performance in actual patient care situations. In addition, the theories and models of clinical judgment that are to be used as standards are highly debatable. Students will choose to perform (or choose not to perform) a given test for a variety of reasons. The development of a strict mathematical model to quantitate the usefulness of the test has entailed oversimplification of the decision process. The decision as to when is the appropriate time to make a definitive diagnosis is based on a multitude of different factors in real life and the simulation of this decision point in a test situation neglects such issues as the possible presence of multiple diseases, the cost of a misdiagnosis (e.g. the cost of missing a treatable disease), and the social and economic implications of a diagnosis.

In conclusion, we feel that this approach of measuring clinical problem-solving ability using a computer-based simulation of a clinical situation has an exciting potential. Obviously this technique can never serve as the single method of measuring clinical judgment. However, it may be possible to develop the approach to the point where it does serve a useful function as an objective, unbiased, definable, reproducible technique of evaluation of one aspect of clinical problem-solving ability.

## REFERENCES

1. Feinstein, A. R.: *Clinical Judgment.* Baltimore, Williams & Wilkins Co., 1967.
2. Weed, L. L.: *Medical Records, Medical Education and Patient Care.* Cleveland, Press of Case Western Reserve University, 1969.
3. Gorry, G. A.: Modelling the diagnostic process. *J Med Educ, 45:*293–302, 1970.
4. Gorry, G. A. and Barnett, G. O.: Experience with a model of sequential diagnosis. *Comp Biomed Res, 1:*490–507, 1968.
5. Gorry, G. A. and Barnett, G. O.: Sequential diagnosis by computer. *JAMA, 205:*849–854, 1968.
6. Greenes, R. A., Pappalardo, A. N., Marble, C. W. and Barnett, G. O.: Design and implementation of a clinical data management system. *Comp Biomed Res, 2:*469–485, 1969.

## APPENDIX

Grading the computer-based examination is intimately linked to the underlying theoretical model of clinical problem solving. The classification component of this model is a simple Bayesian one in which the current view of the patient is given by the following probability distribution:

$$\{P(D_1), P(D_2), \ldots, P(D_n)\}$$

where $P(D_j)$ is the probability of the patient's having disease $D_j$. Here it is required that the following is true:

$$\sum_{j=1}^{n} P(D_j) = 1$$

which means that the list of diseases is exhaustive while the individual diseases are mutually exclusive. By means of Bayes' Theorem, the model updates its current view of the diagnosis for each new attribute as illustrated below.

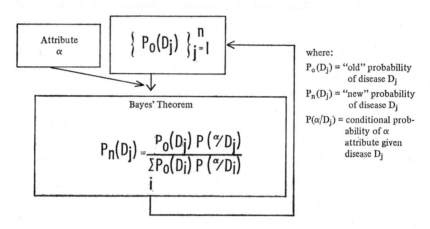

where:

$P_o(D_j)$ = "old" probability of disease $D_j$

$P_n(D_j)$ = "new" probability of disease $D_j$

$P(\alpha/D_j)$ = conditional probability of $\alpha$ attribute given disease $D_j$

The model's information gathering component is slightly more complicated. Its role is to assume a fixed strategy of test selection and use it to select that test to perform on the patient at each stage of the diagnosis which will be of greatest value in crystallizing the diagnosis. After considering a number of approaches to test selection strategy, we decided there are two factors which should be given weight in evaluating a test. First, the discriminating power of a test should in large measure determine its value. We take it as axiomatic that a test which will distinguish between two diseases $D_1$ and $D_2$ is more valuable than a test which does not discriminate. Besides discrimination, however, our model places value on a test for which a "positive" response supports the most likely diagnosis held in the current view. The definition of a "positive" response is arbitrary but relatively straightforward. Thus the test—"location of pain"—has no positive attributes; the tests—"Is the pain area sensitive to touch?" and "Has there been a recent injury to the chest?"—may have positive answers. These latter two tests are useful in confirming the diagnosis of muscular-skeletal disease as the cause of the chest pain.

In this light we consider the following two quantities in evaluating tests:

$$A(T) = \sum_{\substack{\text{all} \\ \text{attributes} \\ \alpha \text{ of test } T}} | P(\alpha/D_1) - P(\alpha/D_2) |$$

$$B(T) = \sum_{\substack{\alpha \text{ is a} \\ \text{positive} \\ \text{attribute}}} P(\alpha/D_1)$$

where $D_1$ and $D_2$ are respectively the first and second most likely diseases. $A(T)$ is a measure of how well test T distinguishes between the disease $D_1$ and $D_2$ while $B(T)$ indicates whether T is a good test to choose for the purpose of confirming the diagnosis $D_1$. A test T is by definition a good test if both $A(T)$ and $B(T)$ are large.

The following example illustrates how tests are selected: Suppose we are examining a patient who either has angina (call it $D_1$) or a muscular-skeletal disorder (call it $D_2$) with $D_1$ currently being considered the more likely. Consider the following three tests:

|  | $D_1$ | $D_2$ |
|---|---|---|
| T1: Does sour acid material come up into the patient's mouth? | | |
| 1. Yes | .05 | .05 |
| 2. No | .95 | .95 |
| | | |
| T2: What is the relation of the pain to exercise? | | |
| 1. Starts immediately after beginning | .10 | .30 |
| 2. Starts soon after beginning | .75 | .40 |
| 3. No relation to exercise | .15 | .30 |

T3: **Is the pain relieved by**
     **nitroglycerin?**

| | | |
|---|---|---|
| 1. Completely | .55 | .02 |
| 2. Partially | .10 | .05 |
| 3. No | .05 | .08 |
| 4. Patient doesn't know | .30 | .85 |

In these tables the decimal numerical entries represent conditional probabilities of the various attributes given the diseases. Observe the following:

$$A(T1) = 0 \qquad A(T2) = .70 \qquad A(T3) = 1.18$$
$$B(T1) = 0 \qquad B(T2) = .85 \qquad B(T3) = .65$$

where $B(T2)$ and $B(T3)$ are calculated by assuming the first two attributes in tests T2 and T3 are positive. T1 is clearly a useless test from every point of view. We have $B(T2) > B(T3)$ indicating that T2 is slightly more likely to result in a positive finding if $D_1$ is in fact present. $A(T3)$ is so much greater than $A(T2)$, however, that T3 must be considered the superior test.

Using this clinical problem solving model we have created an examination which grades individuals on the basis of how well they can mimic its performance. All examinees are given 100 initial points at the outset of each case. As they proceed through the case, selecting tests to perform on the simulated patient, they have points subtracted from their initial score for each test T for which the values of $A(T)$ and $B(T)$ are below a certain threshold. In addition, the student loses a large number of points if he chooses the incorrect diagnosis and a smaller number of points if he chooses the correct diagnosis at a point in time when the actual probability for that diagnosis is too low. In this situation the student has not accumulated sufficient information to justify the diagnosis and is penalized for guessing. Thus the final point total on each case reflects both the examinee's ability to select tests and his ability to arrive at a reasonable final evaluation of the results of these tests.

Chapter 13

# THE DIAGNOSTIC PROCESS VIEWED AS A DECISION PROBLEM

ALLEN S. GINSBERG

## INTRODUCTION

THERE ARE AT LEAST two fundamentally different ways to view the diagnostic process: as a classification problem or as a decision problem. The former views the physician's task as a two step process—the classification of the patient into one of many diagnostic categories and the subsequent decision as to the appropriate therapy for this category and this patient. Viewed as a decision problem, the physician's task is to "decide what to do." That is, he can perform one or more diagnostic tests, he can initiate any one of a number of courses of therapy, or he can simply do nothing and wait to see what develops. After the results of the first step become known, the physician may be faced with a new decision problem. Thus, the process is a sequential decision problem and in contrast to the first view there is no distinction, either in time or in kind, between diagnosis and treatment. In contrast to most of the work in this area, I will adopt the latter view.

Up to a point, both views are capable of yielding useful tools for the diagnostic process. Both of them can conveniently incorporate the uncertainty inherent in diagnostic testing via Bayesian techniques. However, when one wishes to consider the risks and costs in the diagnostic process, adoption of the latter view is extremely helpful and may even be a necessity.

This paper develops an approach to solving the *patient management* problem which relies heavily on the concepts of decision analysis.[1] *Patient Management* is defined here as the process of sequential decisions that must be made by a physician (or other medical workers) in determining the course of action to follow in treating a patient with a particular set of signs and symptoms, i.e. a syndrome.* Most of the possible courses of action open to the physician (e.g. he may perform diagnostic tests, administer therapies, or wait and do nothing) involve uncertainties and/or risks. He attempts to weigh these uncertainties and risks with the possibility of gaining information, the economic costs, and the likelihood of restoring the patient to normal health. Since in the vast majority of clinical encounters the starting point is some minimally described set of signs or symptoms, the problem of deciding what steps to take is of primary concern—even more than that of diagnosis (determining the patient's disease) or of selecting a treatment.

The proposed method relies heavily on the concepts of decision analysis and is *prescriptive* rather than *descriptive*. The present state of the art in decision analysis and in many aspects of clinical medicine appears to make such a procedure possible and workable. Further, many physicians have expressed the need for a patient-management decision-making tool.

## PROBLEM DEFINITION

Before presenting the proposed model and methods, we shall define explicitly which of the many problems faced by the physician will be addressed in this study. *Patient Management* includes both the problem of how to go about the diagnostic process and the interaction of this process with other decisions, such as when to start treatment. Thus, the problem addressed starts when a patient presents a syndrome to the physician. This syndrome may consist solely of patient-discovered symptoms; it may consist solely of a sign (or signs) found by a physician on a routine medical examination; or it may consist of some combination of signs and symptoms. The physician is now faced with a decision: What action should be performed right now? He can elect to take a com-

---

* A *sign* is a physician-discovered abnormality (e.g. a heart murmur); a *symptom* is discernible by persons with no medical training (e.g. pain, shortness of breath). The tern *syndrome* is often defined as a well-recognized set of signs and symptoms, but throughout this paper it is used to represent *any* set of signs and symptoms.

plete history and perform a physical examination, he can order one or more diagnostic tests, he can prescribe a course of treatment, or he can elect to do nothing and "wait to see what develops." After the initial decision is implemented, the problem may be solved—that is, the patient's signs and symptoms may disappear or the patient may die. If the former occurs, good medical practice may dictate that the physician follow up on the patient to make sure that he is truly cured or to properly manage a chronic disease, but his situation will not be directly addressed here. More frequently, the first step does not solve the problem, and the physician faces another decision with another set of alternative options (which may be the same as were available in the first stage) ; and this process may recur at the third, fourth, and subsequent stages.

The next question is, What factors does or should the physician take into account in making the decisions outlined above? Extensive discussions with physicians indicate that the following factors represent the major considerations encountered in actual clinical practice:

1. The risks of complications associated with a diagnostic test or a treatment, including the possibility of death.
2. The dollar costs of the tests and treatments.
3. The diagnostic value of a test, i.e. the amount of information the test will contribute toward identifying a specific disease entity (or a specific treatment action) .
4. Patient characteristics such as sex, age, economic status, and general health.
5. The possible spontaneous changes in the state of the patient following an action which requires a non-zero amount of time or when no action is taken (e.g. if the patient has a particular disease and no action is taken within a specified period, the patient may die) .
6. The patient's feelings about the desirability of the various possible outcomes, both medical and economic.

Other considerations, such as costs of malpractice suits, desire for teaching and/or research, and payment by third parties may also affect physician decisions. However, we choose to regard these as second-order considerations whose effects on the patient-management decision can be evaluated separately.

The final step in defining the patient-management problem is to identify the physician's objective(s) and determine how the above factors would be synthesized to achieve this objective. This would appear to require that we move completely from the descriptive to the prescriptive, since even if we could define a physician's objective and the way in which he synthesizes the factors, the differences among physicians are likely to be so great as to make any such statements of little use. Therefore, we propose that the patient-management problem can be addressed utilizing the concepts of decision analysis (variously known as decision theory or statistical decision theory), with the assumed objective of maximizing the expected utility of the actions taken to achieve the synthesis of the major factors. In its present form, the proposed methodology is suitable for use on an experimental basis; it has not yet been tried experimentally and thus is not ready for widespread use. Furthermore, it is not intended to replace the physician or to simulate his behavior. Rather, it is a prescriptive technique, intended to serve as a decision aid for the physician in the very complex problem of patient-management.

## A HYPOTHETICAL EXAMPLE

Decision analysis is a well-documented technique for solving decision problems under uncertainty. A number of books and articles have been published dealing with both the theoretical [2-5] and the applied [6-8] aspects of decision analysis; therefore we shall not attempt to expound on it here. There has been considerable debate in the literature over the assumptions in parts of this theory, over the basic utility axioms, and over some of the philosophies underlying its usage. In this study, we have subscribed to the axioms, assumptions, and philosophies espoused by Howard,[1] Raiffa,[5] Savage,[2] and Von Neumann and Morgenstern,[9] all of which seem to be in general agreement (except for the concept of subjective probability, which is not used by Von Neumann and Morgenstern). A rudimentary knowledge of probability theory [10,11] and of utility theory [2,9] should be sufficient for an understanding of what is to follow.[*]

---

[*] The concept of utility is explained briefly on p. 209.

A simplified, hypothetical example will be used to illustrate the main ideas of the approach used in this work. For clarity, the example ignores most of the practical problems encountered in a realistic patient-management problem; and it is stated in abstract terms in order to obviate consideration of medical questions.

The patient-management problem starts when the patient, exhibiting a particular syndrome, comes to the physician. This particular syndrome is indicative of a set of possible disease states, and a set of diagnostic tests are available that can provide information about the signs associated with these disease states. (For the present, a *disease state* may be thought of as being synonymous with *diseases*, as defined in common usage. A more rigorous definition will be given in the following section.)

### Acts and Outcomes: The Decision Tree

The decision process starts at the first decision, or stage. In this example, the $n^{th}$ *stage* is taken to be the point in time when the $n^{th}$ decision, in any sequence of decisions, is to be made; the choices at each stage are called *acts*; and the results from any act are referred to as *outcomes*. Fig. 13–1 shows the "decision tree" for the syndrome in question. The feasible alternative acts at the first stage of the decision process (the horizontal lines at the left of the tree) are as follows: *

- Perform test 1
- Treat disease state 1†
- Wait for 2 days
- Perform test 4

If test 1 is performed, one of three possible outcomes will result; for simplicity, only one path through the tree will be followed here. Test 1 requires two days for the results to become known, at the end of which time, stage 2 of the decision process for this path starts. The feasible acts at stage 2 for the outcome assumed in this example (outcome 2) are the following:

- Perform test 1 again

---

* The manner in which the possible disease states are determined, the tests enumerated and the feasible alternatives selected at each stage are discussed in the next section.

---

† It is assumed that there is a single best treatment course for each state.

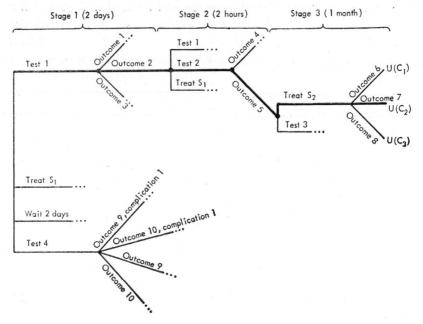

Figure 13–1. A hypothetical decision tree.

- Perform test 2
- Treat state 1

Test 2, the act implemented in this path, takes two hours and has two possible outcomes, denoted as 4 or 5. The result of outcome 5 leads to the alternatives at stage 3:

- Treat disease state 2
- Perform test 3

If state 2 is treated, then one month later, one of outcomes 6, 7, or 8 will be the final result of this path.

It is now possible to define a *consequence* as the set of events (acts and outcomes) along a particular path of the decision tree, where each of these events makes some contribution (usually negative) to the desirability of the path. For example, consequence 1, labeled $C_1$ in Fig. 13–1, consists at least of the costs of tests 1 and 2, the cost of the treatment for state 2, the resulting outcome 2 (e.g. cure, death, etc.), and the passage of two months' and two days' time, with, say, three weeks of this time spent in a hospital. As illustrated in the stage 1 application of test 4, a test result may also include a complication, such as an allergic reaction; this is shown in Fig. 13–1 by combining complication 1 with the two normal outcomes of test 4. This complication may be a direct result of performing the test, or it may arise naturally from the disease state of the patient during the time it requires to apply and interpret the test. It would form a part of the consequences of all paths emanating from the first two branches of test 4.

## Choosing a Strategy

The first step in choosing the best path (i.e. best strategy) — best in the sense of maximizing the expected utility—through the decision tree is to assign a number called the *utility* to each end consequence on the tree, this utility, $U(C_i)$, satisfies the usual axioms, or one of their equivalent variants, as stated by Savage,[2] and has the property that $U(C_i) > U(C_j)$ if and only if consequence i is preferred to consequence j. Thus, utility is a number that tells something about the relative preferences for things or outcomes, but it also has the important property that if the decision-maker is offered a "lottery" which gives him a chance of $C_i$ occurring with probability p, and $C_j$ with probability 1–p, then he will be indifferent between accepting this lottery and a sure consequence $C^*$ if and only if

$$U(C^*) = p \cdot U(C_i) + (1 - p) \cdot U(C_j)$$

The right-hand side of this equation is called the expected utility of the lottery. The decision-maker will prefer $C^*$ if and only if $U(C^*)$ is greater than this expected utility, and vice versa.

To illustrate how the probabilities of occurrence of the outcomes in the decision tree are calculated, devices called *nature's trees*[1] are displayed in Fig. 13–2. Each tree represents one of the three acts performed at each of the three stages in the completed path of the decision tree in Fig. 13–1. The first two branches on the first tree for test 1 in Fig. 13–2 represents the events that the patient is either in state 1 or state 2. The probabilities of these events, $p(S_1)$ and $p(S_2)$, called the prior probabilities, are a quantification of the physician's belief about the state of the patient, given the incidence of the states in the population, and the

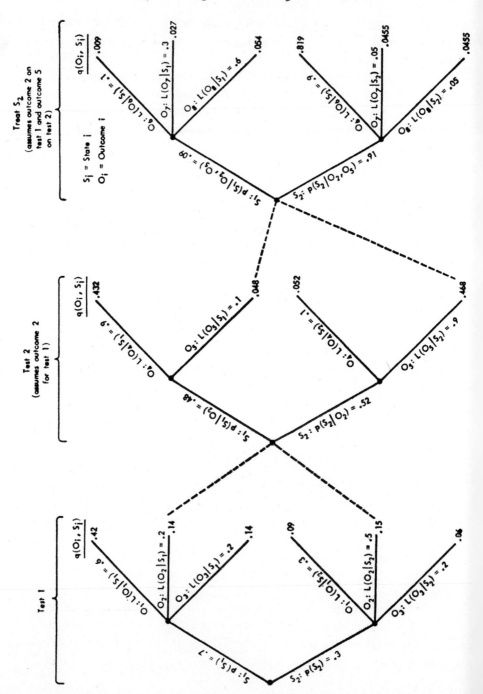

results of the history and physical examination of this patient.* The next two sets of three branches each represent the three possible outcomes of test 1. The probability of outcome i, given the patient is in state j, written $L(O_i/S_j)$ and herein referred to as a *likelihood*, is displayed on each of these branches. To be complete, we should talk of $L(O_{it}/S_j)$ where $O_{it}$ is the $i^{th}$ outcome on the $t^{th}$ test, but where no confusion will result, the test subscript will be omitted. Thus, in this example, there are two sets of likelihoods, one for each sate. Using the rules of conditional probability, we can compute the probability of outcome i by the following formula:

$$q(O_i) = \sum_{\text{all } j} p(j) \cdot L(O_i|S_j) \qquad \text{for all outcomes i} \qquad (1)$$

Here, $q(O_i)$ is referred to as the *preposterior distribution function*. To compute the posterior probabilities (the probabilities of the states given each outcome), we apply the discrete version of Bayes' rule:

$$P(S_j|O_i) = \frac{p(S_j) \cdot L(O_i|S_j)}{\sum\limits_{\text{all } j} p(S_j) \cdot L(O_i|S_j)} = \frac{p(S_j) \cdot L(O_i|S_j)}{q(O_i)} \qquad (2)$$

Referring to the probabilities displayed in Fig. 13–2, and using Equation 1, we see that the probability of outcome 2 occurring is as follows:

$$q(O_2) = p(S_1)L(O_2|S_1) + p(S_2)L(O_2|S_2) = .7 \times .2 + .3 \times .5 = .29$$

Therefore the new probabilities of the states, given outcome 2, are as follows:

$$P(S_1|O_2) = \frac{p(S_1) \cdot L(O_2|S_1)}{q(O_2)} = \frac{.14}{.29} = .48$$

and

$$P(S_2|O_2) = \frac{p(S_2) \cdot L(O_2|S_2)}{q(O_2)} = \frac{.15}{.29} = .52$$

---

* Methods for arriving at estimates of these probabilities are discussed in the next section.

These posterior probabilities now become the prior probabilities $p(S_1)$ and $p(S_2)$ for the second stage of decision, in which the alternatives test 1, test 2, and treatment $S_1$ are available (from Fig. 13–1). Similar calculations carried through for test 2 at the second stage and for treatment $S_2$ at the third stage yield the final outcome probabilities of $q(O_6) = .828$ (i.e. $.819 + .009$); $q(O_7) = .0725$; and $q(O_8) = .0995$. All of these calculations assume independent likelihood—for example, it was assumed that

$$L(O_4|S_1) = L(O_4|S_1, O_2) \tag{3}$$

i.e. the probabilities of the outcomes of the tests (or treatments) depend only on the state of the patient, and results from previous acts do not affect these probabilities. (This assumption is discussed in the next section and suggestions for relaxing it are given.)

Returning to the decision tree in Fig. 13–1, we can now assign expected utilities to the alternatives and choose the decisions at each stage which will maximize the expected utility. If $O_{i,k}$ represents the $i^{th}$ outcome of the $n^{th}$ alternative act $A_{n,k}$ at stage k, and $U(A_{n,k})$ is the utility of act $A_{n,k}$, then the expected utility of this act is defined as the following:

$$E[U(A_{n,k})] = \sum_{\text{all } i} q(O_{i,k})E[U(O_{i,k})] \tag{4}$$

where i ranges over all outcomes emanating from $A_{n,k}$, and

$$E[U(O_{i,k})] = \max_{\text{all } n} E[U(A_{n,k+1})] \tag{5}$$

where n ranges over all alternatives emanating from $O_{i,k}$. Also, if K is the last stage of decision on a particular path, then

$$E[U(O_{i,K})] = U(C_i) \tag{6}$$

Therefore, in order to compute the expected utilities of all alternative acts at each stage, we must start at the far right, or last stage, of each path and for each alternative at this stage assign utilities to the outcomes, according to Definition 6, compute the expected utility of the alternatives as in Equation 4, and assign an expected utility to the outcome preceding these alternatives, according to Equation 5.

The example in Fig. 13–1 will be used to illustrate this process. The sketch below represents the top branch of the decision tree of Fig. 13–1. The numbers in parentheses are arbitrarily assigned expected utilities which represent results of calculations on the parts of the branch not shown in the example.

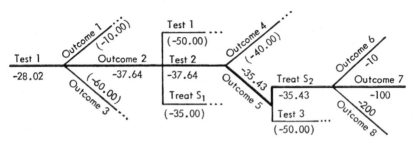

Assuming the utilities of consequences $C_1$, $C_2$, and $C_3$ are $-10$, $-100$, and $-200$, respectively, and using the probabilities calculated on the nature's trees, the expected utility of the action, treat $S_2$, can be computed as

$$U(\text{treat } S_2) = (.099 + .819)(-10) + (.027 + .0455)(-100) \\ + (.054 + .0455)(-200) = -35.43$$

Since $-35.43$ is greater than the $-50.00$ hypothetical expected utility of test 3, the expected utility of outcome 5 is assigned this value. The expected utility of test 2 is then computed as follows:

$$U(\text{test } 2) = (.432 + .052)(-40) + (.048 + .468)(-35.43) = -37.64$$

This result is greater than both of the expected utilities of test 1 and treat $S_1$, so it is assigned as the expected utility of outcome 2. The expected utility of test 1 is the following:

$$U(\text{test } 1) = (.42 + .09)(-10.00) + (.14 + .15)(-37.64) \\ + (.14 + .06)(-60) = -28.02$$

If we assume that this utility, $-28.02$, is greater than the expected utility of all other actions at stage 1, then one optimal strategy would be

1. Do test 1
2. If outcome 2 results, perform test 2
3. If outcome 5 results, treat $S_2$

In order to specify a complete decision strategy, similar calculations would have to be performed for all other paths in the decision tree. Because of the way in which the calculation proceeds, i.e. in a recursive manner from the last stage to the first stage, this process of evaluating the branches of the decision tree is referred to as *folding back* the tree.

## CONSTRUCTION OF THE GENERAL MODEL FOR A SYNDROME

This section describes the detailed steps and procedures required to build a decision model for a given patient syndrome. To provide an overview of the process, these steps are summarized below:

1. Define the syndrome.
2. Define all disease states and their
    a. Treatment of choice,
    b. Untreated time course and associated probabilities,
    c. Treated time course and associated probabilities.
3. List all relevant tests and their
    a. Time required,
    b. Costs, complications, and associated probabilities,
    c. Outcomes and associated likelihood probabilities.
4. Construct the decision tree:
    a. Choose the starting point,
    b. Prune the width,
    c. Limit the depth.
5. Construct the utility model:
    a. Define the components of a consequence,
    b. Postulate and test for special relationships among components,
    c. Define assessment procedures.

### Step 1: Define the Syndrome

Theoretically, any syndrome can serve as a starting point of a decision analysis. However, syndromes having certain characteristics tend to be more amenable to analysis or easier to fit into a general decision framework, or both. Some of these characteristics are the following: it must occur frequently enough in clinical practice to make the development of the decision model and data economically justifiable; it must have a relatively limited number of possible associated acts (of the order of magnitude of 50–100) in order to prevent the decision tree from becoming unmanageably large; it must present a challenging decision problem rather than having only one or two possible disease states; and relevant medical information relating to the associated disease states and diagnostic tests must be readily available.

### Step 2: List the Disease States

In order to construct a decision tree and perform the calculations described in the previous section, it is necessary to compile a list of disease states which could be associated with the syndrome. This, in turn, requires that the concept of a *state* be clearly defined. One natural definition is to postulate a one-to-one correspondence between states and a well-accepted taxonomy of diseases such as the *Standard Nomenclature of Diseases and Operations*.[12] However, for an action-oriented decision procedure intended to maximize expected utility, such as we are proposing, this definition is not workable—from the point of view of actions, it is nonoperational, and from the point of view of assigning utilities to outcomes, it is ambiguous. Both of these deficiencies occur because the categories delineated in most classifications of disease each may include different treatments, different prognoses, and different associated syndromes. To illustrate, consider three well-known disease categories: pneumonia, congestive heart failure, and lupus erythematosis. In pneumonia, the treatment, prognosis, and probabilities of test outcomes all depend on the causative organism; in congestive heart failure, treatment and prognosis depend on the cause of the failure; and in lupus erythematosis, treatment and prognosis depend on the presence of renal lesions. Thus, it is often impossible to associate a single state, so defined. The reverse of this might also occur—it may be unimportant to distinguish between two or more diseases with regard to actions taken or utilities.

Given these objections, it would seem natural to eliminate the intermediate step of mapping from signs and symptoms to diseases, and instead to define the states directly, i.e. define them in terms of constellations of signs and symptoms, rather than giving names to these constellations which may have differing implica-

tions for action and/or prognosis. Though this scheme elimi-
nates much ambiguity, it introduces other problems. The very
large number of possible combinations of signs and symptoms
(i.e. states) makes the task of associating states with treatment actions and prognoses extremely complex, involving many questions
of medical technology. Also, it is convenient to be able to describe
a patient's condition by a single term rather than by a long list
of signs and symptoms.

The classification scheme we have used involves repartitioning
existing disease categories such that all diseases in each new
category have three characteristics in common: (a) the likelihood
probabilities conditioned on the category for all tests, (b) the
treatment, and (c) the prognosis (both with and without treatment). We call these new categories *disease states*. For example,
some disease states associated with the syndrome of pleural
effusion would be pneumococcal or streptococcal pneumonia;
staphylococcal pneumonia; congestive heart failure/myocardial
infarction, and congestive failure due to other causes.

This definition of states gives rise to a very difficult practical
problem. It is possible for two or more related or unrelated disease
processes to be active concurrently in a single patient. For example, a patient may have bronchogenic carcinoma which causes
a pneumococcal pneumonia to develop (a related disease process);
or a patient with rheumatoid arthritis may also have pneumococcal pneumonia (an unrelated disease process). Theoretically,
the multiple-disease phenomenon can be allowed for by simply
allowing for combinations of the simple disease states in the
classification scheme (e.g. defining a state called bronchogenic
carcinoma-pneumococcal pneumonia). However, if all possible
combinations of simple disease states are to be considered, the
solution of the decision problem can become computationally intractable.* Therefore, the set of states to be considered in a given
problem must, at times, be limited in some manner. The problem

---

* If n is the number of simple disease states (i.e. associated with a single
process), then the total number of possible states is $N = \sum_{i=1}^{n} \binom{n}{i}$. If $n = 10$, $N = 1265$.

of selecting a subset from the totality of subsets is somewhat akin to a pattern-recognition problem, and since machines have thus far proved notoriously inadequate to deal with the latter,[13] it might be necessary to have the physician perform the selection, both in general (i.e. with no particular patient in mind) and considering a specific patient. This scheme would by no means be foolproof—the physician might inadvertently omit the one state which is the true state of the patient, and additionally, the selection could require too much of the physician's time.

It is suggested that the simplified method applied in Ginsberg [14] which assumes that only "single" disease states are possible, can handle most problems adequately. Some of the more frequent combinations of which one state causes the other, like bronchogenic carcinoma/pneumococcal pneumonia, are added as extra "single" states. This procedure will work in most cases, but it is of limited help to the doctor in deciding on a course of action for patients with several concurrent disease states. Even in such patients, however, decision analysis of some well-defined syndrome may lead to wise conclusions about the management of the case. Also, if the physician feels that multiple disease processes are operating, he may be able to modify the recommended strategies and/or the basic data of the analysis in accord with considerations introduced by the secondary processes. The procedure may also be used to identify test results that indicate a high probability of more than one disease being present. (This potential capability has not been tested as yet, however.)

After a complete list of disease states is compiled, additional information is required about each state. For simplicity, it can be assumed that a single treatment exists for each state. (Generalization to the case of multiple possible treatments is a straightforward process.) The time course for each disease state, both untreated and treated, must be specified—the time course being defined as changes in the state of the patient, including complications arising spontaneously from the disease state or resulting from the treatment. It is possible to treat time as a continuum, but doing so creates unwarranted computational difficulties. These difficulties are avoided, and little is lost, by breaking time into discrete intervals related to the rapidity with which complications typically arise in a given disease state. Thus for the state of acute myocardial infarction from a coronary occlusion, time should probably be quantized in units of hours early in the time course and in days and weeks in the later stages; the course of pneumococcal pneumonia could be described in terms of days and eventually weeks; and tuberculosis would undoubtedly be measured in weeks and months, because of both the slower development of complications (such as lung abscess) and the longer course of treatment. Though it does not appear that the results of the analysis will be particularly sensitive to definition of the lengths of the time intervals, some investigation of this aspect is undoubtedly desirable.

Since changes of state and occurrence of complications within a time interval are usually uncertain, the probabilities of these events must also be specified. The assigning of numerical probabilities to events is a difficult problem which is encountered in a number of places in the patient-management decision process. We shall not attempt to describe methods for making this assignment for each type of probability; methods applicable to all the probabilities encountered here will be described under *Step 3*. At this point, it is sufficient to state that these probabilities should reflect the decision-maker's beliefs and must have the usual properties of probabilities (i.e. $p_i \geqslant 0$; $\sum\limits_{\text{all } i} p_i = 1$).

### Step 3: List the Relevant Diagnostic Tests

A relevant diagnostic test is defined as one that is capable of detecting any of the signs that can occur in any of the disease states associated with the syndrome under study. For example, the ECG is a relevant test for the pleural-effusion syndrome, since it can detect left ventricular hypertrophy or a myocardial infarction, signs often associated with congestive heart failure, which can cause a pleural effusion. Of course, the ECG can also detect signs associated with other disease states such as pericarditis and myxedema.

A number of characteristics must be determined for each relevant test. The time required to perform the test and interpret the results must be known in order to establish the time scale for each decision path. Though it is theoretically possible to deal with a probability distribution of times, this refinement results in unwarranted computational complexity. Also there is no simple certainty equivalent, such as the mean time; however, a point estimate using some measure of central tendency appears adequate. One difficulty with stating a standard set of values for this time parameter, or any other parameter associated with diagnostic tests, is that the values are likely to vary from institution to institution and even from time to time within a given institution. (This and other problems of implementation are discussed in Ginsberg.[14])

The *real* cost of a test, as stated earlier, consists not only of the dollar cost but also of possible complications or side effects (e.g. death, hemorrhage, days of pain). The probabilities of these complications must be stated in the decision model. In most cases these probabilities are independent of the state of the patient, but where significant differences in the chances of complication exist that are dependent on the state of the patient, these probabilities can be treated as conditional on the state. These probabilities are often not dependent on patient characteristics such as age, sex, etc., but in cases where these characteristics have significant effects, the appropriate adjustments to the probabilities can be made by the physician using the model.

Most important, all the possible outcomes of each test must be listed. The form of these outcomes can be quite different for different types of tests. Tests that result in either a positive or a negative outcome, e.g. the acid-fast sputum smear, have the simplest form. Another class of outcome, still discrete, but more complex than a dichotomy, is that which indicates specific physiological abnormalities (e.g. outcomes of pleural or kidney biopsies). Listing the possible outcomes of such tests usually presents no difficulties, as the possibilities are discrete and finite in number.

Many medical diagnostic tests have outcomes that are measured along a continuous scale. Normally, continuous outcomes present no theoretical difficulties in a decision-analytic model, although they do pose some serious computational problems. However, for the present model it is necessary to have discrete outcomes, because the set of alternative acts at each state is not necessarily exhaustive but may rather be a subset of the set of all possible acts (see *Step 4*) ; the composition of a particular subset is a function of the outcomes that have occurred at the preceding states. Many continuous-outcome scales have already been partitioned by medical practice; for example, "normal values" or "normal ranges" have been established for some tests (i.e. a value below a certain level or within a certain range is said to be normal, and a value above or outside is abnormal). These divisions of the outcome scales are often unsatisfactory for a decision analysis because they may result in the loss of some information. For instance, a result just below the normal value or just outside the normal range may imply something about the patient's state different from that which is implied by a reading far from the normal values. It is not likely that an objective, repeatable procedure for partitioning test outcomes can be developed; however, an observation presented in Ginsberg [14] pp. 28–29, combined with expert medical judgment may enable an adequate job to be done.

To compute the probabilities of the outcomes for a given test, it is necessary to assign numerical values to the likelihood probabilities, $L(O_i/S_j)$, i.e. the probability of outcome i given the patient is in state j. Because of the way in which we have defined disease states, a questionable assumption is implicit in the notation $L(O_i/S_j)$. Since a patient who is in disease state $S_j$ may or may not exhibit a particular symptom or sign, $s_k$ (e.g. the sputum TB culture is not always positive in patients with proven TB), writing $L(O_i/S_j)$ assumes that the probabilities of the outcomes are conditionally independent of any symptom or sign the patient may be known to have. Likewise, other patient factors, such as current drug regimens, are not accounted for (e.g. in proven cases of TB, the probabilities of the outcomes of the TB skin test are grossly altered by the concomitant presence of steroid drugs). Fortunately, the assumption of conditional independence, or a close approximation thereof, is justified in most medical diagnostic tests, largely because the known existence of state $S_j$ usually provides most of the needed information regarding signs and thus outcomes. Even when this is not the case, conditional independence can hold if there exists no causal or statistical relationship, which appears to be the case for many of the tests and outcomes encountered in medical practice. Ginsberg [14] discusses approaches for dealing with cases where conditional independence clearly cannot be assumed.

One further assumption made here is that the likelihood probabilities are constant with respect to the elapsed time since the onset of symptoms. In many disease processes this is clearly an unrealistic assumption—certain signs and/or symptoms are known to appear early in the course of some diseases, while others do not appear until quite late. But given the difficulties involved in determining a patient's status in the course of the disease process, and the almost complete lack of medical knowledge of the time course of signs and symptoms in most diseases, the above assumption is hard to relax at this time. Again, we must rely on the physician's judgment and experience and allow him to set the likelihoods on the basis of his subjective evaluations of the situation.

The methods for quantifying probability distributions described in this section apply to all of the probabilities associated with this model. Broadly speaking, there are two classes of methodologies for quantification: objective and subjective. The objective (or empirical, or frequentistic) approach consists of using historical data to estimate the probabilities via a relative-frequency calculation. This approach, in spite of its "objective" view, however, has a number of serious drawbacks. First, in clinical medicine, the historical data required are simply not available for the vast majority of the probabilities and are not likely to be available in usable form for a long time. In addition, local variation—for example, in the likelihood probabilities—can be great enough to require extensive data collection and reduction efforts at individual institutions, or periodic large efforts within an institution. This problem, combined with the lack of available data for specific occurrences, makes it difficult to obtain sufficiently precise estimates (particularly in the case of nonindependent probabilities).

It seems likely that only a massive, tightly controlled data-collection effort can provide adequate, usable objective probabilities, and such an effort is not likely to receive the required support until the use of decision analysis in patient-management is widely accepted. At least for the present, therefore, it is necessary to use the subjective approach, i.e. subjective estimation of the probabilities, using expert judgment. The data can be expressed in any of several forms. The two most common modes are direct estimation, e.g. stating values for $L(O_i/S_j)$ such that the sum over all outcomes of these likelihoods is 1, or by some form of ratio such as the likelihood ratio, $L(O_i/S_j)/L(O_i/S_j')$. Edwards [15] has collected some evidence that the likelihood-ratio estimation is somewhat easier to understand and produces more accurate estimates of known probabilities. However, a difficulty arises when the conditon of likelihoods summing to 1 is imposed: Since the estimator sees only ratios, it is nearly impossible for him to juggle the ratios so that the sum of the likelihood probabilities (summed over i for each j) is unity. This difficulty can be overcome either by using sophisticated hardware techniques which aid the estimator in producing legitimate probability distributions, or by using only I · J–J of the ratio estimates and the constraint that the sum of the probabilities of the outcomes for each state is 1, in order to compute the probabilities. The ratios not used in the calculation can then be computed and presented to the estimator, who can perform an iterative adjustment until all the ratios reflect his beliefs and the probabilities sum to 1. Whichever method is used to elicit the probabilities, the resulting estimates reflect the beliefs of the decision-maker—the same beliefs he would, or at least should, use in making an unaided decision.

In practical use, the subjective approach may present a difficulty similar to that faced by the objective methods. In most cases of clinical patient management, the number of estimates required is so large as to preclude the supplying of a new set of probabilities for each case encountered. This implies that a set of "standard probabilities" must be used, with the attendant problems of variation from time to time, institution to institution, and physician to physician. However, there is some evidence that these variations are not as wide as those in other areas of decision-making. Ginsberg and Offensend [16] found extremely close agreement between two physicians on a large set of probabilities associated with a particular case. The only discernible differences were in their estimates of the prior probabilities of the disease states. A similar consistency between physicians is noted in the probabilities associated with the pleural-effusion example in Ginsberg.[14] Nevertheless, to allow for variation in subjective probabilities, the model is designed to allow the physician to change any of the standard probabilities that he feels are inappropriate. Further research in methods for assigning probability is needed, but careful use of subjective probability estimation combined with physician understanding of the concepts involved is at least a workable interim measure.

### Step 4: Construct the Decision Tree

The most difficult and time-consuming task in constructing a decision model is the construction of the decision tree, or the set of alternative acts and outcomes at each stage of decision. Theoretically, the decision tree follows immediately from *Steps 1 to 3*. The set of acts at stage 1 are perform diagnostic tests, either singly or in one of the possible combinations for the case being considered; apply any one of the treatments of choice; or wait and do nothing for any one of a number of discrete time periods. The outcomes of each of the acts are defined in *Steps 2* and *3*. The set of stage 2 acts subsequent to each of these outcomes is the same for all outcomes—namely, the same set of acts as at stage 1—and so on through stages 3, 4, etc. It is clear that unless there are very few possible disease states and diagnostic tests, the number of branches and paths in the tree quickly becomes too large to be practical. Another factor which can make the size of the tree intractable is the proliferation of stages; in many of the paths there is no natural termination point at which the decision problem can be considered completed. Thus there is a need to *prune* the theoretical tree both in width (i.e. the number of alternative acts at a stage) and in depth (i.e. the number of decision stages). To avoid the impossible task of constructing the entire theoretical tree and specifying the tremendous amounts of data required, this pruning must be accomplished prior to consideration of a specific patient. Thus no patient-specific data are available to aid in this process.*

---

* For example, if the patient is male, the possibility of ovarian tumor and all its associated tests could be pruned.

One possible alternative is to develop heuristic procedures for automatically pruning the tree. For example, the treatments and tests associated with disease states whose incidence in the population, given the syndrome, is below some cutoff point can be eliminated from the early stages. Or alternatively, those tests whose cost (in terms of money and possible complications) is above a given value can be eliminated in the early stages; or possibly some combination of probabilities and costs can be used. However, it is difficult to evaluate the efficacy of such schemes; and instances can almost always be found where they are particularly unworkable, mainly as a consequence of the inherent rigidity in even the most sophisticated heuristic rule.

However, a device does exist which has proven quite capable of recognizing alternatives that are clearly noncontenders at various stages of a sequential decision process, without the use of formal algorithms: the human mind. It does not take much medical training or experience to predict that a brain operation or a skull angiogram for a patient with headaches will be wholly unworthwhile at an early stage of the decision sequence. With training and experience, much more subtle judgments can also be correctly made, without the explicit use of probabilities or utility functions. This suggests that physicians, preferably expert in the area involved, should perform the initial pruning of the theoretical decision tree. From the limited experience gained in attempting to construct an illustrative decision tree for the pleural-effusion syndrome, we have concluded that a knowledgeable physician, teamed with a decision-analysis expert, can effectively prune the tree to a manageable size. The details of this process are discussed in Ginsberg,[14] in relation to the illustrative example. Here we shall state only the guiding principle under which the pruning is to be carried out: *At each stage, eliminate from consideration those acts whose expected utility, if computed, is highly likely to be less than the expected utility of alternative acts under consideration.*

The pruning process starts with the single set of alternatives at the first stage and can then either proceed along a particular path or be done stage by stage. The expected utilities are *not* computed;

they are only estimated in a very gross sense by the physician and decision analyst, taking into account such relevant factors as the incidences of the disease states in the given syndrome, the total costs of the acts, and the diagnostic worth of the tests (i.e. the test likelihoods). Eliminating an act at an early stage usually reduces the size of the tree more than does a later elimination. Thus, it is likely that pruning within the first few stages of the tree will be sufficient to reduce the tree to a manageable size.

A consideration which emphasizes the need for delimiting the action space is the time required to perform the various acts. The interval between the start and the outcome of many acts is sufficiently long that significant changes in the patient's condition can occur. For example, during the two days' time required to grow a sputum bacterial culture, the patient might spontaneously get well, he might die, or he might develop any of a number of complications, depending mainly on his true underlying disease state. Therefore, the act space in the model must include not only single actions, such as "grow bacterial culture," but also combinations of actions such as "grow bacterial and fungus cultures." Determining which combinations should be included in each set of acts at each stage of decision—a problem that would be clearly unmanageable if complete enumeration were attempted—is the other component of the *a priori* pruning process which must be performed by the physician. Here, at least one formally optimal rule and a number of reasonable heuristic rules can be stated. The formal rule is the obvious one that no acts need ever be combined with an act whose expected utility cannot change during the time required to perform the act. For example, the ECG can always stand alone, since it is reasonable to assume that no changes in the patient's condition will take place during the five or ten minutes it takes to administer and interpret the test. (As in the case of pruning simple acts, the details of the process for deciding when or when not to combine acts are discussed with the example in Ginsberg.[14])

So far, we have considered only the question of limiting the number of acts at each stage. A question which arises independently of considerations of tree size, but which affects both the width and depth of the tree is, where should the formal decision analysis start? The earliest possible point in the decision process at which the proposed methods could be brought into use is when the patient has presented a syndrome and no other information has been obtained. Instigation of the formal analysis at this early stage, however, implies that the act space must include the extremely large numbers of possible maneuvers in a physical examination and questions in a history-taking. If the routine history and physical (H&P) are omitted from the formal decision analysis, with the physician using his unaided judgment to perform them, both the width and depth of the decision tree are decreased substantially. Other economic and psychological considerations also reinforce the conclusion that omitting the H&P from the formal decision analysis at this time is justified. If the H&P are omitted from the formal decision analysis, it is necessary to formulate a way of explicitly incorporating the findings from them into the analysis. Bayes' rule affords a way in which to accomplish this. For example, each maneuver on the physical examination and each question on the history can be considered as a separate test. Given the likelihoods of these H&P tests, the prior probabilities of the disease states (i.e. the relative incidence in the general population), and the likelihoods of the syndrome given the states, we can compute the posterior probabilities of the disease states. Formally, if we let $L(O_{i,t_m}/S_j)$ be the probability of outcome i on test $t_m$, given the patient is in state j, $p(S_j)$ be the prior probability of state j, and $L(Y/S_j)$ be the likelihood of the syndrome Y given state j, and we assume the independence of all probabilities, then the posterior probabilities $p'(S_j)$ of the disease states are as follows:

$$p'(S_j) = P(S_j|Y,O_{i,t_1}, \ldots, O_{i,t_m}) =$$

$$K \cdot L(Y|S_j) \cdot p(S_j) \cdot L(O_{i,t_1}|S_j) \ldots L(O_{i,t_m}|S_j), \qquad (7)$$

where K is the normalizing constant. These $p'(S_j)$'s then become the starting state probabilities for the formal decision analysis. A similar, but more easily implemented approach is to consider all the maneuvers and questions as a single test, say $t^*$, obtain estimates of $L(\overline{O}_{i,t}*|S_j)$ where $\overline{O}_{i,t}*$ is the $i^{th}$ vector of all outcomes in

_not dealing w/ formulation of_
_= initial diagnostic hypoth_

t*, and compute the posterior probabilities as follows:

$$p'(S_j) = K \cdot p(S_j) \cdot L(\overline{O}_{1,t}*|S_j) \qquad (8)$$

This process can be carried out for the general problem, in the absence of any particular patient, in which case it would be necessary to estimate the likelihood distribution for all possible outcome vectors—a potentially gargantuan task. The alternative is to have the physician, after completing the H&P, estimate the likelihood probabilities for the specific outcome vector of that H&P; then Equation 8 yields the starting probability distribution for the analysis.

As stated previously, it is desirable from the standpoint of computation and data specification to limit the depth, or number of stages, of the decision process. Some of the paths on the decision tree are naturally self-limiting, in the sense that when one of a certain class of outcomes is encountered, there are no more decisions to make. Examples of end outcomes in this class are death and cure.* A path may also be terminated when a specific treatment is applied to a patient whose true disease state is the one for which the treatment is designed, but the patient neither dies nor is cured. This can occur, for instances, in the treatment of bronchogenic carcinoma, where the patient lives for only three or four years after start of treatment; however, the *decision process* is finished after the treatment is applied. If, in this example, the patient's true state is not bronchogenic carcinoma, the possible outcomes are generated by the untreated courses of the other disease states. This latter situation gives rise to the possibility of paths with an infinite, or at least a very large, number of stages. Numerous repetitions of the same diagnostic test also result in the same problem.

It appears that some simple heuristic rules combined with expert medical judgment and numerical sensitivity testing can help to resolve these questions. The objective of these approaches is to

---

* In some instances, it is difficult to say the patient has been "cured' 'in the full sense of the word. For example, the disease process may have caused sufficient damage by the time it is arrested that the return of the patient to his previous state of health is impossible. Thus, *cure* is used here to mean arresting the disease process.

make the size of the tree manageable and to minimize the effects on the resulting decision strategy of arbitrarily limiting the length of some paths. The details of these methods are discussed herein.

### Step 5: Define the Utility Structure

The computation of the maximum expected utility strategy requires that a real number, called the utility, be assigned to each end outcome, or consequence, of the decision tree.† As defined earlier a *consequence* is the set of events that occur on a particular path of the tree, where each event makes some contribution to the desirability of the path. A consequence can include the costs and outcomes of tests and treatments, and the natural progression of the disease process. The principal problem in assigning a utility to consequences arises from a characteristic common to many types of decision problems: The consequence consists of two or more attributes or variables which may not be commensurate and/ or independent. For example, suppose that, in the medical context, the events in all consequences can be described in terms of three variables: dollars spent, x; days in bed, y; and days of pain, z. The consequence C can then be represented as the following:

$$C = (x, y, z)$$

The task is to determine the decision-maker's utility function U which maps C into utility numbers possessing the properties described in the hypothetical example.

We speak of the *decision-maker's* utility function, because in a realistic usage of the decision aid proposed here, the utilities employed must principally reflect the preferences of the person responsible for the decisions—in most cases, the physician. To be sure, the utilities must also at times reflect the preferences of the patient, and in some cases possibly those of society. Rather than getting bogged down in the quite valid question of whose utilities should be used, it will be assumed for purposes of this discussion that the utility function is that of the physician, appropriately modified for the case being considered. Operationally, it is undoubtedly too time-consuming for each physician to completely

---

† Note that since the paths and consequences have one-to-one correspondence, we could also speak of assigning the utility to the path.

assess the U function for each patient. Therefore, it will probably prove desirable to provide a set of "standard" utilities with the model, arrived at by experts looking at typical cases; however, the using physician will be able to change those components of the U function which he considers incorrect or inappropriate for the particular patient he is managing.

The judgments required to assess the U function or to make changes in it are by no means easy ones. But they force an explicitness and a consistency which are to a large extent absent in the action choices that physicians currently make. In choosing a management plan (without analytic aids), the physician is in fact implicitly stating a utility function; the philosophy of decision analysis is to force the decision-maker to state the utility relationships explicitly. Some of the appeal of this scheme stems from the fact that it is easier to argue and agree, or agree to disagree, about the *utilities* than about the *choices of action,* because the utilities are but one of many considerations in the choice of action.

Ginsberg [14] discusses the approaches to the problem of multidimensional utility functions that might be used in this context drawing heavily on the work of Raiffa.[17] Two interrelated steps are required to produce one-dimensional utilities with the required properties: the translation of the components of a consequence into a single measure, and the conversion of this measure into a utility. Though it is theoretically possible to deal with dimensions which are not strictly additive, i.e. are not independent, the complexities introduced are great enough to encourage use of the assumption of simple additivity. This assumption can be approximated in practice by defining the components with the objective of independence in mind. The method recommended in Ginsberg [14] suggests defining the components of a consequence as follows:

1. *Out-of-pocket dollar costs*—all actual money spent along the path of the consequence, including costs of treating temporary complications and lost income, if any, from items 2, 3, 4, 6, and 10 below.
2. *Days in bed with no pain*—all days either at home or in a hospital with essentially no pain or discomfort,

3. *Days in bed with mild pain*—all days with moderate pain or discomfort requiring little or no sedation (e.g. headache, mild pleuritic or abdominal pains, mild respiratory distress not requiring artificial breathing assistance).

4. *Days in bed with severe pain*—all days with near continuous severe pain or discomfort requiring heavy sedation.

5. *Days to diagnosis or definite action*—days until the patient can be told, with some degree of certainty, what the problem is (assumed to be days until first treatment action is taken).

6. *Permanent complications*—events that persist for all or most of the patient's remaining life (e.g. loss of limb, blindness, paralysis, fibrothorax).

7. *Temporary complications*—events arising as a result of a test or treatment, or as a result of the disease process itself (e.g. hemorrhage from a pleural tap, drug reaction, meningitis). *Temporary* implies that the complication is either self-limiting or curable, though it may indirectly lead to a permanent complication or death.

8. *Short-term severe pain*—five or ten minutes of severe pain caused by a procedure such as a liver or kidney biopsy, pleural tap, etc.

9. *Long-term mild pain*—three or four days of mild pain with little or no loss of function (e.g. a necrotic ulcer resulting from a skin test, or the aftereffects of a liver biopsy).

10. *Days of restricted activity*—days during which the patient is unable to function at a normal level (e.g. due to shortness of breath, tiredness).

11. *Death*—painless death in periods ranging from one month to five years, with no pain or disability prior to death.

These components are defined so as to (a) provide a natural and understandable set of variables, (b) completely describe all events that affect the desirability of a consequence, and (c) attempt to create components having independence relationships that simplify the transformation of the multiattributed consequences to scalars. The success of the latter cannot, of course, be evaluated until extensive testing has been carried out.

Assuming utility independence of these components, the decision-maker can translate each of these components into a common scale. For reasons of simplicity and familiarity, it is suggested that the common scale be the first component, dollars. Thus the person whose utilities are to be used is asked, what is the most you would be willing to pay to avoid each of the components? (e.g. two days in bed without pain, four days in bed without pain, two days in bed with mild pain, etc.). By use of standard lottery comparison techniques, (see Raiffa [17]) the decision-maker's utility function for money can be determined and the desired utilities are thus achieved. Two exceptions to this procedure are temporary complications which are translated into appropriate amounts of the other components, and permanent complications for which a different approach is used. Since it may be difficult or even impossible to estimate directly tradeoffs for certain permanent complications, (e.g. loss of limb or sight) death, or pain, a lottery comparison method appears to be more appropriate for these determinations (see Reference 14 for details of the complete process).

### AN APPLICATION TO THE SYNDROME OF PLEURAL EFFUSION

To demonstrate the feasibility of the above approach to the patient management problem, the author, with the generous help of Dr. Glen Lillington, M.D., of the Palo Alto Medical Clinic, has applied these concepts to the pleural effusion sign,* the details of which are put forth in Ginsberg.[14] The model and data described therein are intended only to demonstrate the feasibility and desirability of the technique, and as a vehicle for experimentation, not to provide a ready-to-use clinical tool. The probability and utility data obtained do not represent a definitive set of numbers, they do, however, demonstrate that at least some physicians can and are willing to estimate the quantitites involved; provide a data base for future discussion, modification, and experimentation; and provide some evidence, albeit very scanty, that the differences among physicians' beliefs regarding the probabilistic data

---

* Pleural effusion is a collection of fluid in the space between the pleural surfaces (the double-walled lining of the lungs). It is a sign, *not* a disease.

are small enough that general agreement can be reached on most points.

Together the author and Dr. Lillington defined 43 disease states associated with pleural effusions, the untreated and treated time courses of the states (both short- and long-term in the latter case), the treatment costs (in dollars and days with pain), and the 54 relevant diagnostic tests and their times, costs, complications, and likelihood probabilities. The rules and principles used in constructing the decision tree are discussed, and a sample portion of the resulting tree is displayed. To demonstrate the utility estimation approach outlined above, four subjects, three physicians and a secretary, were presented with the direct estimation questions and lottery comparisons. In addition, one physician, Subject C, was asked to estimate the secretary's (Subject D) values, the results designated as Subject E. The principal observations from experimental data in Table 13–I are as follows:

1. Though the subjects found the decisions difficult, they were able to give answers for all situations except direct estimation of payments to avoid quadriplegia and death. Subject D, in fact, stated that she would be willing to sacrifice all current and future assets to avoid all events except chest scar and pain.

2. The payments on each of the events are at least of the same order of magnitude for all subjects and, in most cases, are only negligibly different. The exceptions to this are Subject D's extreme aversion to blindness and Subject C's estimates for Subject D. These payments were considerably below all others, mainly as a result of Subject C's belief that D would be more risk-preferring and of his low estimate of her financial state.

3. In the few reliability checks made in the lottery method, the subjects proved to be quite consistent (the sample correlation coefficient for three pairs of observations for each subject is .86).

4. The agreement between the lottery estimates and the direct estimates is amazingly close for all subjects. The individual sample correlations are $r_A = .997$, $r_B = .983$, $r_C = .998$, $r_E = .878$, and the overall correlation is .928. Considering the involved calculations necessary to translate the answers to the lottery choice situations into dollar amounts, and the large number of estimates the sub-

## TABLE 13-I
### DOLLAR TRADEOFFS FOR PERMANENT COMPLICATIONS, PAIN, AND DEATH

Maximum Payments (thousands of dollars)

| Event [a] | Subject A | | Subject B | | Subject C | | Subject D | | Subject E | |
|---|---|---|---|---|---|---|---|---|---|---|
| | Lottery | Direct | Lottery | Direct | Lottery | Direct | Lottery | Direct | Lottery | Direct |
| Chest scar | 0 | .020 | .075 | 0 | .150 | .100 | .050 | .200 | .050 | .100 |
| Short-term pain | .020 | .025 | .150 | .150 | .400 | .250 | .450 | .100 | .060 | .500 |
| Long-term pain | .020 | .025 | .150 | .150 | .300 | .250 | .100 | .050 | .100 | .750 |
| Loss of one hand | 10 | 10 | 22 | 25 | 16 | 10 | 57 | b | 5 | 10 |
| *Loss of one hand* | *14* | : | *17* | : | *6* | : | *52* | : | *12* | : |
| Loss of both hands | 53 | 60 | 45 | 50 | 40 | 38 | 67 | b | 11 | 25 |
| *Loss of both hands* | *50* | : | *135* | : | *48* | : | *65* | : | *9* | : |
| Loss of both arms | 58 | 75 | 139 | 175 | 64 | 65 | 80 | b | 12 | 50 |
| *Loss of both arms* | *61* | : | *161* | : | *75* | : | | : | *13* | : |
| Total blindness | 77 | 100 | 87 | 75 | 84 | 85 | 119 | b | 13 | 85 |
| Quadriplegia | 113 | b | 247 | b | 116 | 110 | 94 | b | 18 | b |
| Death in 5 years | 106 | b | 230 | b | 155 | b | 87 | b | 19 | b |
| Death in 3 years | 107 | b | 232 | b | 205 | b | 100 | b | 20 | b |
| Death in 1 year | 113 | b | 247 | b | 234 | b | 107 | b | 20 | b |
| Death in 6 months | 119 | b | 273 | b | 250 | b | 110 | b | 20 | b |
| Death in 3 months | 121 | b | 288 | b | 260 | b | 113 | b | 20 | b |
| Death in 2 months | 121 | b | 300 | b | 263 | b | 114 | b | 20 | b |
| Death in 1 month | 121 | b | 308 | b | 264 | b | 114 | b | 20 | b |
| Discounted net worth | | | | | | | | | | |
| @ 6% | 620 | | 602 | | 550 | | 115 | | 115 | |
| @ 10% | 424 | | 391 | | 377 | | 85 | | 85 | |

*Note:* [a] Events and values in italics are reliability checks.
[b] Subject unable to estimate.

jects were required to make, this agreement is indeed far better than was expected.

5. If discounted net worth (current assets plus the present value of all future income) is considered as a reasonable measure of the maximum anyone can pay for any consequence, the subjects' estimates appear reasonable; that is, they are all below the estimates of discounted net worth. A plausible hypothesis for the fact that Subjects A, B, and C were not willing to sacrifice their entire net worth in order to avoid death is that they were unwilling to strip their families of all assets. Subject D, who has no family to support, gave answers to the lottery choices which resulted in maximum payments almost exactly equal to her net worth discounted at 8 percent. It should be noted that none of the subjects were told their "estimated net worth" prior to the experiment, with one exception: Subject C's direct estimates were very high in relation to his lottery estimates and the numbers for all other subjects. When told his net worth (assumed for this experiment) and given the options of changing his direct estimates, he revised them considerably downwards.

6. Subject C's estimates of Subject D's payments are very much lower that what D was willing to pay, and Subject C was unable to anticipate her extreme aversion to blindness. These observations, if true in general, emphasize the need to develop better means for introducing the patient's preferences into the decision-making process, both in current practice and in developing and using decision aids such as the one proposed here. One possible way to accomplish this end might be to prepare a small number of standard sets of dollar tradeoffs based on a number of crucial independent variables, such as age, sex, current and future financial state, occupation, etc. The tradeoffs for a particular patient would then be selected on the basis of these variables, possibly modified to account for any major deviations from the hypothesized trade-offs implied by the patient himself, or because of special knowledge the physician may have regarding the case.

## IMPLEMENTATION

It seems reasonable to assume that some kind of man-computer interactive system will have to be developed before the techniques proposed here can be implemented in *clinical practice.* Such a system will be necessary for several reasons: (a) the physician will have to be presented with large amounts of information (e.g. the decision tree, probabilities, and utilities) ; (b) the physician will need to transmit large amounts of information (e.g. pruning the tree, prior probabilities, other probabilities, and utilities) ; and (c) large amounts of computations will need to be accomplished (e.g. computing probabilities and expected values and folding back the tree) . To demonstrate how these requirements arise, we shall describe one possible way in which the techniques could be implemented. The steps in this implementation are summarized below:

1. Prune dominated alternative acts (based on H&P and x-ray results) .
2. Supply state probabilities (based on H&P and x-ray results) .
3. Adjust probabilities where necessary (e.g. likelihoods, treatment outcomes) .
4. Adjust utility tradeoffs and assessment where necessary.
5. Compute strategies (fold back tree) .
6. Perform sensitivity tests (optional) .

First, the physician must perform the H&P.* Using the results of these, he interacts with the computer system to *supply* two kinds of information: (a) identification of alternative acts that are clearly dominated, and (b) estimates of the probabilities of the states in the case being considered, based on the H&P. The dominated acts are identified† and pruned to reduce the size of the decision tree and thereby reduce both the amount of data that must be verified and the volume of computation in subsequent steps. As in the pruning performed prior to applying the analysis to a particular patient, pruning only the act spaces at the first few stages will usually produce sufficient reduction. The state-proba-

---

* For the pleural-effusion syndrome, he must also perform and interpret the x-rays.

---

† For example, if the patient is male, the pelvic pneumogram used to detect an ovarian tumor is clearly dominated; or if the patient is a child of five, the tests associated with the signs of various malignant states (e.g. sputum or pleural-fluid cytology, bronchoscopy, etc.) are probably not reasonable contenders, particularly in the early stages.

bility estimates can be supplied directly or can be given as odds. Supplying this information for all possible states can be very time-consuming, but since many of the states can usually be ruled out with near certainty by the physician on the basis of the H&R, the following procedure appears adequate. Restrict the sum of the probabilities of the states that a physician wishes to consider explicitly to a number near 1.0 (say .90), then divide the remaining probability equally among the possible but unlikely states. This assures that even if the physician considers a state extremely unlikely, the computational process could still point to that state if the evidence so indicated.*

A complete set of the necessary probabilities are stored in the computer. Even though these probabilities have been determined as accurately as possible—by a consensus of expert judgment and/or from objective data—they cannot all be appropriate in all situations. For example, if the patient is under steroid therapy, the likelihood probabilities for the TB skin test must be adjusted; or if he is old and debilitated, it may be necessary to adjust the probabilities of the outcomes of treating the various states. To illustrate the influence of exogenous factors on likelihood, a list of conditions under which the test likelihoods would need to be adjusted and a physician's estimate of the direction and qualitative magnitude of the changes (i.e. small, medium, or large) for various tests are given in Ginsberg.[14]

The physician wishing to adjust the probabilities either has to name the particular probabilities or choose those to be changed from a list of all the probabilities. Since the former method requires intimate knowledge of the model and the latter will generally take too much time, some combination of the two modes may be appropriate. For instance, the computer could display all the tests and ask the physician which ones are likely to exhibit out-of-the-ordinary behavior because of some symptom, sign, or historical fact concerning the patient. It could then display those probabilities separately, and the physician could call for modifications. The same general pattern could be used for the other types

---

* Assigning a zero prior probability to a state will exclude it from consideration regardless of the evidence that may build up subsequently.

of probabilities as well. Undoubtedly, in the future, more sophisticated data bases and processing rules will enable the computer to make these adjustments automatically, using the input of the basic patient data.

Again, the physician cannot be expected to state explicitly all the tradeoffs and/or utility functions required for the analysis for each patient. But he is very likely to want to adjust any set of standard utilities that might be supplied with the model. One possible way to conserve the physician's time and yet allow him to reflect his and his patient's utilities adequately was described previously.

After the physician is satisfied that the probabilities and utilities accurately reflect his views, the computer computes the optimal strategies (*Step 5*) and displays the results. The physician can then elect to follow the strategies exactly as suggested; he can modify his choice at any particular stage, based on factors he feels were not accounted for in the model; or he can choose to ignore the suggested management plan completely.

If there is a question or doubt in the physician's mind regarding any of the probabilities and/or utility numbers used in the calculations, he can test the sensitivity of the computed strategies to changes in these data by indicating the changes he wishes to make, then returning to *Step 5*. This process constitutes *Step 6*.

This illustrative application emphasizes one important requirement of the computer system (hardware and software) to be used: *It must be capable of rapid and smooth interaction with the physicians who use it.* In *Steps 1, 3, 4,* and *5* the system must be able to present large amounts of information to the user in reasonably short periods of time, and in *Steps 1, 2, 3,* and *4* the user must be able to communicate somewhat smaller amounts of information to the computer system smoothly and rapidly. With carefully designed software, the newest currently available hardware (e.g. high-speed time-shared computers, remote electronic displays, light pens, tablets, high-speed printers, etc.) should be capable of accomplishing these tasks. The system, if properly planned, can accumulate vast amounts of data relative to construction of the decision tree and to the probabilities and utilities when it is in use; these data can, in turn, be used to improve the quality and efficiency of the decision system.

Though we have described the proposed methods as an aid to physicians, it is equally likely that they could also serve to augment the decision-making capability of other health workers. For example, the scope of responsibility of physician assistants could be widened if they had similar tools available. The physician assistants' decision trees might be different in character (i.e. they would contain numerous alternative acts suggesting referral to various physician specialists), but the basic principles would be unchanged.

## CONCLUSIONS

The analytical techniques developed in this study appear to be a potentially valuable aid to the physician in patient-management decision problems. This technique is unique, to the best of our knowledge, in that it includes all five of the following desirable characteristics of decision analysis:

1. *Use of probability theory to deal with uncertainty.* Uncertainty is inherent in the patient-management problem, and the rational way of dealing with uncertainty is through the use of probability theory. In the proposed method, probability theory is integrated with the other aspects of the problem in a simple and explicit manner.

2. *Use of utility theory to deal with personal values and preferences.* Personal values and preferences are also inherent in the patient-management problem, and a rational and widely accepted way of dealing with these is through the use of utility theory. In the proposed method, utility theory is also integrated with the other aspects of the problem in a simple and explicit manner.

3. *Explicit consideration of relevant factors.* The major considerations encountered in actual clinical practice (see p. 205) can all be explicitly taken into account with this technique.

4. *Flexibility.* Because of its relatively simple mathematical structure, the technique is quite flexible, allowing useful and practical modifications. A prime example of this is the use of expert judgment in prepruning the decision tree.

5. *Ease of understanding.* The natural formulation of the de-

cision problem, which is similar to the way in which many physicians view the problem, allows a quick and easy understanding of the technique.

These characteristics, combined with the fact that preliminary efforts to formulate the problem as a formal dynamic-programming model and as a control-theory model have been unsuccessful, support the conjecture that the methods proposed here are currently the most promising for the problem at hand.

It is generally acknowledged that the clinical patient-management problem is one of the most complex and important decision problems being faced today. In this study, we have attempted to bring together the technologies of medicine and quantitative decision-making to produce a tool that can aid men in making these decisions. Human judgment still plays an important role in this methodology, but the processing of the complex considerations and data has been reduced to an algorithmic procedure. Though in no sense can the procedures be said to produce the *best* decisions, they appear to be capable of suggesting decision strategies which are more consistent and, in most cases, better (in the sense of higher expected utility) than those obtained by any other methods in existence today. Deep research into the components of the proposed model or into other methods of aiding the decision-making process might produce a better tool, but in view of the immediacy of the needs, we feel that the proposed technique could be of great near-term value.

## REFERENCES

1. Howard, R.: The foundations of decision analysis. *IEEE Trans Systems Science and Cybernetics, SSC–4:* September 1968.
2. Savage, L. J.: *The Foundations of Statistics,* New York, John Wiley & Sons, 1950.
3. Chernoff, H., and Moses, L.: *Elementary Decision Theory.* New York, John Wiley & Sons, 1959.
4. Pratt, J. W., Raiffa, H. and Schlaifer, R.: *Introduction to Statistical Decision Theory,* Preliminary Edition. New York, McGraw-Hill Book Company, 1965.
5. Raiffa, H.: *Decision Analysis.* Reading, Massachusetts, Addison-Wesley Co., 1968.
6. Edwards, W.: *Bibliography: Decision Making.* University of Michigan, Ann Arbor, Engineering Psychology Laboratories, 1966.

7. Edwards, W. and Tversky, A. (Eds.) : *Decision Making.* Baltimore, Maryland, Penguin Books, Inc., 1967.

8. Schlaifer, R.: *Analysis of Decisions Under Uncertainty.* Preliminary Edition. New York, McGraw-Hill Book Company, 1967.

9. Von Neumann, J. and Morgenstern, O.: *Theory of Games and Economic Behavior,* 2d ed., Princeton University Press, 1947.

10. Hadley, G.: *Introduction to Probability Theory and Statistical Decision Theory.* San Francisco, Holden-Day, 1967.

11. Feller, W.: *An Introduction to Probability Theory and Its Applications,* Vol. 1. New York, John Wiley & Sons, 1957.

12. Thompson, E. T. and Hayden, A. C. (Eds.) : *Standard Nomenclature of Diseases and Operations,* American Medical Association. 5th ed. New York, McGraw-Hill Book Company, 1961.

13. Dreyfus, Hubert: *Alchemy and Artificial Intelligence.* The Rand Corporation, P–3244, December 1965.

14. Ginsberg, A. S.: *Decision Analysis in Clinical Patient Management With An Application to the Pleural Effusion Syndrome.* The Rand Corporation, R–751–RC/NLM, July 1971.

15. Edwards, Ward: *Nonconservative Probabilities Information Processing Systems.* Technical Documentary Report No. ESD–TR–66–404, Air Force Systems Command, Hanscom Field, Bedford, Massachusetts, December 1966.

16. Ginsberg, Allen and Offensend, Fred: An application of decision theory to a medical diagnosis-treatment problem. *IEEE Trans Systems Science and Cybernetics. SSC–4:* September 1968.

17. Raiffa, Howard: *Preferences for Multi-Attributed Alternatives.* The Rand Corporation, RM–5868–DOT/RC, April 1969.

## Chapter 14

# SOME APPROACHES TO COMPUTERIZED MEDICAL DIAGNOSIS

T. Allan Pryor
Homer R. Warner

T HE CLASSIFICATION OF A patient into a disease category having therapeutic and prognostic usefulness may be viewed as a stepwise procedure. One step represents the reduction of raw data into a set of parameters. A second step might deduce from these parameters a classification of these test values (i.e. ECG waveform), and a final step arrive at a diagnosis from the set of test classifications. As an example of steps 1 and 2, we will present a discussion of some approaches to ECG classification. Step 3 will be illustrated by examples of patient diagnosis using both binary and distributed information.

During the past six years, four methods of classifying electrocardiograms using the computer have been tried at the Latter-day Saints Hospital. In each case, a modified Frank lead system was used to generate an X, Y, Z lead. The first method used Markov sequences. The present state of the sequence was defined as the last N sampled points of a waveform. From this state the next state or M points on the waveform was predicted. The sequences were constructed by sampling waveforms from known classifications and generating frequency distributions for the changes from one state to the next. With this information the final predictive matrices for each category could be generated. The number of possible states is $l^{dn}$, where l is the number of values each point may assume and d is the dimension of the waveform and n is the number of points back in time (Fig. 14–1). Two waveforms were used. The first was the spacial velocity generated by the X, Y, and Z values, i.e. $S.V. = \sqrt{\dot{x}^2 + \dot{y}^2 + \dot{Z}^2}$. In this case d is equal to 1. Hence, the

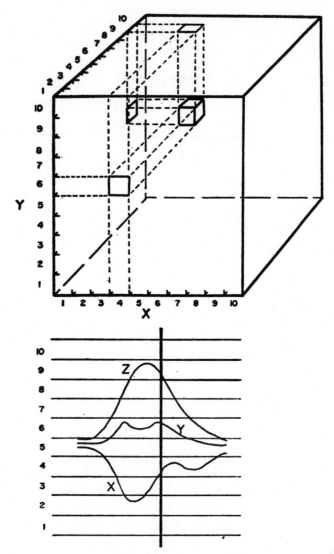

Figure 14–1. Three dimensional histogram for ECG interpretation.

state matrix could contain several points back in time and fit within available computer memory. In the second application of the predictive histogram the actual sampled X, Y and Z values were used. Here, d is equal to 3 and the values of X, Y and Z were digitized into only 10 possible values. With just one point backward in time, the matrix size is 1000 cells and for two points backwards in time, the size of the matrix increases to one million cells. Reductions, however, could be made in the size of the matrix since the values at any one point cannot vary over the complete range of values due to the continuous nature of the waveform. None the less, the problem remains the same, that is, the size of the matrices. To classify a waveform, the points of the waveform were successively used to predict a point on a theoretical curve. This was done using the state information from each of the matrices of known classification. The theoretical curves could then be correlated against the actual to determine the class in which the unknown belonged. The major problem with this technique results from the size of the matrices necessary to store the state information. That is, if the number of points backwards in time was small, say one point, then the changes predicted were only local changes with time. This caused the generation of similar waveforms from each state matrix giving no discrimination between the classes. If more points back in time were used the size of the matrices and time for computation became excessive.

The second method continued the use of histograms. However, in this case, rather than being predictive histograms, they were in fact three-dimensional amplitude histograms. Again the known waveforms were sampled and each sample in time was used to develop the histogram for that class. To diagnose a waveform it was sampled, a histogram generated from this waveform and this histogram was correlated against the various class histograms. A probability was assigned to each class by the following equation:

$$P_i = \frac{C_i}{\Sigma C_j} \tag{1}$$

$C_j$ is the correlation of the unknown histogram to that of the j in class. A wide variety of wave shapes in one class resulted in a smoothing of the histogram. Hence, if all possible shapes from one classification were included in the generation of a single histogram the resulting histogram would correlate equally well against any unknown waveform. As a result, a method of adaptive generation of the histogram was tried. Here, as new cases were considered, a correlation against its histogram and the known histograms were determined. If the correlation was greater than .80 the new waveform was added into the histogram of that particular class. Unfortunately, this criteria resulted in the generation of an arbitrarily large number of different classifications and histograms.

At this point the histogram technique was dropped and linear discriminant analysis was tried. The program used was the standard Bi-Med discriminant analysis program contained in the Bi-Med program series. This program performed the ECG classification from a set of parameters measured from specific components of the sampled ECG waveforms. Thus, for the first time in the project it became necessary to derive parameters from the original data before proceeding to step 2 as defined in the introduction.

With this program the question, of course, arises of which parameters are most significant in discriminating among the various classifications. Again, variations within the classes presented a problem. Since many of the original parameters did not discriminate between certain classes, they tended to lessen the discrimination among the classes. A technique of weighting various parameters under certain classifications was considered. This, in fact, results precisely in the tree logic which is presently being used. Statistics were generated on the parameters from the discriminant function program to determine individually their discriminatory value among the classes. With this information available it was then possible to develop the present program which follows a tree structured diagnostic logic where the waveform is checked against certain parameters, and if the test is positive the waveform is classified into that category, and if not, a new category is checked by looking only at those parameters important to that particular classification. This program is being used routinely on approximately 50 patients per day at two hospitals in Salt Lake City, and represents one source of input data for a more general diagnostic program (step 3).[1] Table 14–I gives the results of a study using the program.

The original work in medical diagnosis done here was in 1961 and applied Bayes' Theorem to the diagnosis of congenital heart

TABLE 14–I

RESULTS OF COMPUTER ANALYSIS OF ELECTROCARDIOGRAM

| | *N* | *AI* | *II* | *LI* | *LVH* | *RVH* | *LBBB* | *RBBB* |
|---|---|---|---|---|---|---|---|---|
| *N* | 58 | 1 | | | | | | 2 |
| *AI* | | 20 | | | | | | |
| *II* | 1 | | 7 | | | | | |
| *LI* | | | | 2 | | | | |
| *LVH* | 1 | 1 | | | 6 | | | |
| *RVH* | | | | | | 1 | | |
| *LBBB* | | | | | | | 5 | |
| *RBBB* | | | | | | | | 4 |

disease.[2,3] Thirty-three diseases were considered and 50 symptoms. Equation 2 gives the form of Bayes' Theorem used.

$$P_{D_i \, s_1 s_2 - s_i} = \frac{P_{D_i} \cdot \prod\limits_{j=1}^{n} P_{s_j | D_i}}{\sum\limits_{k=1}^{e} P_{D_k} \cdot \prod\limits_{j=1}^{n} P_{s_j | D_k}} \qquad (2)$$

This form of the equation assumes that the symptoms are independent within a given patient; that is, if a patient has symptom 1 he is no more likely to have symptom 2 than if he did not have symptom 1. The equation also assumes that the patient will have one and only one of the diseases in the set. This means that any possible combinations of the diseases that can occur in a single patient must be included as a separate disease. In spite of the fact that many of the symptoms indeed are independent, the method still proves useful since one of two courses can be taken. First, if the two symptoms prove to be highly dependent upon another they may be included as a single symptom. For instance, cyanosis and clubbing of the fingers occur together almost invariably if the cyanosis is severe. Thus, these two symptoms can be made one under the term "severe cyanosis." On the other hand, if the dependence is not a strong one, it may be better to include two not quite independent symptoms as though they were independent, since the amount of information contributed by each is significantly greater than the loss of information incurred if one of the symptoms is ignored. This can be tested empirically by examining the diagnostic performance of the system with and without the symptom in question.

A program was developed which allowed this system to be run from a time-shared computer station at which the symptoms were entered in response to a series of lists of symptoms on the oscilloscope. The physician simply presses the appropriate keys at the console to indicate which of the symptoms presented were actually present in the patient under examination. Those attributes were then used in making the diagnosis. The ability of this computer program to complete the logical process and arrive at the correct diagnosis was tested against the physician who collected the initital data; thus both physician and computer used exactly the same data upon which to make their deductions. The physician was asked to enter his differential diagnosis on the back of the entry data sheet and list by each entry a probability. A system for scoring the physician's performance against the computer was derived using the product of two terms. The first term represents the fraction of times that the computer or physician gave the patient the correct diagnosis with a probability of at least 1 percent. The second term reflects his confidence in the correct diagnosis when he made it and consists of the probability that he assigned to the correct diagnosis. In over 200 cases diagnosed by both physician and computer, the computer program clearly performed better than the physician in all cases except one doctor who was an experienced pediatric cardiologist. He and the computer performed equally well from the same information.

In 1966 another approach to the diagnosis of congenital heart disease was tried in fulfillment of a master of science degree in the Computer Science Department of the University of Utah.[4] This approach used discriminant functions derived from the assumption of multivariant normal distribution of the symptoms. The discriminant functions are given by the following equation:

$$g_i(x) = C_i - \tfrac{1}{2}(X\text{-}M_i)^t \, \Sigma^{-1}(X\text{-}M_i) \quad i=1,\ldots R \qquad (3)$$

where

$$C_i = \log p(i) - \tfrac{1}{2}\log|\Sigma_i| \qquad (4)$$

This function defines the disease which maximizes $g_i(x)$ as the most probable disease that these symptoms represent. The use of this equation requires the generation of the covariant matrix $(\Sigma_i)$ and the mean matrix $(M_i)$ for each disease. These matrices are generated using selected cases of known diseases. In the test which was run, 508 cases were available. Three hundred of these were used as learning observations to generate the covariant and mean matrices for each disease. In those diseases where there were less than 20 cases, the same observations were used over again until at least eight observations were available for each disease considered. Of the 33 diseases which were to be considered, only 28 had any data available. Table 14–II shows a comparison on selected diseases between the multivariate program and the Bayesian diagnostic program. As can be seen from the table there were in some instances improvements using the multivariate analysis, and in some instances the results were not as good. Ex-

TABLE 14–II
COMPARISON OF BAYES' PROGRAM VS MULTIVARIATE PROGRAM
(BINARY SYMPTOMS)

| Disease | Number of Cases | Number Correct (MULTI) | Number Correct (BAYES) | Improvement in % of Correct Cases |
|---|---|---|---|---|
| Normal | 93 | 68 | 70 | 1 |
| Atrial Septal Defect | 85 | 57 | 65 | −1 |
| Atrio-ventricular Communis | 18 | 15 | 14 | 5 |
| Pulmonary Stenosis Gradiant < 40 mm Hg | 34 | 5 | 11 | −12 |

amining the overall performance of the program, the multi-variate program gave the correct diagnosis 80 percent of the time and Bayesian program 60 percent. Whether this indicates a significant improvement is questionable. It is true, however, that the multivariate program as it presently stands is certainly no worse than the Bayesian approach, the major disadvantage being in the time required to perform the analysis. Since no significant improvement in the majority of diseases were shown using this method, the techniques here have not been continued on this application. This decision is based primarily on the simplicity of the Bayesian approach, the amount of data to be stored and updated in the case of the multivariate analysis and the time required to perform the analysis. The time necessary for one diagnosis of the multivariate is two minutes, whereas for the Bayesian equation the time was in the order of milliseconds. Thus, the Bayesian approach has the advantage of easy implementation as an on-line program than can be run from any terminal on the system.

Since the majority of information available to the physiologist or physician comes not in terms of discrete data as used in the congenital heart diagnosis program, but in terms of continuous data, it was necessary to develop a technique for including within any diagnostic program data of a continuous nature. Examples of this might be pressures within a heart chamber in determining acquired heart disease, volume of packed red cells in determining polycythemic states, etc. A technique has been developed for combining both discrete and continuous data in a Bayesian approach to diagnosis. In order to do this, data from each symptom in a given disease was fit to probability density function. In particular, a lag normal distribution was used as the most simple distribution which fit the continuous data. This distribution was originally studied on an analog computer to describe the distribution of transit time of dye particles in the circulation. The function was generated by taking a normal density curve and running the output through a first order lag circuit. The equation of the lag normal curve is as follows:

$$g(x) = f(x) - \tau g'(x) \quad \text{where } f(x) = \frac{1}{\sqrt{2\pi}} e^{-(x-\mu)^2/2\sigma^2} \tag{5}$$

This equation can be shown to be a density function under the condition that tau be positive. With this restriction, only curves which are skewed to the left are generated. However, in practice a transformation may be applied to the original data before attempting to fit the data to this curve if the data is skewed to the right. This is done by inverting the curve about its mean value, i.e. subtracting each value from twice the mean value. This equation also has the property that the mean is equal to $\mu+\tau$ where $\mu$ is the mean of the normal density function in the equation. The variance of the curve is equal to $\sigma^2+\tau^2$ where again $\sigma^2$ is a variance of the normal density function. The data which has been collected for a particular symptom in a given disease is fit to a particular lag normal distribution with $\mu$, $\sigma$, $\tau$, being determined for that fit. These values are then stored as part of the a priori probability matrix to be used subsequently in the conditional probability calculations. This is done for each symptom in each disease under consideration. Fig. 14–2 shows a fit of a symptom.

For a given diagnosis then, an actual probability for that symp-

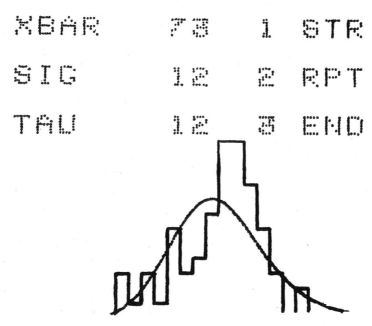

Figure 14–2. Fit of a lag normal curve to a histogram.

tom (test value) given a particular disease is calculated from the stored parameters for the symptoms and diseases. This is done by integrating under the theoretical distribution curve about the measured value of the symptom. Since for each symptom and for each disease there is a probability curve, the probability of finding any particular symptom (test) value in any disease can be determined. This term is then the $P_s/_{(o)}$ for that symptom used in the Bayesian formula.

The first application of this program was in 1967 for diagnosis of rheumatic heart disease.[5] In this instance, six disease categories were considered. They were normal, mitral insufficiency, mitral stenosis, mitral insufficiency and mitral stenosis, aortic insufficiency, and finally, aortic stenosis. The symptoms considered were pulmonary artery mean pressure, pulmonary artery wedge mean pressure, change in pulmonary artery mean pressure from rest to exercise, total pulmonary resistance and fractional change in cardiac output from rest to exercise. The data values of 171 patients were used to determine the lag normal distributions for each of the symptoms and disease patterns. An attempt was made by the program to diagnose diseases of the left heart chambers when only data from the right heart were measured. This was done to determine if these diseases could be diagnosed using only the right heart data, thus eliminating the necessity of the left heart study when these defects were suspected. However, it was found that aortic stenosis and aortic insufficiency could not be differentiated from the right heart symptoms chosen for the study. There was also a problem in the diagnosis of the mitral insufficiency and mitral stenosis. The patients diagnosed by the cardiologists who had one of the defects were often diagnosed by the program to have both defects. Even though some of the results of this study were discouraging, they did point out the possible effectiveness of the technique as a tool for medical diagnosis.

A second application of this program proved to be highly successful. This application diagnosed polycythemic states using hematological findings on patients.[6] It should be noted here that in the case of normal individuals the normal distribution curve ($\tau = 0$) was the most accurate in fitting the data, whereas in those having polycythemia rubra vera, the lag normal distribution curve

TABLE 14–III

COMPARISON OF PERFORMANCE OF PROGRAM WITH HEMATOLOGISTS
AND GENERAL PRACTIONERS ON 103 CASES WITH
POLYCYTHEMIA RUBRA VERA OR NORMAL

|  | *Correct* | *False Positive* | *False Negative* |
|---|---|---|---|
| Program | 95 | 2 | 3 |
| Hematologists | 76 | 2 | 22 |
| General Practioners | 65 | 1 | 34 |

was the best fit. Table 14–III shows the results of this study on
103 cases with polycythemia rubra vera or normal. As seen from
the table, the program was able to diagnose 95 of the cases correctly where experienced hematologists correctly diagnosed 76.
The general practitioners were able to diagnose only 65 of the
cases correctly. It is of note that three of the symptoms used are
interdependent to various degrees—the volume of red packed
cells, blood count, and the hemoglobin concentration. To assess
the effect this has on the ability of the program to make a correct
diagnosis, the three combinations of two red cells parameters
were used to the exclusions of the third, in three trial runs. The
results of these trials can be seen from Table 14–IV.

A data collection system has been developed which has made it
possible to accumulate a large and varied data base on patient's
entering two hospitals in Salt Lake City. A computer-based medical record is developed on each patient entering the hospital. Each
elective admission is sent through a screening procedure on entry
where the following data are collected and entered through a
keyboard: vital statistics, such as height, weight, age and sex. A
self-administered history is performed by each patient using a

TABLE 14–IV

COMPARISON OF PROGRAM PERFORMANCE WHEN SELECTED
MEASUREMENTS OF RED BLOOD CELLS ARE USED
ALONG WITH NON-RED CELL PARAMETERS

| *Measurement Used* | *Correct* | *False +* | *False −* |
|---|---|---|---|
| VPRC RBC Hgh | 95 | 2 | 3 |
| RBC Hgh | 93 | 4 | 3 |
| RBC VPRC | 93 | 5 | 2 |
| VPRC Hgh | 90 | 6 | 4 |
| Hgh | 89 | 3 | 8 |

device with which the patient punches a hole in a prepunched card corresponding to each question he wishes to answer in the affirmative. The questionnaire consists of 280 questions. All the answers, plus the patient's identification number, can be punched on a single card.

After this information is entered into the computer through a card reader, a history is printed consisting of a formatted set of positive statements corresponding to the questions answered in the affirmative by the patient. These questions are concerned with a system review, past history, family history, and a history of drug intakes and allergies, and is used primarily for the physician as a screening procedure prior to his investigation of the present illness in depth.

Blood and urine samples are drawn and sent to the laboratory where the blood is analyzed automatically through a 12-channel autoanalyzer and entered directly into the patient's computer-based medical record. Routine hematological and urinalysis data are entered manually from a keyboard in the laboratory.

Spirometry parameters are measured directly from a potentiometer connected to the spirometer into which the patient performs a forced vital capacity. ECG data is analyzed on-line, using a vector approach and the analysis system described above. If either procedure results in an abnormal diagnosis, the test is repeated immediately.

This data, along with other test procedures such as heart catheterization, cardiac output, and other hemadynamic data from intensive care wards, subsequent ECG analysis and follow-up chemistry data are entered automatically into the patient's record. At the time of discharge the patient's diagnosis is coded into his computer record, using a key word approach to generate the codes. Once the diagnosis has been entered, the patient's record is transferred from the active file on magnetic disc to the library tape which may then be searched for statistical purposes.

The first program in the search routine allows the operator to specify any logical combination of diseases to categorize a group of patients. The records satisfying these logical diagnostic codes are then copied from the master tape onto a subtape which can then be further searched to extract the specified data for subsequent analysis. The kind of data and the set of diseases, of course, are determined by the particular diagnostic matrix the operator wishes to generate. For example, he may wish to look at the distribution of total leukocyte counts in patients with leukemia. After completing such a search, a histogram is generated showing this distribution. The operator then enters his first approximation to tau of Equation 5. The computer solves this equation and superimposes the solution over the experimental histogram. If the fit is not optimal from visual inspection the operator may ask for another solution using a different tau value. Once tau is specified, the other two parameters, $\sigma$ and $\mu$, are determined from the first moment and variance of the experimental data using the relationship described earlier. Thus, a set of lag normal distributions are generated in three parameters for describing the distribution of each variable in each disease and these parameters are stored in a matrix for subsequent use.

The general approach currently being tested is an attempt to first classify the organ system most likely responsible for this set of clinical data obtained at time of admission on each patient. Having once found the most likely organ system involved, a second matrix specifying the nature of the disease involving that organ system may then be tested using some of the same data plus some additional types of tests to achieve this classification.

Of course, most of the patients entering the hospital as elective admissions will already have a primary diagnosis established. The purpose of this screening procedure and the associated diagnostic effort is to find and classify secondary illnesses from which the patient may be suffering and of which the patient's doctor should be aware before initiating treatment for the primary illness. Although some preliminary matrices have been established, critical tests of this approach have not as yet been performed.

Based on the approaches to computerized medical diagnosis presented in this chapter and in other papers, the future holds the exciting promise of continued reliability and improvement of these techniques.

## REFERENCES

1. Pryor, T. A.; Russell, R.; Budkin, A. and Price, W. G.: Electrocardiographic interpretation by computer. *Comp Biomed Res, 2:* (No. 6)

Dec. 1969.

2. Warner, H. R.; Toronto, A. F.; Veasy, L. G. and Stephenson, R.: A mathematical approach to medical diagnosis. *JAMA, 177:*177–183.

3. Warner, H. R.; Toronto, A. F. and Veasy, L. G.: Experience with Bayes's Theorem for computer diagnosis of congenital heart disease. *Ann NY Acad Sci, 115:*558–567, July 31, 1964.

4. Reynolds, D. N.: Learning program for computer diagnosis of congenital heart diseases. Master of Science in Computer Science Thesis, Univ. of Utah, 1966.

5. Christensen, J. A.: The lag normal density function applied to computer diagnosis of rheumatic heart diseases. Master of Science in Computer Science Thesis, Univ. of Utah, 1967.

6. Bishop, C. R. and Warner, H. R.: A mathematical approach of medical diagnosis: Application to polycythemic states utilizing clinical findings with values continuously distributed. *Comp Biomed Res, 2:* 486–493, Oct. 1969.

Chapter 15

# WISCONSIN COMPUTER AIDED MEDICAL DIAGNOSIS PROJECT*—PROGRESS REPORT—

David H. Gustafson
Robert L. Ludke
Paul J. Glackman
Frank C. Larson
John H. Greist

## INTRODUCTION

THIS RESEARCH SEEKS to develop and evaluate a computer-aided medical diagnosis system which combines judgments by physicians with information from past cases. The proposed system uses Bayes's Theorem to make the best use of data from these two sources, and adds information on the patient's symptoms* to produce a diagnosis.

We believe that one reason why some computer-aided diagnostic systems have not worked well is that they do not make use of physicians' knowledge and experience. We hoped these qualities, in combination with a computer's ability to use large amounts of data quickly, would produce superior results.

At this stage, we have focused on thyroid cases because they seem suited to the development of such a program and because of the valuable cooperation of physicians in this field at the University of Wisconsin Medical Center.

Briefly, our method is to complement subjective estimates about

* This research was supported by grant CH–00401–01 from the National Center for Health Service Research and Development.

* Symptom is always used here to refer to history symptoms, physical signs or laboratory findings.

symptom disease relationships with estimates of these same relationships based on medical record data. A smaller medical record data base or a smaller variance between professional's subjective estimates will both lead to more weight being given to the subjective estimates and vice versa. These estimates are essentially the probabilities that each symptom would be present in a given disease condition.

Among the reasons for taking this approach are evidence that subjective estimates can be useful in diagnosis when used with Bayes' Theorem,[1] and that physicians' estimates used in Bayes' Theorem can be good predictors of length of hospital stay.[2]

In our study, several methods of arriving at a diagnosis are compared, including the approach described above. They are as follows:

1. *Subjective Bayesian.* This method evaluates a patient's symptoms entirely on the basis of subjective estimates by physicians. In general, the procedure is for several physicians to estimate the likelihood ratios for conditionally independent symptom complexes.* For each symptom complex they will respond to the following questions: (a) Is the patient more likely to have the symptoms given in the symptom complex $S_i$ if he is euthyroid or if he is hyperthyroid? and (b) How much more likely?

The results will be estimates of the likelihood ratio:

$$\frac{P(S_i|\text{Euthyroid})}{P(S_i|\text{Hyperthyroid})}$$

The same question will be asked of a comparison between Euthyroid and Hypothyroid yielding the following:

$$\frac{P(S_i|\text{Euthyroid})}{P(S_i|\text{Hypothyroid})}$$

The likelihood ratios of all symptom complexes will be estimated subjectively.

The progress report contained in this paper is largely concerned with developing and testing methods of getting good estimates from physicians.

---

* "Symptom complexes" refer to one or more symptoms that have been grouped together due to conditional dependence.

2. *Actuarial Bayesian.* The primary difference between this method and method 1 is the determination of the likelihood ratios. In this method likelihood ratios are relative frequency estimates, calculated from medical record data. Method 2 is actually composed of four actuarial Bayesian models, each one differing only in the size of the data base used in calculating the actuarial estimates. These four methods will be compared because the size of the data base influences the accuracy of the estimates.

Model 2a will use the symptom's likelihood ratio based on actual data whenever the data base contains at least 50 observations. This submethod will use all the actuarial data it can in estimating likelihood ratios and should be the best actuarial method we can develop.

In order to estimate the size of the data base needed before the actuarial methods could reliably replace subjective methods, three other models will be developed. They will employ a specific data base size. Model 2b will use exactly 50 observations, model 2c will use exactly 200 observations, and model 2d will use exactly 500 observations to calculate each likelihood estimate.

3. *Hybrid Bayesian.* In this model actuarial data will be used to revise subjective estimates. This can be done by assuming a distribution on each of the subjective estimates (we will have estimated the mode and the 95 percent confidence limit) and using Bayes' Theorem as a mechanism for revising these estimates on the basis of the actuarial data.

4. *Contemporary Diagnostic Methods.* In order to compare the experimental methods with more commonly used techniques, we will request four physicians from the University Hospital's Thyroid Clinic to give their diagnoses of all appropriate patients. Also, residents will review the same patient information (history, physical examination, and laboratory data) as is used in the Subjective Bayesian method. For each patient they will (a) rank the thyroid diagnoses (hyperthyroid, hypothyroid, euthyroid) from the most to least likely, and (b) estimate how much more likely the favorite diagnosis is than each of the other two. The latter can be converted into a posterior probability estimate for each diagnosis.

## EXPECTED RESULTS FROM THE FOUR SYSTEMS

We hypothesize that the relative effectiveness of the four systems will be as shown in Fig. 15–1. We expect the Subjective Bayesian method (curve B) will be superior to the other methods when very little actuarial data is available. As more data are obtained, the actuarial estimates will become more accurate and the Actuarial Bayesian method (curve C) should gradually improve. We would expect the performance of the Contemporary Diagnostic method (curve A) to remain essentially constant as the amount of data increases. The Hybrid method (curve D) should initially perform as well as the Subjective Bayesian method (since they are identical until actuarial estimates become accurate enough to modify and/or replace the more easily obtained and initially more accurate subjective estimates). Then the Hybrid method, employing estimates of both the subjective and actuarial methods should perform more accurately than all other methods.

The specific questions we want to answer are the following:
(a) Which of the five diagnostic systems will be most accurate?
(b) How large must the actuarial data base be before the system

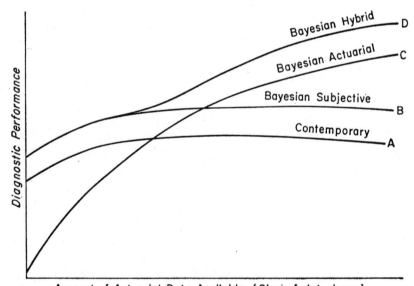

Figure 15–1. Hypothesized relative effectiveness of the methods.

performs as well as the subjective system? (c) How precise should the likelihood ratio based on actuarial data be before it can replace the subjective counterpart in the hybrid model? (d) How does a non-uniform prior probability distribution as opposed to a uniform one influence the performance of a Bayesian diagnostic model? and (e) What are the relative setup and operational costs of the actuarial and subjective systems?

## Measures of Effectiveness for Methodology

Two measures of effectiveness will be used in comparing the four methods. First, the results of the diagnosis will be classified as follows:

1. correct hyperthyroid
2. correct euthyroid
3. correct hypothyroid
4. hyperthyroid—euthyroid estimated
5. hyperthyroid—hypothyroid estimated
6. hypothyroid—euthyroid estimated
7. hypothyroid—hyperthroid estimated
8. euthyroid—hypothyroid estimated
9. euthyroid—hyperthyroid estimated

For each method the number of diagnoses in each of the classifications will be divided by the number of cases where diagnoses were attempted. These percentages and severity of each error for each method will be compared to find significant differences. The second measure is based on the final probability assigned to the correct diagnosis. Each method will arrive at a posterior probability estimate of all possible diagnoses. The probability assigned to the "true" diagnosis will be compared between methods and significant differences determined.

## Methods for Determining True Diagnosis

The results of specific laboratory tests such as Iodine 131 uptake, Serum PBI, or Murphy Pattee, will not be available for Bayesian and Experimental Physician methods. The results of these highly diagnostic tests along with the consensus opinion of the team of endocrinologists, using all available data, will provide one phase of obtaining correct diagnoses. The other phase involves the patient after his evaluation in the clinic. If he receives treatment at the clinic, a team of endocrinologists using all available data will select, by consensus, the correct diagnosis six months after the patient's evaluation.

## PROGRESS REPORT

Three major problems had to be solved before the diagnostic systems could be implemented: (a) How could the independence assumption of the Bayesian requirements be met without making the model too complex to handle—that is, how could we correctly group symptoms together? (b) How could we obtain the subjective estimates for the diagnostic model? and (c) How could we collect and organize the patient data necessary to test these systems? Research described below developed answers to these questions.

### Independence—Grouping of Symptoms

Bayes' Theorem assumes the data to be aggregated are conditionally independent. (Calculation errors of course are proportional to the degree to which this assumption is violated.) Statistical techniques which might be used to determine degree of conditional dependence require massive amounts of data that are unavailable or too costly, so this part of the research evaluated the effectiveness of four techniques that were available to us for subjectively classifying data into conditionally independent complexes or clusters.

Sixty undergraduate students at the University of Wisconsin used these four methods to cluster 25 factors characterizing their fellow students. These factors included income aspiration, educational aspiration, mother's education, father's income, college qualifying test scores, ACT-SAT percentile score, responsibility, sociability, etc. They were chosen because we had a correlation matrix for evaluating subject performance.

First, subjects were introduced to the concepts of dependence and independence of data and then randomly assigned one of the four methods. Fifteen subjects were in each group.

A card-sorting technique (method A) was one approach for subjectively classifying data into independent clusters. Each factor was listed on a separate index card and subjects were instructed to arrange these cards into piles representing the clusters.*

The other three methods involved working with lists of factors rather than cards. In one case (method B), all factors were presented on a single list and subjects divided the data into separate groups so all factors within the same group were strongly related to each other.

The second list method (C) involved three fewer lists (than the total number of factors). The first list contained all of the factors. The second list had all of the factors except the first and

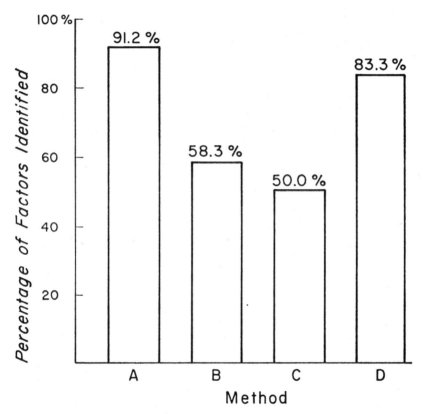

Figure 15–2. Percentage of factors identified by methods A, B, C, D as belonging in a cluster when correlation was above .48.

---

* Data within the same pile was considered to be strongly dependent and any data in a pile by itself was considered independent.

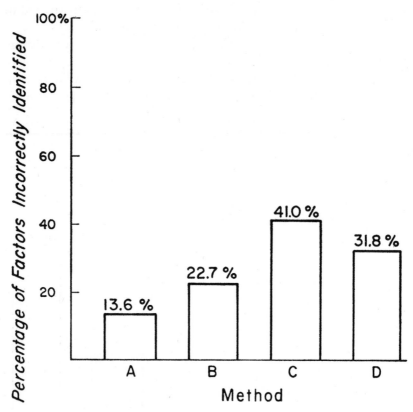

Figure 15–3. Percentage of factors incorrectly put into a cluster when correlation coefficient was .02 or below.

each successive list had one additional factor removed until the last list had only the three factors. We instructed the subjects to examine each list and mark those factors that were strongly related to the *first* factor on that list. With this method, all factors marked on a single list must be interdependent.

The last method (D) was the same as C except each factor marked need only be related to the top factor on the list.

Two criteria were used in comparing the performance of these four methods: (a) If any two factors had a correlation coefficient of .48 or above, we would expect them to be put into the same cluster; and (b) Any two factors with correlation coefficients of .02 or below should not be put together. The comparison of the four techniques according to these criteria is given in Figs. 15–2 and 15–3.

We also evaluated methods according to the time they took. The first two methods (card-sorting and single list) took under half an hour and the last two, with the pages of lists, took 45 minutes to an hour.

We chose the card-sorting technique (method A) to classify signs, symptoms, and laboratory data because it was both fast and accurate.

Having developed this method for clustering, we then used it to cluster thyroid symptoms.

Initially we developed a list of about 125 physical signs, history symptoms, and lab tests for the thyroid diagnosis study. This list came from textbooks, records of thyroid patients, other thyroid diagnosis studies, including the data set used by Williams,[3] and the opinions of physicians.

We deleted symptoms that were, in the opinion of the chief residents and faculty in the department of medicine, rarely used in diagnosis. We placed the final symptom list of 70 into conditionally independent clusters. Being interested only in identifying very strongly dependent relationships, we expected many of the symptoms would remain independent and would not be clustered with others.

Four fourth-year medical students and eight medical residents worked individually to cluster symptoms, then discussed the results with three other physicians from the group. After discussion, they again individually clustered the symptoms using the card-sorting method. These results are in Table 15–I.

### Likelihood Ratio Estimation

There are two approaches to obtaining likelihood estimations. The first is to develop "direct" likelihoods by estimating the probability of a symptom given a particular disease. The second is to estimate the likelihood ratio (a ratio of the probability of a symptom given one disease to the probability of the same symptom given another disease). Research by Edwards and others[1] indicates that likelihood ratios estimated on a logarithmically cali-

TABLE 15–I
THYROID SYMPTOM CLUSTERS DEVELOPED FROM RESULTS
OBTAINED BY MED STUDENTS AND RESIDENTS USING
CARD SORTING METHOD

| *Symptom Complexes* | *Independent Symptoms* |
| --- | --- |
| Lid lag | Age |
| Increased palbebral fissure | Flow murmur |
| Exophathalmos | Skin texture |
| Body temperature | Nail texture |
| Change in temperature tolerance | Onycholysis |
| Skin temperature | Pregnancy |
| Skin moisture | Hair texture |
| Perspiration | Appetite change |
|  | Weight change |
| Bruit over gland | Eyelid condition |
| Thrill over gland | Decreased convergence |
| Cardiac arrhythmias | Myxedema |
| Heart palpitations | Tongue size |
|  | Voice quality |
| Cardiomegaly | Dyspnea |
| Congestive heart failure | Blood pressure |
| Change in muscular strength | Precordial pain |
| Wasting of muscles | Muscular condition |
|  | Splenomegaly |
| Concentration ability | Tendon reflexes |
| Restlessness | Fine tremor |
| Menstrual flow | Anemia |
| Irregularity of menstrual periods | Bowel movement (diarrhea or constipation) |
| Generalized lymph adenopathy | Family history of goiter or thyroid disease |
| Lymphocytosis | Goiter |
| I-131 | Change in general activity |
| PBI | Change in fatigability |
| Murphy Pattee | Psychosis |
| Dilantin | Clinical estimate of intelligence |
| Iodine and birth control |  |
| Pulse rate | Hearing |
| Heart rate or ECG rate | Speech |
|  | Increased anxiety |
|  | Sleep |
|  | Sex |
|  | Serum cholesterol |
|  | Glucose tolerance test |

brated scale of odds tend to reduce conservatism * better than direct likelihood estimates.

The task of developing a means of getting good likelihood ratio estimates from physicians—of getting them to tell us in terms we could use what symptoms are likely to be associated with particular disease states—is a major topic of this paper. The work can be described in roughly four sections:

1. Deciding what training method would best prepare the physicians, and what sort of interactions a group of physicians should have with each other to make the best estimates.

2. Developing the training procedure in detail and testing it on students.

3. Training the doctors, using what has been learned, and briefly testing their training.

4. Developing in detail the individual and group actions the physicians would take to make estimates for thyroid conditions.

### Deciding on Training Method and Group Process

Other research also seems to indicate that training is important in developing effective likelihood ratio estimators.[4] However, we did not know whether training transfers from one topic area to another. Our study requires estimates from several physicians, but we didn't know the best group process to use. The purpose of the research summarized in this section was to evaluate the effects on likelihood ratio estimation of four group processes for obtaining estimates and of three processes for training.

Behavioral research in small group theory has given us several precepts as a base for our research. First, we know that groups have a tendency to take greater risks than individuals,[5] so we compared the effect on likelihood ratio estimation of group versus individual estimators. We also know that consensus does not appear to be necessary to lead to greater risks, and in fact, may be undesirable [7] so we decided not to force consensus. The research work on Delphi techniques indicates [7] that face-to-face contact should be avoided and so we evaluated a process that involved only written feedback between estimators with no opportunity for face-to-face contact. Finally, from small group theory, we know

---

* "Conservatism" is a tendency to underestimate the diagnostic value of important symptoms and overestimate the diagnostic value of unimportant symptoms.

that we can reduce the face-to-face problem [7] by estimation before and after discussion, and so we selected a procedure that involved estimation, structured discussion, and then a reestimation by the individuals. Summarizing then, we prepared four different group processes:

1. individual estimates (E)
2. interacting group [committee approach] (TE)
3. estimation, written feedback, and then reestimation (EFE)
4. estimation, discussion, and then reestimation (ETE)

In the same study, we compared the effectiveness in estimating likelihood ratios of groups with the following:

1. no training
2. training on another data generating process (transfer training)
3. direct training on the data-generating process from which they would be estimating

The experiment was conducted as follows: 288 undergraduate students from the University of Wisconsin were divided into groups of four, and six groups of these students were assigned to each of the following categories:

| Category | Group Process | Training |
|---|---|---|
| 1 | E | No training |
| 2 | E | Transfer training |
| 3 | E | Direct training |
| 4 | TE | No training |
| 5 | TE | Transfer training |
| 6 | TE | Direct training |
| 7 | EFE | No training |
| 8 | EFE | Transfer training |
| 9 | EFE | Direct training |
| 10 | ETE | No training |
| 11 | ETE | Transfer training |
| 12 | ETE | Direct training |

We compared the group geometric mean of the posterior odds to the true posterior odds obtained from demographic records. The topic used was the sex of an individual given his height or weight.

To transfer train, we asked the students to estimate the posterior odds that it would rain or be dry on a particular date in Madison given information about what had happened the day before. In direct training, the question was to guess the sex of an individual from a different age category than that used in our evaluation of the training. Height and weight were given.

We found type of training to have a profound effect on ability to estimate likelihood ratios (Fig. 15–4). Both transfer training and direct training did increase ability. However, direct training, using the data-generating process under consideration, was more effective.

As a result of this study we decided to (a) begin training our subjects on topics unrelated to the diagnostic situation under consideration, but ones easily understood by both experimenters and

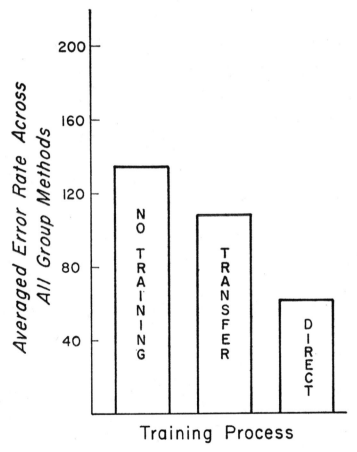

Figure 15–4. Effect of training process on subjective estimation.

the physician estimators and (b) then to move to a topic more directly related to the matter at hand.

Our study also found (Fig. 15–5) that among group processes evaluated, the worst procedure was the estimate-feedback-estimate one involving written feedback but with no discussion. The second best technique appears to be the interacting group. The estimate-talk-estimate procedure gave superior results and was selected to estimate our likelihood ratios.

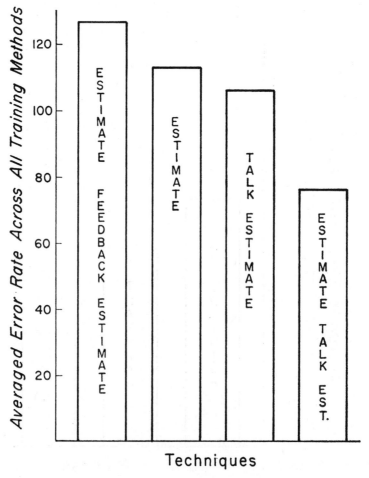

Figure 15–5. Comparison of group process effect on subjective estimation.

## Further Development and Testing of the Training Process

Once we had settled on our general approaches both for training the physicians to estimate likelihood ratios, and for the group process that they would use to make and refine their estimates, we had to actually train the physicians. Before doing this, however, we worked out and tested the training program on four senior-year medical students. The following paragraphs describe this test and in doing so show development of our training program in more detail.

Most people, physicians included, have difficulty in quantifying their judgments, even though they understand the situation under consideration. Therefore, an important part of this work is our two-step program for training the physician (or, at this stage, student) to accurately describe in terms of likelihood ratios his feelings of the relationships between symptoms and disease states of thyroidism.

In the first step, called pretraining, we provided information on the basic definitions, concepts, and procedures for estimating likelihood ratios, and information about our computer-aided medical diagnosis study. Each subject was asked to read our *Training Manual for Physician Likelihood Ratio Estimators* and was given the option of reading our *Information Manual of the Computer-Aided Medical Diagnosis Study for Physician Likelihood Estimators*.

In the second step, groups of four physicians met with us. We reviewed the manuals and equipment used in estimates and then asked the subject for likelihood ratio estimates of several kinds of problems.

We decided to use the following four measures to evaluate the medical students' training program:

1. We determined accuracy in estimating likelihood ratios by comparing individual and group geometric means of their estimates with the actual likelihood ratio for each problem. We hypothesized that accuracy would increase during training.

2. The level of confidence a student had in estimates was determined by the width of the interval of estimation the student placed around his likelihood estimate. The level was calculated

by taking the difference between the upper and lower limits of the interval and dividing by their mean. We hypothesized that the student would also become more confident in his estimates during training.

3. We calculated the log variance by taking the variance of the log of the estimates from the log of the geometric mean of the estimates for each problem.

4. Finally, we sought the reactions and comments of the students at the end of each session.

The only data analyzed so far is the accuracy of the students' estimates. Fig. 15–6 is a plot of the difference between the actual and estimated posterior probabilities of the most likely hypothesis for each problem. The graph is divided into four sections to differentiate between the four types of subject matter we made use of: heights, Cushing's Syndrome, gastric ulcers, and thyroid conditions.

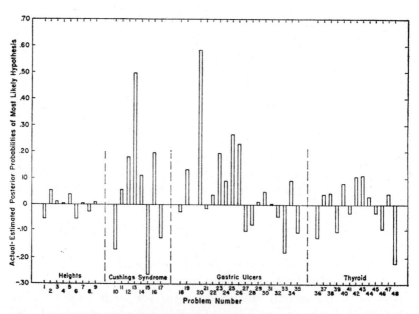

Figure 15–6. Results of medical students training program: actual-estimated posterior probabilities of most likely hypothesis vs. problem number. Probabilities are calculated from the geometric means of the final likelihood ratio estimates.

For problems 1 through 9, the students estimated heights of American men and women in various age groups. The average heights for men and women in each group were given. Because this subject was well understood, the accuracy of the estimates became very good as the students became familiar with the data generating process and the procedures.

For problems 10 through 17, the students made estimates using possible symptoms for Cushing's Syndrome. For these, the population used was not defined, and as can be seen in Fig. 15–6 this had a significant impact on accuracy. The students first had difficulty in quantifying the relationships between the symptoms and the unclear states, so there was a large difference between estimated and actual. Also they could not clearly interpret the feedback (the values of the actual likelihood ratios), and thus did not learn and improve.

For problems 18 through 35, the students made estimates for symptoms and benign-malignant states of gastric ulcers. The population for this data was defined, but not all symptoms were. This also had a significant effect, as can be seen in problems 20, 25, 26, and 27. Except for these and problem 23, the accuracy was fairly good until problem 33, because the process was understood and well-defined populations enabled good feedback. The inaccuracies in problems 23, 33, 34, and 35 may have occurred because these involved groups of three or four symptoms.

Students also made estimates for symptoms and states of thyroid disease (problems 36–48). Though not actually part of the training program, these problems were used to test the effects of different populations on the accuracy of the estimates and to determine the students' ability to make estimates for thyroid disease. For problems 36 through 44, the students were instructed to consider the population from which the data was taken, whereas for problems 45 through 48 are the same as problems 36 through 39. The accuracy of estimates was determined using the same data. It appears that how the population is defined does have an effect, but no conclusive results can be stated from this small sample. Also, except for problem 48, the accuracy of the estimates is fairly good.

Without having prior estimates for the thyroid problems, we cannot conclude that training had a positive effect on the accuracy of the medical students' thyroid estimates. However, from these results we can conclude that definitions of the populations from which the feedback data and of the symptoms must be clearly stated in order to acquire reasonable estimates. We can also conclude that when the data generating process is clearly defined and understood, such as the case with the heights problems, the medical students can provide very accurate estimates.

### Training of Physicians to Estimate Likelihood Ratios

At this stage we had some confidence in our procedure for training physicians and so went ahead with the method we had used on the four students, although we eliminated the work with Cushing's Syndrome because of the difficulties with it.

In training our residents, we made another test; this one to see how effective the training was for them. Our test was to ask them to make likelihood ratio estimates of six thyroid symptoms, both before and after the training. To compare these two sets of estimates and therefore see the value of our training, the same four measures were used as in the medical students' training.

The only data analyzed at this time is the accuracy of the residents' estimates. Fig. 15-7 is a plot of the difference between the actual and the estimated probabilities for each problem to illustrate the accuracy of the estimate over time (increasing problem numbers). The graph is divided into four sections to differentiate between the different types of problems: the thyroid pretest, heights, gastric ulcers, and the thyroid post-test. It should be noted, however, that the problems were not the same for the medical students and the residents training program.

For the thyroid pretest, problems 1 through 6, the residents were given a brief orientation to the procedures and equipment to be used in the estimation task, but were given no training or no feedback. However, they were given a detailed definition of the thyroid population they were to make estimates for. These results verify that even though physicians may fully understand the situation they are making estimates for, they have difficulty in accurately quantifying their true feelings.

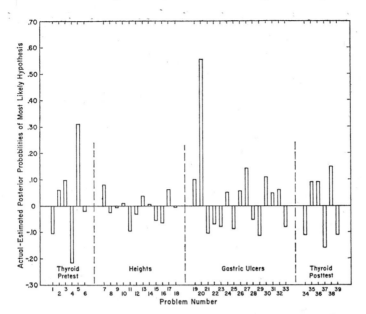

Figure 15–7. Results of resident's training program: actual-estimated posterior probabilities of most likely hypothesis vs. problem number. Probabilities are calculated from the geometric means of the final likelihood ratio estimates.

Problems 7 through 33 consist of the training program in which the populations were defined for each type of problem and feedback was given on each problem. As with the medical students, the residents made very accurate estimates for the height problems. Also, with the gastric ulcer problems, the effect of not having clearly defined uniform symptom definitions on accuracy is illustrated; for example problem 20. However, for problems 30 through 33 where the residents were asked to make estimates for symptoms containing more than one symptom, there does not appear to be an increase in error as there was with the medical students. This may be due to the resident's greater experience.

Problems 34 through 39, the thyroid post-test are the same as problems 1 through 6. As with the pretest, the population was clearly defined and no feedback was given to the residents. Comparing the pretest and post-test, it appears that the training had some effect, but did not increase the accuracy greatly. We are currently investigating this fact. From the results of the heights, we know that when the data generating process is well understood, the residents give very accurate results, yet the results for the thyroid problems are not as accurate. This may imply that experienced endocrinologists rather than residents must make the estimates. We plan to test this hypothesis soon.

### Development in Detail of Individual and Group Actions for the Physicians Making Estimates

With physicians trained by the method above, and having developed a general outline of the group process they would follow in giving estimates, we are able to develop the details of getting the best estimates from them in a short amount of time.

First, we had them respond to the following questions for each thyroid symptom and cluster:

1. Which patient would be more likely to have the symptoms given in the symptom complex $S_i$, one who is hyperthyroid (or hypothyroid) or one who is euthyroid?

2. How much more likely?

The results of these questions will be estimates of

$$\frac{P(S_i|\text{Euthyroid})}{P(S_i|\text{Hyperthyroid})}$$
(or Hypothyroid)

Each physician also defined an interval around each of his likelihood ratio estimates. This interval was merely a range of possible likelihood ratios in which the physician was confident that the "true" likelihood ratio would fall, assuming the "true" likelihood ratio was known. To obtain this we included the following three items:

1. I would be extremely surprised if the "true" likelihood ratio was greater than ————:1.

2. I would be extremely surprised if I was told that my answer to the question of which patient would be more likely to have the symptoms in $S_i$ was incorrect. YES——— NO———

3. I would be extremely surprised if the "true" likelihood ratio was less than————:1.

The second question was asked to determine whether the physician was expressing the lower limit of his interval of estimation in terms of the most likely hypothesis (which patient was more likely to have the symptoms).

The interval of estimation was used as a measure of the physician's confidence. If for a particular estimate the physician's interval of estimation was smaller than the intervals for his other estimates, it would imply that the physician is more confident than usual. Such an estimate should be given more weight.

For the physicians to make the most accurate likelihood ratio and interval estimates, two pieces of equipment are used. The first of these was a problem-estimate card designed to provide the pertinent information about the problem and a place to record estimates. Fig. 15–8 is an example of a problem-estimate card used in the thyroid data collection program.

The second piece of equipment was the log-odds scale. Each time a physician made a likelihood ratio estimate, he was actually defining a numerical relationship between two hypotheses. That is, he was saying that one hypothesis was so many times more likely to occur than the other. The log-odds scale allows one to actually see the relative importance given to different values on

```
COMPLEX NO._____ PHYSICIAN _____ DATE_____

    1.  WHICH PATIENT WOULD BE MORE LIKELY TO HAVE THE SYMPTOMS:




        ONE WHO IS HYPERTHYROID OR ONE WHO IS EUTHYROID?

            HYPERTHYROID_____ EUTHYROID _____

    2.  HOW MUCH MORE LIKELY?        _____:1

    3.  I WOULD BE EXTREMELY SURPRISED IF THE TRUE LIKELIHOOD RATIO
        WAS GREATER THAN _____:1

    4.  I WOULD BE EXTREMELY SURPRISED IF I WAS TOLD THAT MY ANSWER
        TO STATEMENT #1 WAS INCORRECT.

            YES _____        NO _____

    5.  I WOULD BE EXTREMELY SURPRISED IF THE TRUE LIKELIHOOD RATIO
        WAS LESS THAN _____:1
```

Figure 15–8. Example of a problem-estimate card used in the thyroid data collection program.

the scale. The scale also shows that as the value of the estimates becomes larger, it is more difficult to make fine distinctions.

During the estimation task, scales were mounted in a frame with three movable magnetic pointers. Each physician was given one and asked to make his estimates on it before recording them. He did this by placing the middle pointer at the likelihood ratio estimate for his most likely hypothesis and placing the end pointers to show his interval of estimation.

The physicians, meeting in groups of four, were asked to individually make estimates of the likelihood ratio and the intervals of estimation for a problem. After group discussion they each reestimated.

Currently, we are collecting from the residents their estimates of the relationships between the symptoms and various states of thyroid disease. The residents make estimates in groups of four using the estimate-discussed-reestimate process. Once the subjective estimates have been collected the diagnostic systems will become operational.

### Patient Data Collection

To evaluate the effectiveness of our four diagnostic techniques, information will be used from patients at the University of Wisconsin Endocrine Clinic. Information on these patients will be processed by the computer in order to reach a probabilistic value. In order to do this, an effective means was needed for collecting information not only on the presence of the certain symptoms, but also on the absence of symptoms. Slack's work [8] indicates that both the patients and physicians view his computer-based history and physical system as both enjoyable and useful. Slack's work led to the development of a computer-based history and physical routine for thyroid disease that could be useful as both an aid to the physician and as a tool to collect a uniform set of patient data for our diagnostic project. Dr. Larson, in conjunction with other members of the medical staff developed these routines based on history and physical information of interest in the diagnosis and treatment of thyroid disfunction. Currently, patients with suspected thyroid disease are referred to the interviewing room where a computer-based history interview is conducted in an interactive mode. The history information is then forwarded to the attending physician and an additional copy is referred to us. At this time, all patients with suspected thyroid disease who enter the endocrine clinic participate in the computer-based history interview. The computer-based displays are needed first.

In summary then, a computer-based history and physical examination have been developed. The history routine is in use at University Hospitals collecting information for the physicians and for this diagnostic project. The physical examination is in its final revision state. Any information collected here will be then used in the diagnostic system once it is completed.

## SUMMARY

The Computer-Aided Medical Diagnosis Project has completed several fundamental research endeavors necessary to develop the diagnostic systems. First, the technique for clustering symptoms into conditionally independent complexes has been developed and patient information has been clustered. Secondly, a technique has been selected for training physicians to be likelihood ratio estimators and the physicians have been trained. Estimations of the likelihood ratios are being obtained now. Histories are being taken on the LINC computer on a routine basis. Physician examinations will need to be done by hand, but a computer system is in the final stages of completion. An empirical data base has been developed through information obtained from the University of Florida Endocrine Clinic and through information being extracted from the University Medical Records at the University of Wisconsin. Within the next year the diagnostic systems will be implemented. We are presently working on likelihood estimations and the computer routines for processing and analyzing data.

## REFERENCES

1. *IEEE Trans. Human Factors in Electronics, HFE–7:* March 1966.
2. Gustafson, D. H.: Evaluation of probabilistic information processing in medical decision making. *Organizational Behavior and Human Performance, 4:* (No. 1), March 1969.
3. Fitzgerald, L. T. and Williams, C. M.: Modified programs for computer diagnosis of thyroid disease. *Radiology, 82:*237, February 1964.
   Overall, J. E. and Williams, C. M.: Conditional probability for diagnosis of thyroid function. *JAMA, 183:*307–313, February 2, 1963.

4. Goodman, Barbara: Group decision making in situations of risk. The University of Michigan, 1970.
5. Van de Ven, A. and O'Brien, D.: The decision-making effectiveness of differentiated group processes on solution-synthesis problems. Unpublished research proposal, College of Engineering, University of Wisconsin, Madison, Wisconsin, 1970.
6. Dalkey, N. C. and Helmer, Olaf: An experimental application of the Delphi method to the use of experts. *Management Science,* g, 1963.
7. Dalkey, N. C.: "The Delphi method: An experimental study of group opinion. *Memorandum RM–5888–PK,* June 1969.
8. Slack, W. V.; Hicks, G. P.; Reed, C. E.; Van Cura, L. J. and Carr, W.F.: A computer-based medical history system. *N Engl J Med, 274:*194–198, January 27, 1966.
9. Slack, W. V.; Peckham, B. M.; Van Cura, L. J. and Carr, W. F.: A computer-based physical examination system. *JAMA, 200:*224, April 17, 1967.

## Chapter 16

# COMPUTER-AIDED DIFFERENTIAL DIAGNOSIS OF HEMATOLOGIC DISEASES (A BAYESIAN PROBABILITY MODEL)*

RALPH L. ENGLE, JR.
MARTIN LIPKIN
BETTY J. FLEHINGER

$\mathbf{A}$T THE FIRST MEETING on The Diagnostic Process held in 1963 Dr. Martin Lipkin summarized most of the work of our group up to that point.[1] I now have the opportunity of bringing you up to date on our more recent activities. Ours is a group effort. In addition to Dr. Lipkin, Dr. Flehinger, and myself, significant contributions to the work being discussed have been made by Drs. Leo Leveridge, B. J. Davis, and Richard Friedman.

Many of you will recall that we were working with a diagnostic model in which significance values and weights were assigned by physicians to each finding in each disease. Given a set of patient's findings, diseases were selected by calculating ratios called *weighted averages* which, in essence, compared the weighted findings of the patient under consideration with the weighted findings of a typical or classical patient with a particular disease. More recent versions of this model, using 540 findings in 76 hematologic diseases, have been reported in the *Digest of the 7th International Conference on Medical and Biological Engineering* in 1967 [2] and in the *Annals of the New York Academy of Sciences* in 1969.[3] We do not feel that any of these models have been rigorously tested. However, so that we will have some feel for the effectiveness of these significance models, as we call them, I would like to mention

---

* From the Department of Medicine, New York Hospital–Cornell Medical Center, New York, New York and the I.B.M. T.J. Watson Research Center, Yorktown Heights, New York.

briefly some of our reported results. In a single experiment, findings from 144 individual patients with hematologic diseases obtained from the records of the New York Hospital were analyzed using this model and a differential diagnosis obtained for each patient. The same records were reviewed by a hematologist who arrived at a diagnosis and divided the patients into two categories:

1. Reasonably typical and straightforward diagnoses (51 patients)

2. Difficult diagnoses often with atypical features (93 patients)

In the first category (typical) the computer diagnosis agreed with the hematologist's diagnosis in 48 of the 51 patients or 92 percent, while in the second category (atypical) the computer diagnosis agreed with the hematologist's diagnosis in 60 of the 93 patients or 65 percent. Among those patients where the correct diagnosis was not made by the computer as the first diagnosis were eight patients where the correct diagnosis was listed second, three patients where the correct diagnosis was listed third, and ten additional patients where the correct diagnosis was included among the first ten diagnoses listed by the computer.

I do not want to go into any further detail about the significance model since I want to spend the remainder of the time on the Bayesian model we have been developing for the past three years. Early in our work we had elected not to use a Bayesian model because we were concerned that diseases and findings of low incidence might get overlooked, concerned that findings in patients are not independent as assumed in Bayes formula, and concerned that diseases are not mutually exclusive as assumed. We were, of course, aware of the importance of probability in the decision making process and with the early work of Ledley and Lusted [4] and of Warner [5] who suggested and used the Bayesian approach to decision making in medical diagnosis.

In 1967 Dr. Betty Flehinger, a statistician, joined our group. She stressed the similarities between certain Bayesian approaches and our significance model and suggested that a Bayesian model could be built on the foundation of the significance model affecting a sort of merger of the two approaches. Under her direction we have used a model similar to that reported by Nugent,

Warner, Dunn, and Tyler [6] for Cushing's disease which was presented by Nugent [7] at the first meeting on the Diagnostic Process. However, we believe that there are some significant differences in the way in which we use the model.

The principle of the Bayes's formula we use may be best seen in a scheme modified from Cliffe [8] (Fig. 16–1). I hope statisticians will forgive this elementary approach. It should be useful to those of us not well grounded in mathematics. In a population of 400 represented by the large rectangle, 20 percent have disease A and 80 percent do not have disease A. They may have other diseases or be normal. Sixty of the 80 people or 75 percent who have disease A also have a particular finding while 58 of the 320 people or 18.125 percent who do not have disease A have the same finding. The figures in the blocks are the frequencies that are known or that are capable of being estimated. The probability of disease A given the finding is equal to the number of people with disease A who have the finding divided by the total number of people in the population who have the finding or, in this model:

$$\frac{60}{60+58}$$

We may substitute known or estimated quantities for the 60 and 58. The 60 is 75 percent of 20 percent of the total population of 400 and the 58 is 18.125 percent of 80 percent of the total popula-

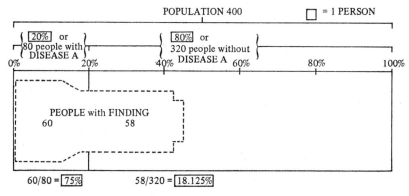

Figure 16–1. The principle of Bayes' formula seen in a scheme modified from Cliffe.

tion. The total population of 400 cancels out. Another way of writing this is as follows:

$$\frac{[.20x.75x400]}{[.20x.75x400]+[.80x.18125x400]}$$

If we now generalize these figures we find that the expression is equal to the following:

$$\frac{P_A \text{ x } p_{Aij}}{P_A \text{ x } p_{Aij} + (1\text{-}P_A) \text{ x } q_{Aij}}$$

$P_A$ = probability of occurrence of disease A in the clinical population.

$P_{Aij}$ = probability that patient who has disease A has finding j for symptom or descriptor i.

$q_{Aij}$ = probability that a patient in the clinical population who does not have disease A has finding j for descriptor i.

If we now wish to consider multiple findings which are selected to be essentially independent we are able to insert the products of the p's and q's as seen in the formula:

Probability [disease A, given a patient's findings] =

$$\frac{P_A \underset{\substack{\text{patient's} \\ \text{findings}}}{\Pi} p_{Aij}}{P_A \underset{\substack{\text{patient's} \\ \text{findings}}}{\Pi} p_{Aij} + (1\text{-}P_A) \underset{\substack{\text{patient's} \\ \text{findings}}}{\Pi} q_{Aij}}$$

Nonmathematicians may need to know that the capital pi stands for product. We realize, of course, that findings in patients are rarely if ever completely independent, even if carefully selected. This is a compromise which we make.

In our Bayesian model we attempted to build on and to correct many of the deficiencies in our previous work and to develop a decision program capable of automatically improving itself as data accumulate. We first defined the total population to be hematology patients seen as inpatients or outpatients at the New York Hospital. We then took the following five steps with reference to each disease:

First, preparation of a list of signs, symptoms, and laboratory procedures (hereafter called *descriptors*) pertinent to the disease utilizing as much information as possible from our previous significance model. In defining descriptors, a strenuous effort was made to keep them independent. Consider, for example, hemoglobin, hematocrit and red blood cell count. These are obviously highly dependent. We therefore combined them into one descriptor called "red blood cells."

Second, for each descriptor, preparation of a list of those findings which, relative to the given disease, were thought to be significantly different. It was required that these findings be mutually exclusive and exhaustive, i.e. for every patient tested, one and only one finding for each descriptor be selected. This was a difficult task. After a lengthy discussion about the descriptor, red blood cells, we finally arrived at the following set of ten significantly different findings:

Descriptor: Red Blood Cells

| Findings: | | | |
|---|---|---|---|
| 1. | Hgb < 7 | MCV > 94 | MCH > 30 |
| 2. | Hgb < 7 | MCV 80–94 | MCH > 30 |
| 3. | Hgb < 7 | MCV < 80 | MCH > 30 |
| 4. | Hgb < 7 | MCV < 80 | MCH < 30 |
| 5. | Hgb 7–13 | MCV > 94 | MCH > 30 |
| 6. | Hgb 7–13 | MCV 80–94 | MCH > 30 |
| 7. | Hgb 7–13 | MCV < 80 | MCH > 30 |
| 8. | Hgb 7–13 | MCV < 80 | MCH < 30 |
| 9. | Hgb 13–17 | RBC 3.5–6 | PCV 30–55 |
| 10. | Hgb > 17 | RBC > 5 | PCV > 50 |

In order to analyze all the diseases from one list of findings it was important that wherever possible a descriptor relevant to more than one disease be subdivided into the same findings for all the diseases concerned. As the number of diseases analyzed increased, this became an increasingly difficult task, often requiring redefinition of findings in diseases previously analyzed.

Third, for each finding of each descriptor a group of physicians and the statistician estimated the prior distributions of the following two probabilities based on judgment and available incidence data:

1. $p_{Aij}$, the probability that a patient who has disease A has finding j for descriptor i.

2. $q_{Aij}$, the probability that a patient who does not have disease A has finding j for descriptor i.

The estimates of these probabilities were entered as ratios of two numbers. For any given ratio, the degree of certainty associated with the estimate is represented by the values of the numerator and denominator. For example, if a given finding is thought to occur 50 percent of the time, an entry of 5/10 indicates less certainty than an entry of 50/100 which in turn indicates less certainty than an entry of 500/1000.

It was necessary that the estimates of $q_{Aij}$ be consistent from one disease to another. This became increasingly difficult as the number of diseases increased.

The ratio $p_{Aij}/q_{Aij}$ indicates the relevance of a finding to a disease. If $p_{Aij}/q_{Aij}$ is greater than 1, the finding favors the diagnosis of the disease. If the ratio is less than 1, the finding is against the diagnosis of the disease.

The process of estimating the $p_{Aij}$'s and $q_{Aij}$'s was a difficult one. Information about the p's was sometimes available from the significance model, sometimes in textbooks, but more often the judgment of the physicians had to be exercised. The q's had to be based almost entirely on judgment. It was always necessary to bear in mind that the p/q ratio had to be consistent with the physician's judgment of the significance of the finding in the diagnosis of the disease.

The model allows these prior distributions to be automatically and simply modified as data accumulate. Each time the diagnosis of a disease is confirmed for a patient, the distributions of p's for that disease and q's for all other diseases will be revised.

For example, for the disease polycythemia vera and the descriptor blood pressure the initial estimates of p and q for three findings are shown below:

Disease:        Polycythemia Vera
Descriptor:     Blood Pressure
Findings:

$$p_{Aij} \qquad\qquad q_{Aij}$$

|              |          |          |
|--------------|----------|----------|
| Hypertension | 42/100   | 10/100   |
| Normal       | 57/100   | 88/100   |
| Hypotension  | 1/100    | 2/100    |

If one patient with a confirmed diagnosis of polycythemia vera and two with other diseases all have hypertension, the values are modified as follows:

|              | $p_{Aij}$ | $q_{Aij}$ |
|--------------|-----------|-----------|
| Hypertension | 43/101    | 12/102    |
| Normal       | 57/101    | 88/102    |
| Hypotension  | 1/101     | 2/102     |

In this model the values of the less certain ratios are modified more rapidly than the more certain.

Fourth, estimation by physicians of a prior distribution of probability $P_A$ of occurrence of a given disease in the clinical population based on hospital experience with relative frequency of various hematologic diseases. As in the case of the p's and q's

TABLE 16–I

COMPUTERIZED PARTIAL LISTING FOR ONE PATIENT OF FINDINGS
RELEVANT TO ALL DISEASES IN THE SYSTEM

Clinical Pathology
    Blood count—HGB<7
    Blood count—HGB<7,MCV80–94,MCH>30
    Leukocyte count 10–50000
    Lymphocytes 20–40%
    Lymphocytes Atyp. in PB—None
    Monocytes <=5%
    Eosinophil % – <3%
    Granulocytes (Neut, Eosin, Basophils) 50–70%
    Neutrophils, Hypersegmented—Absent
    Granulocytes (Immature) in PB
    Blasts, Promyel., Prolymph. in P.B. <10%
    Anisocytosis, Etc.—Absent
    Target cells—Absent
    Nucleated Erythroid cells in PB
    Spherocytes in P.B.—Absent
    Platelet count 150–400
    Sickle cell preparation—Positive
Bone Marrow
Lab IA
    Urine color—Normal
Lab III
    Bun elevated

TABLE 16–II

COMPUTERIZED LIST OF ELIMINATED DISEASES OF ONE PATIENT
WITH A $p_{Aij}$ OF 0

Eliminated Diseases
    Megblast. A. of Preg.
        Sex—Male
        Pregnancies—None
    Erythroblastosis fetalis
        Age 20–30 yrs.
Diagnosis on basis of pathognomonic data
    None

this probability was entered as the ratio of two numbers indicating degree of certainty and the numbers can be automatically modified as data accumulate.

Fifth, for each disease, the estimated prior probability $P_A$, the list of possible findings relevant to the disease, and the associated $p_{Aij}$'s and $q_{Aj}$'s were stored on a computer disk. The Bayes Theorem algorithm already shown was programmed for computing the probability that the patient has the given disease from his findings.

A questionnaire relevant to this model was generated by computer from the merged lists of findings relevant to all the diseases in the system. This questionnaire was organized in a form useful either for recording the findings of patients actively being treated in the hospital or for extracting old records. After this form was filled out, the data were key-punched and read into the computer. The following is then printed out:

1. An organized summary of the patient's findings. A sample partial listing for one patient is shown in Table 16–I.

TABLE 16–III

COMPUTERIZED LIST OF ALL DISEASES OF ONE PATIENT IN ORDER OF
PROBABILITY

Differential Diagnosis

| | | |
|---|---|---|
| 1 | Sickel cell anemia | 0.10D 03 |
| 2 | D I Hemolytic anemia | 0.76D 02 |
| 3 | L.E. disease | 0.55D 02 |
| 4 | Multiple myeloma | 0.32D 02 |
| 5 | Hodgkin's disease | 0.31D 02 |
| 6 | Anemia of liver disease | 0.85D 01 |
| 7 | Chronic myelogen. leuk. | 0.79D 01 |
| 8 | Sickle cell trait | 0.59D 01 |
| 9 | Lymphosarcoma | 0.15D 01 |
| 10 | Hemochromatosis | 0.11D 00 |

TABLE 16–IV

COMPUTERIZED LIST OF ONE PATIENT'S FINDINGS WHICH FAVOR
AND ARE AGAINST DIAGNOSIS P/Q>1 IN ORDER OF P/Q

1  Sickle Cell Anemia            0.10D 03

| Patient findings that favor this diagnosis | P/Q |
|---|---|
| Sickle cell preparation—Positive | 20.08554 |
| Joint complaints—Plain alone | 16.44465 |
| Skin color—Jaundice | 14.87973 |
| Blood count—HGB<7, MCV80–94, MCH>30 | 12.18249 |
| Race—Negro | 9.97418 |
| Leg ulcer—Present | 8.16617 |
| Abdomen—Hepatomegaly only | 8.16617 |
| Fever | 4.48169 |
| Cardiac murmurs—Present | 3.00417 |
| Age 20–30 yrs. | 1.53726 |
| **Patient findings that are against this diagnosis** | **P/Q** |
| Priapism—Absent | 0.97142 |
| Bone tenderness—Absent | 0.95983 |
| Convulsions—Absent | 0.95218 |
| Lymphadenopathy—Absent | 0.83527 |
| Abdominal pain—Absent | 0.68386 |

2. A list of those diseases which were eliminated because one of the patient's findings has a $p_{Aij}$ of 0 (Table 16–II). Note that in this example the reasons given for disease elimination are very obvious. This could be made less absolute by using a $p_{Aij}$ of 0 to 0.01.

3. A list of those diseases which were definitively diagnosed because one of the patient's findings had a $q_{Aij}$ of 0. This, too, could be made less absolute by using a $q_{Aij}$ of 0 to 0.01 (Table 16–II).

4. A list of all diseases in order of probability together with the probability score (Table 16–III). The probability score is the probability of each disease x 100. The score for sickle cell anemia is read .10 x $10^3$ or 100. The estimates of the p's and q's when inserted into the formula sometimes allow a score very close to 100, particularly if the disease in question is of very high probability. In rounding off to two decimal places this may appear as 100 in the printout.

5. Analysis of each of the first five (sometimes ten or 15) diseases in the probability list including: (a) List of patient's findings (Table 16–IV) which favor the diagnosis (p/q>1) in order of p/q (Shown for the first disease in Table 16–III). (b) List of

TABLE 16–V
COMPUTERIZED LIST OF FINDINGS TO TEST IN ORDER OF P/Q

| Symptoms to test | P/Q |
|---|---|
| Hemoglobin electrophoresis—Hemoglobin S | 99999.99999 |
| Bilirubin $>=10$ MG% | 148.41316 |
| Reticolocyte count $>10\%$ | 54.59815 |
| Bilirubin 5–10 MG% | 49.40245 |
| BM—Hypercellular | 20.08554 |
| X-Ray, skull, vertical striation | 9.97418 |
| Thymol turbidity (TT)—Increased | 8.16617 |
| X-Ray, gall bladder, stones—Present | 6.04965 |
| X-Ray, heart—Enlarged | 5.47395 |
| Bilirubin 1–5 MG% | 4.95303 |
| Reticulocyte count 5–10% | 4.48169 |
| ESR 0–9 | 1.11628 |
| ESR 9–15 | 1.08872 |
| X-Ray, skull, no vertical striation | 0.90937 |
| X-Ray, gall bladder, stones—Absent | 0.73345 |
| Thymol turbidity (TT)—Normal | 0.53259 |
| X-Ray, heart—Normal | 0.18268 |
| Bilirubin $<1$ MG% | 0.11080 |
| ESR $>15$ | 0.10026 |
| Reticulocyte count 1–2% | 0.04505 |
| BM—Hypocellular | 0.02024 |
| Reticulocyte count $<1\%$ | 0.01228 |
| BM—Normal | 0.00111 |
| Hemoglobin electrophoresis—Hemoglobin SA | 0.0 |
| Hemoglobin electrophoresis—Hemoglobin AA | 0.0 |

patient's findings (Table 16–IV) which are against the diagnosis $(p/q<1)$ in order of p/q. This should be in reverse order so that the findings most against the diagnosis are listed first (Shown for the first disease in Table 16–III). (c) List of findings to test (Table 16–V) in order of p/q. (Shown for the first disease in Table 16–III).

We do not yet have a satisfactory comparison between the Bayesian model and the significance model. However, I can tell you about some very preliminary experiments. The comparison has been made more difficult because of modifications we have continued to make in the significance model, modifications which we thought should result in its improvement.

After completing 31 diseases with 534 findings in the Bayesian model we compared it with this new significance model I just mentioned. A total of 36 cases (eight new patients from the wards of the New York Hospital and 28 cases from the records of the New York Hospital) were abstracted and prepared for entry into the two models by filling out the two questionnaires required. Thirty-one of these patients including the eight new patients were tested in both models and the results compared. After each case was analyzed by the work group, a subjective judgment was made concerning how well the model performed as an aid to the physician in decision-making. The ratings were excellent, good, fair, poor, and unable to evaluate. The results of the evaluation are summarized as follows:

Comparison of Evaluations

| | New Significance (No. of Cases) | Bayes (No. of Cases) |
|---|---|---|
| Excellent | 8 | 14 |
| Good | 10 | 7 |
| Fair | 5 | 1 |
| Poor | 4 | 3 |
| Not evaluable | 4 | 6 |
| | — | — |
| Total | 31 | 31 |

Although the number of cases was few, the Bayesian model had appreciably more excellent ratings and fewer fair and poor ratings than the new significance model. It was therefore concluded that the Bayesian model, even though it was tested with only 31 cases for only 31 diseases, was probably an order of magnitude better than the new significance model.

Since 23 of the cases tested in the new significance model were the same cases tested in the old significance model, a direct comparison of these cases in the two models could be performed. Value judgments were made as described in the last experiment. The results are summarized as follows:

Comparison of Evaluations

| | New Significance (No. of Cases) | Old Significance (No. of Cases) |
|---|---|---|
| Excellent | 6 | 5 |
| Good | 8 | 9 |

| | | |
|---|---|---|
| Fair | 4 | 5 |
| Poor | 3 | 4 |
| Not evaluable | 2 | |
| Total | 23 | 23 |

Despite all the adjustments made in the old significance model, the new significance model was given essentially the same ratings as the old. It was concluded that by making adjustments in the model new aberrations appeared, making it difficult to make further improvements in this model.

Aided by our experience we are able to compare the requirements and attributes of the Bayesian model with those of the significance model and draw conclusions which are shown in Table 16–VI. "Considered" refers to the fact that the requirement is considered by the physician at the time he assigns the significance ratings to the findings. Asterisks pinpoint those attributes which are more difficult to deal with in the significance model and which are relatively easily handled by the Bayesian model. Automatic learning refers to the dynamic process by which the Bayesian

TABLE 16–VI

COMPARISON OF DECISION-MAKING MODELS

| | *Significance Model* | *Bayesian Model* |
|---|---|---|
| Definition of population | Considered | Yes |
| Definition of descriptors and findings | | |
|   (Selection and arranging) | Yes | Yes |
|     Independence vs. Clusters | Considered | Partial solution |
|     Mutually exclusive | Considered | Yes |
|     Exhaustive, including absence of finding | Considered | Yes |
| Frequency of disease | Considered | Yes, $P_A$ |
| Recorded frequency of finding in patients with and without this disease | Considered | Yes $\rbrace$ $p_{Aij}$ |
| Physicians judgment about importance of finding for diagnosis of this disease | Yes | Yes $\rbrace$ and $q_{Aij}$ |
| Diseases mutually exclusive | No | No |
| Automatic learning | *Difficult | Yes |
| Sequential diagnosis possible | Yes | Yes |
| Allowance for uncertainty | Considered | Yes |
| Internal consistency | *Difficult | Yes |
| Algorithm | *Empirical | Defined |

model continually updates and improves the frequency estimates used in the formula. This process is difficult to build into the significance model. Internal consistency is difficult to maintain in the significance model because of the many parameters which must be considered by the physician as he assigns significance ratings to findings. This is not required in the Bayesian model. The algorithm for the significance model has a large empirical component since the weight values of the significance ratings used in the formula are modified by physicians until optimal results are obtained. The Bayes formula is entirely defined. It seems clear from this analysis then that the Bayesian model we are using, which incorporates many of the advantages of the significance model, has in turn some important advantages over the significance model alone.

We plan to pursue this Bayesian model. In developing our ideas we have asked ourselves what the physician does in his decision-making which is not taken into consideration in the Bayesian model we are using. Some of these considerations might be incorporated into future models. We have considered the following parameters:

1. Time relationships. When in the course of time did certain findings appear? This is extremely difficult though not impossible to incorporate into a model. It greatly complicates data entry and data analysis.

2. Dynamic consideration of population. The physician dynamically modifies the total population frame of reference as he makes a decision. Multiple Bayesian models, one for each frame of reference, might simulate this.

3. Dynamic consideration of variability of interdependency of findings from one disease to another. The physician makes allowances for variations in degrees of dependency between two findings in two different diseases. Bayesian models could be developed to partially simulate this, possibly by varying arrangement of descriptors and findings.

4. Use of micro- and macrodecisions in the diagnostic process. Physicians often break large decisions down into smaller and sometimes sequential decisions. This may be due to limitations of

human brain. If these micro- and macrodecisions are desirable and identifiable, they too might be simulated.

5. Maximizing certain diagnoses because of treatment prospects, urgency, severity, prognosis, subjective impact on patient, and cost-risk considerations. These, too, could be incorporated into a Bayesian model.

6. Intuition, as yet undefinable by classical logic.

It seems possible, then, that future models might be developed which would simulate even more closely the diagnostic process as performed by a physician, thereby enhancing the model's effectiveness as an aid to differential diagnosis.

In summary, although we have made some attempts to improve the significance model previously reported for aiding in the differential diagnosis of hematologic diseases, our most recent work has been the development of a Bayesian decision-making model based on the significance model. In a sense, this Bayesian model combines the best features of the significance model with the classical Bayesian approach. Before the model is completely operative it is necessary for physicians to estimate the parameters required for Bayes' formula. This is done so as to be consistent with the physician's judgment of the significance of the various findings in the diseases. Once the model is operative, it is capable of learning the parameters which are then used in the formula. Preliminary experiments indicate that this Bayesian model is probably an order of magnitude better than the significance model alone as an aid to diagnosis.

## REFERENCES

1. Lipkin, M.: The role of data processing in the diagnostic process. In J. A. Jacquez (Ed.) : *The Diagnostic Process.* Ann Arbor, Michigan, Malloy Lithographing, Inc., 1964, pp. 255–280.
2. Engle, R. L., Jr.: Computer-aided differential diagnosis of hematologic diseases. *Digest of the 7th International Conference on Med and Biol Engineering,* Abstract 11–18. Stockholm, 1967, p. 194.
3. Lipkin, M.; Engle, R. L., Jr.; Flehinger, B. J.; Gerstman, L. J. and Atamer, M. A.: Computer-aided differential diagnosis of hematologic diseases. *Ann N.Y. Acad Sci, 161:*670–679, 1969.
4. Ledley, R. S. and Lusted, L. B.: Reasoning foundations of medical diagnosis. Symbolic logic, probability, and value theory aid our understanding of how physicians reason. *Science, 130:*9–21, 1959.

5. Warner, H. R.; Toronto, A. F.; Veasey, G. and Stephenson, R.: A mathematical approach to medical diagnosis. Application to congenital heart disease. *JAMA, 177*:177–183, 1961.

6. Nugent, C. A.; Warner, H. R.; Dunn, J. T. and Tyler, F. H.: Probability theory in the diagnosis of Cushing's Syndrome. *J Clin Endocrinol Metab, 24*:621–627, 1964.

7. Nugent, C. A.: The diagnosis of Cushing's Syndrome. In J. A. Jacquez (Ed.) : *The Diagnostic Process.* Ann Arbor, Michigan, Malloy Lithographing, Inc., 1964, pp. 185–209.

8. Cliffe, P.: Computers in medicine. In D. N. Baron, N. Compston, and A. M. Dawson (Eds.) : Recent Advances in Medicine. London, J. and A. Churchill Ltd., 1968, pp. 1–35.

Chapter 17

# EXPERIMENTS WITH STATISTICAL AND QUASI-STATISTICAL METHODS IN DIAGNOSIS*

JUDITH M. S. PREWITT

## INTRODUCTION

MEDICAL DIAGNOSIS TRADITIONALLY involves evaluation of patient history, symptoms, signs, laboratory tests, and radiological reports in the light of the physician's own knowledge and experience. The physician's logic tends to be sequential, deductive yet informal, and oriented towards recognizing known syndromes and diseases. In the best circumstances, the accuracy of a diagnostic decision is constrained only by the patient's actual and observed condition, and medical knowledge of the occurrence of such observations over the range of possible diseases. However, the physician is hampered in this analysis by his limited ability to uncover complex patterns in mixtures of many interdependent variates, and by his conservatism in estimating probabilities in the presence of redundancy and natural variation.

In contrast, the digital computer, appropriately programmed, can view data simultaneously as well as sequentially, and is especially adept where humans are deficient—namely, in assimilating large collections of mixed-type variates and compensating for complicated correlations among them. To the extent that the diagnostic process can be emulated or described by numeric and logical models, it can be mechanized by computer techniques. Indeed, the digital computer may be indispensible if a great many factors must be considered, yet trustworthy results be obtained soon enough to affect the course of patient care.

To those formal activities which are concerned with emulating the diagnostic logic of the physician we give the name "compu-

294

tational diagnosis." Disciplines which have materially contributed to this area of research include: statistical decision theory, graph theory, pattern recognition, heuristics, numerical taxonomy, and operations research.

The subject matter of computational diagnosis spans a broad spectrum of data structures and objectives. The patient record itself is seldom standardized in content and format. Its constituents comprise nominal and ordinal, qualitative and quantitative, discrete and continuous, subjectively and objectively determined variates. Redundant and irrelevant items, as well as material of questionable accuracy may have been included, whereas diagnostically relevant details may have been unavailable or simply overlooked.

Even differential diagnosis, wherein a patient is evaluated relative to preconceived independent disease alternatives, is subject to complications. The probability distributions of syndromes for suspected diseases, as well as the incidence of these diseases, may represent nonstationary processes in time and in space. For rare diseases, these distributions may not even be ascertainable by sampling. Sometimes diagnostic criteria and disease categories are ill-defined or ambiguous; sometimes the classification scheme for diseases is not as universal as supposed. The totality of possible afflictions is certainly not known, and unlike Mendelyeev's periodic table of the elements, conventional schema for disease classification make no advance provision for yet-to-be discovered maladies.

Many of these between-application differences are idiosyncracies of practice. They can be remedied in principle by more careful and complete data collection, for example. Relevance, redundancy, precision, and consistency can be handled properly with multivariate statistics, particularly by techniques of covariance adjustment. Problems of disease systematics, however, raise conceptual, perceptual, and philosophical issues that are not so readily disposed of.

Yet when model problems, based on adequate patient records and observations are investigated, we surprisingly find that relatively simple algorithms perform well over a broad range of diagnostic situations, even when sufficient conditions for applicability of the methods are patently violated. This empirically verified robustness or insensitivity to superficial between-problem differences encouraged us to develop a library of algorithms which succeeded in many well-defined analyses, and could be extended or generalized quite naturally to more challenging diagnostic material.

This is the evolutionary philosophy we adopted in broaching problems of differential diagnosis and disease taxonomics. This chapter recounts our experiments in computational diagnosis using two different approaches: the first, a method based on classical statistical decision-theory and optimization; the second, a new pattern detection algorithm using quasi-statistical and topological concepts to explicate the notion of a cluster.

In the decision-theoretic approach, the diagnostic process is modelled by optimal classification strategies based on multivariate decision functions or discriminants. Optimization consists of minimizing the expected risk (cost), or alternatively, the probability of "erroneous" decisions. Here error is construed to mean discord between the physician-expert and the computer with respect to a complete set of preconceived and mutually exclusive diagnostic alternatives. Sometimes tolerances are prescribed for the likelihood that a diagnostic decision will be withheld or a critical misclassification made, and the optimization is constrained. The method is considered parametric in so far as the analytical forms of the underlying probability distributions or optimal discriminants are hypothesized in advance. These functions involve constants or population parameters which are statistically estimated, usually under the tutelage of a diagnostician who screens and identifies an exemplary sample. Even when "tuning" of these decision functions is unsupervised, the diagnostician remains the final arbiter of their performance.

However, these statistical techniques are inapplicable when the possible outcomes are not enumerable in advance, when the probability distributions of the variates cannot be specified, when they are computationally intractable, and also when the supply of labelled learning samples is insufficient. In these cases, robust, nonparametric approaches such as cluster analysis may be useful.

The essential components of a non-parametric clustering algorithm are (a) a similarity function defined for all pairs of subjects, (b) a grouping or merger strategy, and (c) a halting criterion. Unlike the statistical approach, neither the nature nor the number of diagnostic classes need be prescribed; the cluster detection proceeds algorithmically, without human intervention or supervision. The advantages of this distribution-free approach, however, are counter-balanced by its inability to lead to strong statistical assertions about the clusters and the error rate.

Although cluster analysis has been used mainly for constructing taxonomies and suggesting evolutionary pathways, it is also germane for prediction. For example, although a classification is defined by grouping on the basis of one set of characteristics, subsequent analysis may reveal other properties that vary systematically over the configuration of categories, and exhibit a similar pattern of between-cluster to within-cluster variation. In these situations, predictions based on the concomittant variables can be made in spite of unavailable primary data, by using the independently determined configuration of clusters. This is the essence of many diagnostic problems.

The basis of each of these two methods will first be described. Background material and results on a diverse set of diagnostic problems will then be presented.

## The Decision—Theoretic Approach in Differential Diagnosis

The decision-theoretic formulation postulates a known set of $N$ diagnostic alternatives and a universe of subjects to which the associated diagnostic labels can meaningfully be applied. A subject is represented by a random vector $X = (x_1, \ldots x_M)$, where each component refers to a specific feature or response, e.g. clinical observation, laboratory test measurement, item of personal history or family background. The M-dimensional vector space $\Omega_M$ spanned by all possible random vectors comprises the feature space or parameter space for the diagnosis problem. Decision theory is used to partition this space into $N$ (usually) mutually exclusive and exhaustive regions, $(R_1, \ldots, R_N)$, corresponding to the $N$ diagnostic alternatives, $(C_1, \ldots, C_N)$. Diagnosis then consists in assigning a subject S to diagnostic category $C_i$ if, and only if, his vectorial representation X falls in the corresponding region $R_i$. The partition is deliberately constructed so that long-term diagnostic performance is optimized in some sense.[8,9,15,26,35]

Sometimes several categories are associated with a single region, or no category is, and no unique decision is forthcoming. This modified approach has favorable implications for the control of error rate, but obviously at the expense of introducing a nonzero rejection rate.[3,4,5,27]

The vectorial representation maps subjects into points and categories into sets, in a space of limited dimensionality. Different selections of variates clearly may lead to topologically diverse descriptions of the universe. Similarly, variants in decision-theoretically relevant details may lead to systems of decision regions which are not homeomorphic. From the point of view of computer implementation, feature spaces in which the images of the various diagnostic categories correspond to compact and well-separated clusters of points are desirable. Part of the motivation for developing feature selection algorithms is to generate such well-behaved configurations in sample spaces of *low* dimensionality.[22]

Desirable diagnostic performance is usually construed to mean consensus between computer and physician. Bayesian optimal decision strategies are suitable formalizations for this because, by design, they maximize the probability of concordance or else minimize the penalties of discordance (computer "error"). The objective function which is optimized (maximized or minimized) is a function of (a) prior probabilities, $p_i$ and $p(X \mid i)$, and (b) a loss matrix $L = (L(D_j \mid C_i))$, specific to the application.

The a priori information consists of (a) the relative frequencies $P = \{p_i: i = 1, \ldots, N\}$ with which the diagnostic labels apply, and (b) the relative frequencies $\{p(X \mid i): i = 1, \ldots, N\}$ of the possible observations within each diagnostic category. In other words, $p_i$ is the prior probability that $C_i$ is the "correct" diagnostic category for a randomly selected subject, and $p(X \mid i)$ is the conditional density for X when the subject does in fact belong to $C_i$. The composite probability density $p(X)$ of the random vector X is a linear combination of these two probability distributions:

$$p(X) = \sum_{i=1}^{N} p(X|i) \, p_i \tag{1}$$

$$p_i > 0 \text{ for } i = 1, \ldots, N \tag{1a}$$

$$\sum_{i=1}^{N} p_i = 1. \tag{1b}$$

Bayes' inversion formula relates these prior distributions to the posterior probability $p(i \mid X)$:

$$p(X)p(i|X) = p_i \, p(X|i) \text{ for all } X \text{ and } i = 1, \ldots, N. \tag{2}$$

Element $L(D_j \mid C_i) \geqq 0$ of the loss matrix expresses the penalty or risk incurred in deciding $D_j$ ($j = 1, \ldots, N$) in favor of category $C_j$, when the subject actually belongs to category $C_i$.

Let $\Psi(j \mid X)$ ($j = 1, \ldots, N$) represent the probability of a decision $D_j$ in favor of $C_j$, conditional on the observation X, and $\Psi(0 \mid X)$ represent abstention $D_0$:

$$\sum_{j=0}^{N} \Psi(j|X) = 1 \tag{3a}$$

$$\Psi(j|X) \geqq 0 \text{ for } j = 0, 1, \ldots, N \tag{3b}$$

The ideal or Bayesian strategy minimizes the expected risk (average loss):

$$\rho(\Psi|P) = \sum_{i=1}^{N} R(\Psi|C_i) \, p_i \tag{4}$$

where

$$R(\Psi|C_i) = \sum_{j=0}^{N} \int \Omega_M \, L(D_j|C_i) \, \Psi(j|X) \, p(X|i) \, du \tag{5}$$

is the average risk for (mis)classifying a member of $C_i$. This is accomplished by favoring the category of least conditional average risk for each individual decision:

$$Y(j|X) = \sum_{i=1}^{N} L(D_j|C_i)\, p(X|i)\, p_i = \sum_{i=1}^{N} L(D_j|C_i)\, p(i|X)\, p(X) \qquad (6)$$

$$= p(X)\, \min\, [\; \sum_{i=1}^{N} L(D_j|C_i)\, p(i|X) : 0 \leq j \leq N]$$

This category is also indicated by the largest discriminant value, $d_j(X) = \ln Y (j \mid X)$.

If a uniform penalty is assigned for erroneous decisions, a uniform bonus is assigned for correct decisions, and indecision is prohibited, then the loss function is represented by a square symmetric matrix:

$$L(D_j|C_i) = 1 - \delta_{ij} = 0,\; i = j \qquad\qquad (7)$$
$$= 1,\; i \neq j$$

Algebraic simplification shows that the average loss is also the probability of misrecognition. The Bayesian strategy favors the most likely category:

$$D_i: X \to C_i \text{ if } p_i p(X|i) \geq p_j p(X|j) \text{ for } i,j = 1, \ldots, N \qquad (8a)$$

or equivalently,

$$D_i: X \to C_i \text{ if } p(i|X) \geq p(j|X). \qquad\qquad (8b)$$

This particular rule can be formulated in terms of the likelihood ratio for categories $C_i$ and $C_j$:

$$\lambda(i,j) = p(X|i)/p(X|j). \qquad\qquad (9)$$

It is the unconditional maximum likelihood decision rule, and is tantamount to the following thresholding operation:

$$D_i: X \to C_i \text{ if } \lambda(i,j) \geq \tau(i,j) = p_j/p_i. \qquad\qquad (10)$$

The well-known (conditional) maximum likelihood decision rule:

$$D_i: X \to C_i \text{ if } \lambda(i,j) \geq 1 \qquad\qquad (11)$$

is the Bayes rule for equal priors ($p_i = p_j$ for all $i,j$). Other useful though suboptimal (non-Bayesian) classification strategies result from varying the likelihood threshold $\tau$; minimizing the maximum probability of mistaken assignment to any one class (minimax strategy of Von Mises); or maximizing the probability of a subject being rightly assigned to one group, when upper bounds are placed on the probability of a subject being wrongly assigned to that group (generalized Neyman-Pearson rule). These variations in objective criterion may be better suited for some diagnosis problems than the classical Bayes approach to optimization.[25]

Linear and quadratic discriminants were used in our studies. They are technically correct when the conditional densities $p(X \mid i)$ are unimodal, ellipsoidally symmetric multivariate densities, and the loss is symmetric, i.e. a decision is forced, and the loss function assigns a standard penalty for erroneous computer decisions, none for correct decisions.[6,7] The discriminants are monotonic functions (logarithms, for example) of the quantity:

$$\alpha_M \, |\Sigma_i|^{-\frac{1}{2}} f[[(X - U_i)^T \Sigma_i^{-1} (X - U_i)]] \, p_i \qquad (12)$$

where $\alpha_M$ is a positive constant depending only on feature space dimensionality M, $U_i$ is the multivariate population mean for $C_i$, $\Sigma_i$ the corresponding dispersion matrix, and f is a monotonically decreasing function of its argument:

$$U_i = E[(X \mid X \varepsilon C_i)] \qquad (13a)$$

$$\Sigma_i = E[(X - U_i)(X - U_i)^T \mid X \varepsilon C_i] \qquad (13b)$$

Multinormal probability densities fall into this category:

$$p(X \mid i) = (2\pi)^{-M/2} |\Sigma_i|^{-\frac{1}{2}} \exp[-\frac{1}{2}(X - U_i)^T \Sigma_i^{-1} (X - U_i)],$$
$$i = 1, \ldots, N. \qquad (14)$$

The robustness of these functions is well-documented [6,27] and they are often used in situations for which they are not strictly optimal.

Were it not for the facts that the probabilities $p_i$ and $p(X \mid i)$ are seldom known, and that the penalties $L(D_j \mid C_i)$ are difficult to quantitate, the discriminant constants could be evaluated, and automated Bayesian diagnosis would become a straightforward computational exercise. In practice, compromise with the strict definition of optimality is unavoidable. Most often, an actual decision rule which approximates the ideal in some sense, and retains the same analytic form, is used. Population parameters or discriminant constants are statistically estimated on the basis of a representative sample consisting of correctly labelled prototypes for each diagnostic category. The process of estimation is called "learning," and the initial data base is called the "learning set." Since explicit external information is supplied, the learning is supervised.

Adaptive and nonadaptive learning techniques each have their advocates. Adaptive learning updates parameter estimates or discriminant constants by using individual observation vectors sequentially. These adjustments are iterated in the hope of generating a sequence of decision rules which gradually improve and asymptotically approach optimal performance.[1] Probabilistic assumptions are not essential when discriminant constants rather than population parameters are updated. Nonadaptive learning, which we favored, uses all the learning samples simultaneously, and when feasible, it is to be preferred, since the question of convergence does not arise.

As an example, in the nonadaptive linear discrimination of two equi-probable Gaussian categories with common covariance, the actual rule is usually the sample analog of the Bayes rule:[8]

$$\text{Ideal: } D_I(X) = X^T \Sigma^{-1}(U_1 - U_2) - \tfrac{1}{2}(U_1 + U_2)^T \Sigma^{-1}(U_1 - U_2) \tag{15a}$$

$$\text{Actual: } D_A(X) = X^T S^{-1}(X_1 - X_2) - \tfrac{1}{2}(X_1 + X_2)^T S^{-1}(X_1 - X_2) \tag{15b}$$

where $X_1$ and $X_2$ are sample means, and $S$ is the pooled sample covariance matrix. (Many authors simply delete the population constant in 15a, and use the analogous actual rule.)

The classification procedure outlined above is a form of statistical hypothesis testing. The discriminants are used as test statistics. The hypothesis: "$X \to C_i$" ($X$ represents a subject S from $C_i$), is accepted whenever $X$ is in the region $R_i$ of maximum $p(X \mid i) \, p_i$:

$$X \to C_i \text{ if } X \, \varepsilon \, R_i = \{X \mid p(X|i)p_i \geqq p(X|j)p_j, \, j = 1, \ldots, N\}. \tag{16}$$

Tie-breaking is unimportant for present purposes. In principle, the Bayes risk or minimum error probability $E_{min}(P)$ can be calculated, given the distribution of the test statistic:

$$E_{min}(P) = \rho(\hat{\Psi}|P) = 1 - \sum_{i=1}^{N} \int_{\Omega_M} \hat{\Psi}((i|X)\ p(X|i)\ p_i\ du$$

$$= 1 - \sum_{i=1}^{N} p_i \int_{R_i} p(X|i)\ du. \qquad (17)$$

Whereas decision rules of the preceding type are easy to implement, it is hard to predict their performance. The expected value of the probability of misclassification is a function of the unknown population parameters not only for the ideal Bayes rule, but for any actual rule as well. As the previous example Equation 15b illustrates, even for the simple case of two Gaussian populations with common covariance, the true error rate of an actual decision rule depends on the very complicated distribution of the random variable $D_A(X)$ ;[11] this is a function of the design sample statistics $X_1$, $X_2$, and S, which in turn are functions of the unknown population means and dispersion, $U_1$, $U_2$, and $\Sigma$. Under these circumstances, performance can at best be estimated. Our preference was to use estimates derived from the observed error rate of a specific actual rule. Although an actual decision rule is inferior to the Bayes rule by definition, estimates based on single experiments tend to be over-optimistic and misleading; the quoted error rates are often based on improper use of the original design sample as the test sample, or else on too small or too homogeneous a test set. However, the actual error rate, (i.e. the observed error rate of a specific actual rule) follows a binomial distribution. Confidence intervals for observed values can therefore be obtained; their lengths, of course, will depend on the size of the test sample.[10]

To supplement the error rate, Wilks' lambda, also a sample statistic, gives a global summary of the discriminatory power of a set of patient variables, relative to the given set of diagnostic alternatives:

$$\Lambda = |\hat{W}| / |\hat{T}| \qquad (18)$$

where $\hat{T}$ is the total sample covariance matrix and $\hat{W}$ is the pooled within-class sample covariance matrix. $\hat{T}$ and $\hat{W}$ are the maximum likelihood estimates of the corresponding population parameters, adjusted for bias. The population parameters are defined by the following:

$$T = E[(X - U)(X - U)^T] \tag{19a}$$

$$W_k = E[(X - U_k)(X - U_k)^T \mid X \; \varepsilon \; C_k] \tag{19b}$$

$$W = \sum_{k=1}^{N} p_k W_k \tag{19c}$$

where $U_k$ are the class centroids and U is the universe centroid:

$$U_k = E[X \mid X \; \varepsilon \; C_k] \tag{19d}$$

$$U = \sum_{k=1}^{N} p_k U_k. \tag{19e}$$

Let $x_{mki}$ represent the $i^{th}$ feature of the $k^{th}$ member of class $C_m$, $X_{m.i}$ the averaged $i^{th}$ feature for $C_m$, $X_{..i}$ the universal average of the $i^{th}$ feature, $N_m$ the number of samples of $C_m$, and N the total number of samples in all G groups. $\hat{T}$ and $\hat{W}$ are matrices with the following elements:

$$\hat{T}_{ij} = \sum_{m=1}^{G} \sum_{k=1}^{N_m} (x_{mki} - X_{..i})(x_{mkj} - X_{..j})/(N - G) \tag{19f}$$

$$\hat{W}_{ij} = \sum_{m=1}^{G} \sum_{k=1}^{N_m} (x_{mki} - X_{m.i})(x_{mkj} - X_{m.j})/(N - G) \tag{19g}$$

for i,j = 1,....,M, and

$$N = \sum_{k=1}^{G} N_k. \tag{19h}$$

$\hat{T}$ can be partitioned into within- and between-class components, $\hat{W}$ and $\hat{B}$, as follows:

$$\hat{T} = \hat{W} + \hat{B} \tag{19i}$$

so that

$$\hat{B}_{ij} = \hat{T}_{ij} - \hat{W}_{ij}, \qquad i,j = 1, \ldots, M. \qquad (19j)$$

Similarly, T can be partitioned:

$$T = \sum_{k=1}^{G} p_k W_k + \sum_{k=1}^{G} p_k \delta_k = W + B. \qquad (19k)$$

$\hat{B}$ is an estimate of its population correspondant:

$$B = \sum_{k=1}^{G} p_k \delta_k. \qquad (19l)$$

The appropriate degrees of freedom are $N-1$ for $\hat{T}$, $N-G$ for $\hat{W}$, and $G-1$ for B. Lambda ($\Lambda$) is the reciprocal of a generalized variance ratio. As a special case, the effectiveness of a single parameter and the effectiveness of a set of parameters for pairwise comparison of classes each reduces to the familiar Fisher's F.[27] (For a discussion of feature effectiveness and feature selection in diagnosis and a selective bibliography see References 22 and 25.)

Since the variables included in a diagnostic study have in effect been pre-screened by the physician, it is not surprising to compute extraordinarily high F-values for single parameters. However, a parameter may be highly significant by traditional statistical standards, yet fail to yield clinically acceptable diagnostic performance. Thus whereas statistical significance commonly connotes discriminatory relevance, the performance requirements in diagnosis are more stringent. To cope with this conceptual disparity, we have introduced new terminology for discussing significance levels in this context (Table 17–I).

## THE CLUSTERING ALGORITHM

Clustering is relevant to diagnosis in two respects. First, it can be used for the *de novo* construction of disease taxonomies, i.e. for delineating distinguishable health states and establishing the corresponding diagnostic characteristics. Second, it can be used for assigning specific diagnostic labels according to the best match between the patient's medical profile and profiles typifying health and disease states. This is merely a restatement of the roles of

**TABLE 17-I**
**SUGGESTED NOMENCLATURE FOR SIGNIFICANCE LEVELS**
**IN TAXONOMIC PROBLEMS**

| Level of Significance for F-Values | Parameter Designation |
|---|---|
| 0.100 | Relevant |
| 0.050 | Important |
| 0.025 | Significant |
| 0.010 | Highly significant |
| 0.005 | Determining |

clustering in classification and discrimination, couched in medical terminology.

A nonparametric cluster synthesis was developed for these purposes, using similarity rather than probability or maximum likelihood as the basis for class membership.[21,23] The algorithm is a three-phase hierarchical procedure which develops a tree of nested clusters in feature space. The essential components of the algorithm are (a) a (dis)similarity function defined for all pairs of subjects and clusters, (b) a grouping or merger strategy, and (c) a halting criterion. The similarity function is dynamic; values change as the clustering proceeds. Cluster formation is governed by optimization of an objective function consisting of all current similarity values.[34] At each iteration, the status of the configuration of clusters is summarized by the current value of an objective measure. The sequence of values of the objective measure can be used for determining a halting criterion or cutoff. Program options permit variation of data normalization, measures of similarity, and clustering strategies.

As long as emphasis is placed on efficient detection of the underlying pattern of classes rather than on perfect assignment of samples to preconceived categories, the hierarchical approach is attractive. Although there is no provision for revoking or revising cluster assignments, many more subjects and variables can be accomodated than in less structured non-hierarchical schemes. Computer time is proportional to the square of the current number of clusters, and decreases with each iteration as clusters are merged. Storage for raw data is proportional to the product of sample size and dimensionality, and storage for the square symmetric (dis)similarity matrix is proportional to sample size squared, clearly the dominant term. Memory is conserved by retaining a triangular sub-array of the dissimilarity matrix for current values of the objective function and the diagonal for mean square cluster radius, leaving the remainder for cluster contributions to the objective measure. The program code itself is parsimonious because data normalization, and likewise cluster fusion, is accomplished by variants of a single transformation.

In the first or preprocessing phase, parameters of the unsorted samples can be transformed by one or more mappings, which are subsumed by the general linear transformation with translation. If X is the original M-vector, and Y the corresponding M'-vector of transformed variates $(M' \leq M)$, then independent linear mappings,

$$Y = A(X - B) \tag{20}$$

where A is an M x M' rotation matrix and B is an M-dimensional translation vector, can be applied successively.

Pure translation results from taking A as the M x M identity matrix, and pure rotation from setting B equal to the null vector in $\Omega_M$. Selected features can be accentuated or de-accentuated by appropriate placement of scale factors in a square diagonal matrix, and they can be suppressed or retained by setting the corresponding diagonal elements to 0 or 1. In a typical application, variables are centered about the universal centroid, and scaled by their standard deviations.

The original variables may also be replaced by a smaller subset which parsimoniously represent their dependence structure and discriminatory information content. For example, uncorrelated, standardized variates can be derived by utilizing special variance-minimizing or cluster-enhancing linear transformations. These mappings can be learned by feature selection based on either principal components analysis, other types of factor analysis, or canonical analysis of a similar, but independent design data set. They are useful for determining the minimum number of independent dimensions needed to adequately account for struc-

tural or discriminatory information latent in the original variables.[13,30] The canonical transformation is potentially useful for
preprocessing since it is not orthonormal, whereas the orthonormal principal components transformation is ineffective for clustering in Euclidian spaces.

Factor analysis is a generic term for correlation-analyzing techniques. The variant known as principal components analysis can
be used to transform to uncorrelated, variance-maximizing variables, which are linear compounds of the original variates. The
transformation matrix V consists of the orthonormalized eigenvectors $v_i$ corresponding to the eigenvalues $\lambda_i$ of the correlation
matrix R:

$$(R - \lambda_i)\ v_i = 0 \qquad\qquad (21a)$$

where

$$v_i^T\ v_i = 1 \qquad\qquad (21b)$$

and

$$v_i^T\ v_j = 0 \text{ for } i \neq j. \qquad\qquad (21c)$$

$\lambda_i$ turns out to be the value of the directionally maximized
variance.

Canonical analysis can be used to obtain uncorrelated, standardized variables for which the ratio of among- to within-class variance is maximized. The transformation matrix V consists of the
eigenvectors of the matrix product $\hat{W}^{-1}\ \hat{B}$:

$$(\hat{W}^{-1}\ \hat{B})\ V = V\ \Lambda \qquad\qquad (22a)$$

where $\hat{B}$ is the sample among-class, and $\hat{W}^{-1}$ the inverse within-
class covariance matrix, and $\Lambda$ is a square diagonal matrix whose
non-zero elements are the eigenvalues $\lambda_i$ of the following:

$$(\hat{W}^{-1}\ \hat{B} - \lambda_i\ I)\ v_i = 0. \qquad\qquad (22b)$$

The compounding coefficients $v_i$ are again subject to normalizing
constraints:

$$v_i^T \hat{W} v_i = 1 \tag{22c}$$

and

$$v_i^T \hat{W} v_j = 0 \text{ for } i \neq j. \tag{22d}$$

$\lambda_i$ turns out to be the maximized generalized variance ratio in the direction of $v_i$:

$$\lambda_i = v_i^T \hat{B} v_i / v_i^T \hat{W} v_i. \tag{22e}$$

Results are relatively immune to moderate perturbations of the transformation coefficients.

Since factor analysis uses no a priori information about class structure, the variance cannot be directly ascribed to natural groupings in the data. Better results are to be expected from empirically learned canonical transformations which explicitly incorporate this type of information. However useful they may be for ovaloid cluster configurations, linear mappings are not a panacea for preprocessing. Sundry interlaced, manifold-like structures do in fact arise in applications, and cannot benefit from this type of cluster-enhancing transformation.

Finally, if the variates have a common range, so that all observation vectors are contained in a definite M-dimensional interval, then the procedure of normalizing a profile $X = (x_1, \ldots, x_M)$ by its elevation and scaling by its scatter, images all profiles on the same M-sphere. Specifically, if each component $x_i$ is adjusted by the mean of all components, $\mu = (1/M) \sum_{i=1}^{M} x_i$, and standardized by the dispersion about this mean,

$$\sigma^2 = (1/M) \sum_{i=1}^{M} (x_i - \mu)^2, \text{ then the following:}$$

$$y_i = (x_i - \mu) / \sigma , i = 1, \ldots, M \tag{23a}$$

is projected on to the hypersphere of radius M:

$$\sum_{i=1}^{M} y_i^2 = (1/\sigma^2) \sum_{i=1}^{M} (x_i - \mu)^2 = M\sigma^2/\sigma^2 = M. \tag{23b}$$

Alternatively, the analysis may proceed directly from dissimilarities or similarities rather than object parameters. Similarities are converted into dissimilarities for programming purposes. These may be normalized to the range 0 to 1, inclusive, so that printed histories of the clustering process retain a manageable format.

The second phase consists of computing a measure of dissimilarity or distance for all sample pairs, using one of a variety of metrics or similarity coefficients. These include Euclidean and other Minkowski metrics, correlation coefficients, nonmetric distance, matching coefficients, generalized Tanimoto distance, and Cattell's measure of nonrandom association. (For a discussion of measures of likeness and numerical taxonomy, see Reference 29.)

The last phase involves iterative processing of the dissimilarity or distance matrix, and merger of the "nearest neighbors" or the "most similar elements" in accordance with the selected clustering strategy. Initially, each sample point is a singleton cluster. At each iteration, the most similar or closest clusters are merged to form a new cluster which replaces them. Dissimilarities or distances between revised clusters and unperturbed clusters are computed. The procedure is repeated until all objects have been subsumed by a universal cluster. A hierarchy or tree of nested clusters, encompassing the entire sample, is generated. The root corresponds to the conjoint partition, branch tips correspond to the disjoint partition, and nodes represent intermediate arrangements.

The triangular array of dissimilarities or distances constitutes an objective function which is minimized at each iteration and drives the formation of clusters. Fusion of clusters, in turn, entails reassessment of intercluster differences and repetition of the entire cycle. This process of dynamic reevaluation involves progressive modification of the dissimilarity matrix by variants of a single transformation which can be activated to emphasize either compactness, connectedness, or central tendency of the resultant clusters.

Let $C_p$ and $C_q$ be distinct clusters which merge to form cluster $C_r = C_p U C_q$ at the $i^{th}$ iteration, and let $C_t$ be any other cluster coexisting with $C_r$ at the completion of this step. We require that the dissimilarity or distance ("difference") $\delta_{tr} = \delta(C_t, C_r)$ between $C_t$ and $C_r$ be a symmetric, nonnegative function of only the differences between $C_t$ and the immediate precursors of $C_r$:

$$\delta_{tr} = \delta(C_t, C_r) = fcn[\delta(C_t, C_p), \delta(C_t, C_q), \delta(C_p, C_q)] \quad (24)$$

with the following properties:

$$\delta_{tr} \geq 0 \quad (24a)$$

$$\delta_{tr} = \delta_{rt} \quad (24b)$$

$$\delta_{tt} = 0 \quad (24c)$$

$$\delta_{tr} = 0 \text{ only if } C_t = C_r. \quad (24d)$$

In practice, the union $C_r = C_p \cup C_q$ inherits the name of the constituent with smaller index: $r = \min[p,q]$.

The minimum function minimizes inter-set distance in the topological sense:

$$\delta_1(C_t, C_r) = \min_{p, q} [\delta(C_t, C_p), \delta(C_t, C_q)]. \quad (25)$$

By linking nearest neighbors, it emphasizes connectedness. The maximum function minimizes resultant cluster diameter, i.e. minimizes the largest intra-cluster distance:

$$\delta_2(C_t, C_r) = \max_{p, q} [\delta(C_t, C_p), \delta(C_t, C_q)]. \quad (26)$$

By recomputing distance on the basis of farthest neighbors, it emphasizes compactness. The compactness and connectedness strategies enjoy the property of being invariant under monotone transformations of the dissimilarity matrix. Thus only rank order of dissimilarities has any operational meaning, and absolute values are not germane. This property is particularly important for clustering nominally scaled variables, which so often appear in psychological studies.

The centrality function supplants two fused clusters by one of four geometric or statistical entities representing a gestalt property of the conglomerate: (a) the cluster average with respect to squared distance, (b) the median, (c) the centroid, and (d) the internal variance minimizer. The first three techniques express the central tendency of the components in the sense of an average position or statistical property. The last technique projects the effect of future mergers on the homogeneity of the resultant conglomerates.

In the first case, the new cluster is represented by a point whose effective squared distance from any coexisting cluster equals the weighted average of squared distances from constituents:

$$\delta^2{}_{31}(C_t, C_r) = (n_p/n_r)\, \delta^2{}_{tp} + (n_q/n_r)\, \delta^2{}_{tq} \qquad (27a)$$

where $n_p$, $n_q$, and $n_r = n_p + n_q$ are the number of objects in clusters $C_p$, $C_q$, and $C_r$, respectively. In the second case, the new cluster is represented by a point midway between the constituents:

$$\delta^2{}_{32}(C_t, C_r) = 1/2\; \delta^2{}_{tp} + 1/2\; \delta^2{}_{tq} - 1/4\; \delta^2{}_{pq}, \qquad (27b)$$

while in the third case, the centroid is used:

$$\delta^2{}_{33}(C_t, C_r) = (n_p/n_r)\; \delta^2{}_{tp} + (n_q/n_r)\; \delta^2{}_{tq} - (n_p n_q/n_r{}^2)\; \delta^2{}_{pq}. \;(27c)$$

The final case postulates effective positions relative to the composite $C_r = C_p U C_q$ so that, should $C_r$ be merged in turn with cluster $C_t$ during the next iteration, the minimum increment in within-cluster heterogeneity (as measured by within-cluster "variance" or sum of squared member-to-member differences) shall ensue:

$$\delta^2{}_{34}(C_t, C_r) = (n_t + n_p)/(n_t + n_r)\; \delta^2{}_{tp} + (n_t + n_q)/$$
$$(n_t + n_r)\; \delta^2{}_{tq} - n_t/(n_t + n_r)\; \delta^2{}_{pq} \qquad (27d)$$

These six strategy-defining formulae are special cases of the following single transformation:

$$\delta^2{}_{tr} = \alpha_p\, \delta^2{}_{tp} + \alpha_q\, \delta^2{}_{tq} + \beta_{pq}\, \delta^2{}_{pq} + \gamma_{tpq}\, |\, \delta^2{}_{tp} - \delta^2{}_{tq}\, | \qquad (28)$$
$$= (\alpha_p \pm \gamma_{tpq})\, \delta^2{}_{tp} + (\alpha_q \mp \gamma_{tpq})\, \delta^2{}_{tq} + \beta_{pq}\, \delta^2{}_{pq}$$

and are obtained by assigning appropriate constant values to the parameters $\alpha_p$, $\alpha_q$, $\beta_{pq}$, and $\gamma_{tpq}$. The correct assignments are automatically made by the clustering program in accordance with the user's selected strategy.

The dynamics of the situation are summarized by successive values of an objective measure which is a generalization of the multivariate within-cluster to total variance ratio, computed in the space of transformed variates. Within-cluster "variance" increases continually as clusters are fused. Since the total "variance" or sum of squared dissimilarities is fixed, there is an inevitable equal reduction in between-cluster "variance." The objective measure therefore is bounded and ranges from a value of 0 for the disjoint partition (no internal heterogeneity) to a value of 1 for the conjoint partition (no external heterogeneity). These changes are computed at the same time that inter-cluster differences are revised. Both the objective function and the objective measure are monotonically increasing functions of the number of clustering events. In general, clusters which are merged because they are currently "the closest" or "the most alike" do not correspond to the smallest possible decrement in between-cluster "variance." However, when the merger strategy of Equation 27d is selected, minimizing the objective function at each iteration coincides with minimizing the objective measure, and cluster formation tends to preserve within-cluster homogeneity or internal structure.

Values of the objective measure are instrumental in selecting significant clusters. In general, the level which seems to correspond to psychological significance is a function of the underlying probability distributions and the cluster merger strategy. Its role as a cutoff criterion is comparable to the role of significance levels in hypothesis testing. In the case of multivariate normal populations with common covariance which are analyzed in Euclidean space, the objective measure equals Wilks' lambda, and it leads to an exact statistical test of significance. In our experiences with diverse data sets, clusters existing at the 0.1 level of the objective measure were persistently in harmony with human judgments.

A variety of displays are available to the user of the program. A summary of preprocessing and processing specifications (input/output formats, data transformations, metrics or measures of similarity, and cluster strategy), and sample statistics (means and covariances), are always provided. A detailed history of cluster formation, giving cluster size and membership, and the current dissimilarity matrix are available on request. Graphs of the objective function and objective measure for the succession of cluster mergers are constructed on the high speed printer. The most important displays are trees showing the hierarchy of clusters with three different ordinates: (a) intercluster distance at time of merger, (b) cluster radius at time of merger, and (c) value of the objective measure at time of merger (Fig. 17–4a-e).

Since the arrangement of clusters is hierarchical and can be described by a tree structure, it is possible to find an ultrametric distance $\delta$ which leads to the same configuration. Values of either the objective function or the objective measure can be used for this purpose, since both sequences are strictly monotonic. The requirement that $\delta$ be a distance implies that the following triangle inequality holds:

$$\delta_{tr} \leqq \delta_{ts} + \delta_{sr}. \tag{29}$$

The stronger ultrametric property requires that the distance from a cluster $C_t$ to a newly formed cluster $C_r = C_pUC_q$ be no greater than its distance to either constituent:

$$\delta_{tr} \leqq \max\ [\delta_{ts}, \delta_{sr}]. \tag{30}$$

Conversely, whenever such an ultrametric is defined initially, a unique hierarchical configuration is generated.

## CLASSIFICATION OF WHITE BLOOD CELLS: A MODEL LINEAR PROBLEM

The objective of the leukocyte study was to distinguish the five types of white cells found in normal human peripheral blood on the basis of computer processing of digitized micro-images. Relevance to automating the differential white cell count and the detection of rare cell abnormalities is immediate, provided that more rapid electro-optical input of slide data is feasible.

For this purpose, stained white blood cells were imaged monochromatically and digitized by a flying-spot microscanner, CYDAC, with high spatial and tonal resolution. Computer programs separated cell images from background, articulated the major morphological units, and generated approximately 80 numeric parameters for describing each white cell image. A leukocyte is represented by a point in a multidimensional vector space in which the coordinate axes are systematically identified with these parameters.[18]

Classification of specimens utilized Bayesian linear discriminants with the maximum likelihood strategy in order to minimize the long-term probability of misclassification. Constants of the linear discriminants were estimated from learning samples labelled by a cytologist. The ideal linear rule is optimal in the sense of Bayes if the multivariate probability densities for the five cell categories are unimodal and ellipsoidally symmetric, and share a common covariance matrix.

The 80 cell parameters varied greatly in their discriminatory relevance and covariance properties, and were highly redundant. In fact, only a small subset was actually necessary for discrimination, and many different sets of four to seven parameters were satisfactory. The best-performing set of variates were not those we would be inclined to pick on the basis of intuitive interpretation of the parameters.[19] As in any discrimination problem, the minimum dimensionality required for acceptable performance levels depended on several factors: (a) the relevance of the available parameters, their resolution and their interrelationships; (b) the number of categories to be distinguished; and (c) the number of learning samples.

In order to condense and optimize the cell representation, relative to the given variates and the linear form selected for the discriminant functions, a feature selection algorithm was used. This procedure directed a stepwise accumulation of predictors in a manner which tries to maximize the between-class to within-class generalized variance ratio (and incidentally, the sample divergence). It would succeed in doing this precisely, were we dealing with multinormal probability densities and independent variates. At each step, the set of already selected parameters is augmented by the as-yet-unselected parameter which gives the maximum, above-threshold increment in the generalized variance ratio, or else is purged of the parameter which makes the least, below-threshold contribution in the context of the remaining parameters.[26,28] The continuous improvement in cluster separability and internal homogeneity is illustrated in Fig. 17–1.

The selection algorithm produced an ensemble of four parameters capable of perfect linear discrimination of the five leukocyte types—that is, able to secure agreement between the computer analysis and the cytologist who provided the labelled learning sample (Table 17–II). That no new information is

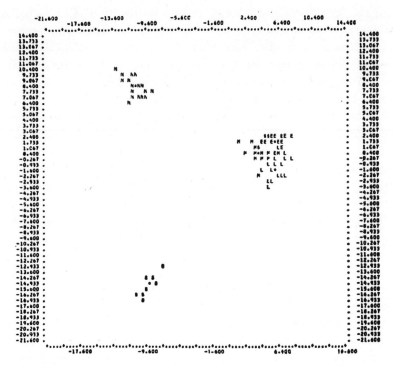

Fig. 17–1A

Figure 17–1. Canonical transformations of leukocyte features. A sequence of canonical spaces for leukocytes based on an increasing number of original variates shows continuously improving separation and condensation of clusters in the best two projections. Individual cell vectors in a sample of 92 are indicated by the letters L, M, N, E, and B, according to their type: lymphocyte, monocyte, neutrophil, eosinophil, and basophil. (A) The best three original variables have been retained, (B) The best five variables are included, and (C) The best 33 variables are included.

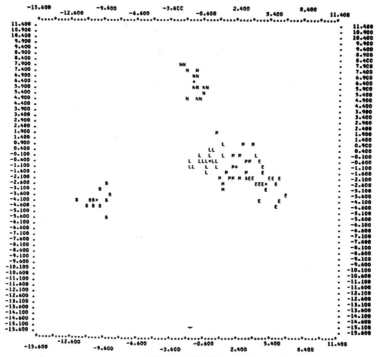

Figure 17–1B.

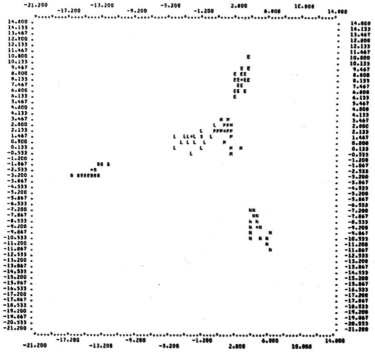

Figure 17–1C.

## TABLE 17–II
### CLASSIFICATION PERFORMANCE FOR CELL DISCRIMINATION
*Percent Correct Classification*

| Iteration | Parameter Added | Cell type | | | | | |
|---|---|---|---|---|---|---|---|
| | | L | M | N | E | B | All |
| 1 | Contrast | 10 | 50 | 100 | 50 | 92 | 58 |
| 2 | Absorbance ratio: nucleus/cell | 80 | 85 | 100 | 100 | 100 | 94 |
| 3 | Mean cell density | 95 | 95 | 100 | 100 | 100 | 98 |
| 4 | Total absorbance | 100 | 100 | 100 | 100 | 100 | 100 |

*Note:* Percent correctly classified in a sample of 92 white cells, with the five categories represented approximately equally in the sample. The letters L, M, N, E, B represent Lymphocytes, monocytes, neutrophils, eosinophils, and basophils, respectively. Iteration refers to the step in the process of feature selection at which the indicated parameter was added to the growing collection of parameters to be used in linear discrimination.

gained with additional variates can also be seen from the essentially linear relationship between inter-cluster distance and dimensionality, using the sequence of best representations generated by the feature selection procedure (Fig. 17–2) .[25]

The five white cell types are represented as well-dispersed, compact clusters even in the space of the three best features (Fig. 17–3a) . If we compute and apply the canonical linear transformation which maximizes between-class to within-class variances in a new coordinate system of standardized and uncorrelated variables, the clustering phenomena are further enhanced (Fig. 17–3b). The intense unimodal clumping and the high degree of separability make apparent the reasons for the success of linear functions, although technically they are not the optimal discriminants.

These demonstrations suggested that the five cell types might be recovered from the data without the need for a learning set or for an analysis based on distributional assumptions, e.g. by a clustering technique. There are also other reasons for seeking a nonparametric or distribution-free approach. Although linear discrimination was effective for unambiguous leukocyte samples, it is likely to prove deficient in dealing with harder-to-distinguish examples. This possibility is further complicated by the fact that the joint probability densities for the several cell types do, in fact, differ in covariance structure and symmetry, and they re-

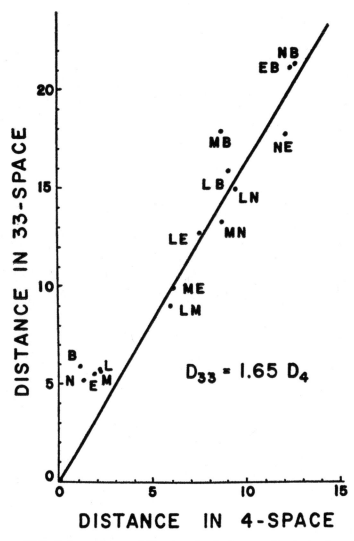

Figure 17–2. Information stabilization in leukocyte discrimination. Inter-cluster distance (mean distance between all member points) and root-mean-square cluster radius in the best four-space for leukocytes, are plotted against the same quantities in 33-space. The almost linear relationship indicates no genuine gain in information as the number of variables increases beyond four. Variables were selected sequentially, using stepwise feature selection based on maximizing the covariance-adjusted increment in between- to within-class variance ratio.

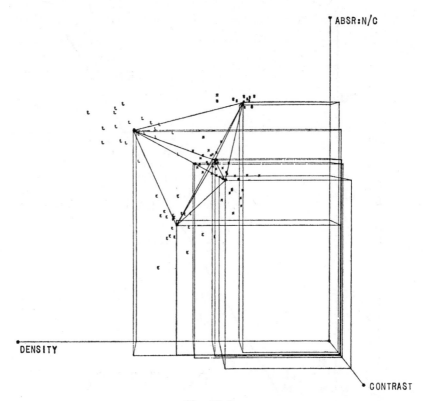

Fig. 17–3a.

Figure 17–3. White blood cell discrimination: best representation.

a. An actual sample of 92 white cells is represented in a perspective view of the space of the three best parameters for discrimination: contrast, nuclear to cell absorbance ratio, and mean cell optical density. Individual cells are indicated by letters L, M, N, E, and B, according to their type: lymphocyte, monocyte, neutrophil, eosinophil, and basophil. Lines connecting group centroids and marking their projections onto the coordinate planes have been introduced as a visual aid.

b. The canonical linear transformation to uncorrelated and standardized coordinates dramatizes the clustering and separability latent in the data for Fig. 17–3a, since this is a space of maximum total to within-class generalized variance ratio, $\Lambda^{-1}$. The between-to within-class generalized variance ratio is maximized automatically at the same time.

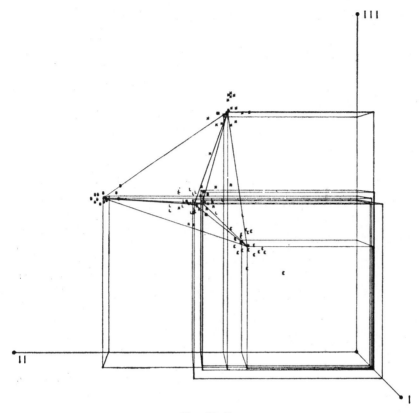

Fig. 17–3b.

spond differently to variations in the preparation and presentation of specimens.

The first application of the hierarchical clustering algorithm was to validating the traditional leukocyte taxonomy which formed the basis of the statistical approach. Using the method as described above, recovery of the five white cell types was completely effective at the 0.1 level of the objective measure (Fig. 17–4a-e) . The five categories were stable over a range of normalization procedures, metrics, and cluster merger strategies. For Minkowski spaces with exponents 1.0, 1.5, and 2.0, classification errors on a sample of approximately 100 cells were only 1, 1, and

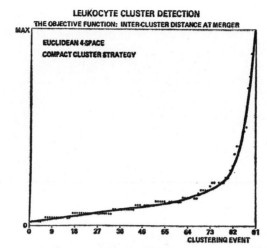

Figure 17–4a

Figure 17–4. White blood cell discrimination: cluster synthesis. The 92 leukocytes of Fig. 17–3 were represented in a Euclidean space using the four parameters which lead to perfect linear discrimination: contrast, nuclear to cell relative absorbance, mean cell density, and total cell absorbance. Compact groups were generated by minimizing cluster diameter at each iteration. Essentially the same configuration was also produced by the centrality merger strategy.

a. The objective function. Inter-cluster distance at time of merger, as a function of cluster event number.

b. The objective measure. Within-cluster to total variance ratio in the metric space of choice, as a function of cluster event.

c. Cluster formation tree. Tree representation with the objective function (intercluster distance at time of merger) as ordinate.

d. Cluster size tree. Tree representation with cluster radius as ordinate.

e. Final cluster tree. Tree representation with the objective measure (generalized variance ratio) as ordinate.

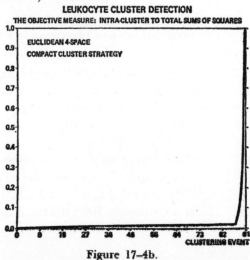

Figure 17–4b.

## LEUKOCYTE CLUSTER FORMATION  TREE: 1

EUCLIDEAN 4-SPACE
COMPACT CLUSTER STRATEGY

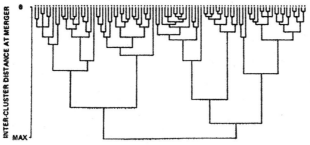

Figure 17-4c.

## LEUKOCYTE CLUSTER FORMATION  TREE: 2

EUCLIDEAN 4-SPACE
COMPACT CLUSTER STRATEGY

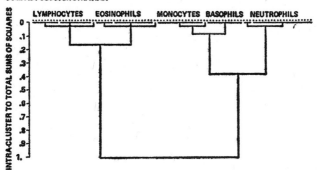

Figure 17–4d.

## LEUKOCYTE CLUSTER FORMATION  TREE: 3

EUCLIDEAN 4-SPACE
COMPACT CLUSTER STRATEGY

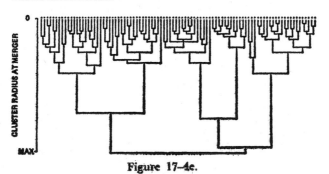

Figure 17–4e.

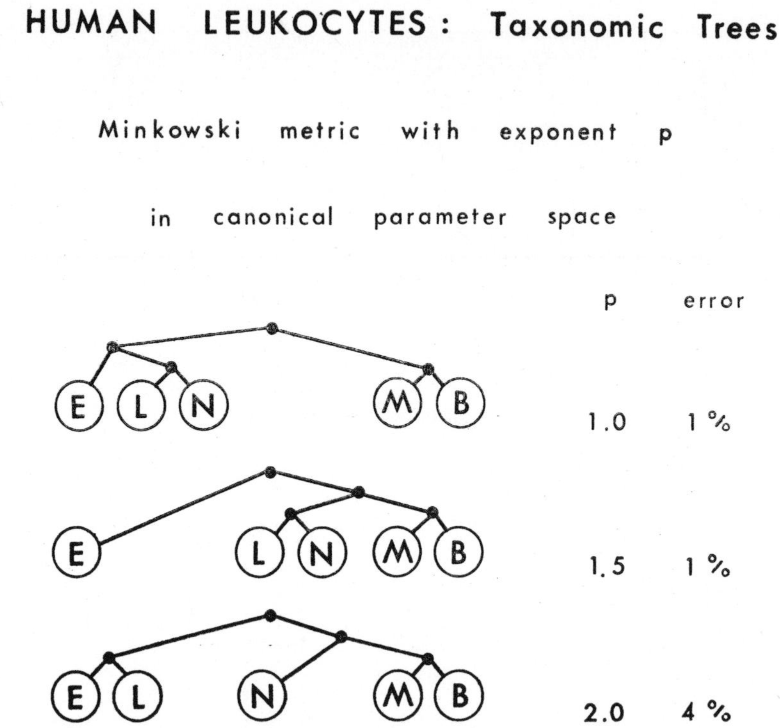

# HUMAN    LEUKOCYTES :   Taxonomic   Trees

Minkowski    metric    with    exponent    p

in    canonical    parameter    space

Figure 17–5. Comparison of several taxonomic trees for the same sample of white blood cels. These trees were computed in different n-dimensional Minkowski spaces by varying the value of the exponent p in the formula for distance between points $X = (x_1,\ldots,x_n)$ and $Y = (y_1,\ldots,y_n)$ :

$$d(X, Y) = \sum_{i=1}^{n} [(x_i - y_i)^p]^{1/p}.$$

All five cell types are detected. They merge at nodes of varying levels for the three trees, but the terminals representing them maintain their left-to-right pattern. The trees for p=1.0 and p=1.5 reconstitute the cytologist's classification of the test sample with less error (1 percent) than the trees in Euclidean space (4 percent).

4 percent, respectively. The nodal positions marking merger of the main cell types varied with the metrics, but the categories maintained a regular pattern of relationship (Fig. 17–5).

Thus taxonomic consistency was established between the un-

# THE DENVER CLASSIFICATION OF HUMAN CHROMOSOMES

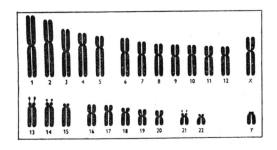

| | 1 | 2 | 3 | 4 | 5 | 6 | 7 | 8 | 9 | 10 | 11 | 12 | X |
|---|---|---|---|---|---|---|---|---|---|---|---|---|---|
| Short | 41.5 | 31.6 | 30.8 | 16.6 | 16.0 | 20.6 | 18.6 | 15.3 | 16.2 | 13.8 | 15.0 | 12.4 | 19.9 |
| Long | 44.7 | 49.1 | 36.9 | 45.7 | 42.2 | 34.9 | 31.5 | 31.2 | 29.2 | 30.7 | 28.5 | 29.9 | 35.2 |

| | 13 | 14 | 15 | 16 | 17 | 18 | 19 | 20 | 21 | 22 | Y |
|---|---|---|---|---|---|---|---|---|---|---|---|
| Short | 4.8 | 5.2 | 4.8 | 12.1 | 9.0 | 6.4 | 9.6 | 9.3 | 4.2 | 3.9 | 2.0 |
| Long | 28.9 | 28.8 | 27.1 | 18.4 | 20.5 | 19.2 | 13.9 | 12.2 | 12.4 | 11.6 | 15.7 |

Figure 17–6. Idealization of the Denver chromosome classification. Pooled values of arm lengths and total lengths from several sources have been combined. The sketch highlights prominent morphological features such as centromeres and satellites. (From Penrose, 1966)

verbalized discriminatory criteria used by the morphologist, and the feature space based on computer-generated, tonally oriented leukocyte parameters. By this we mean that the morphologist's classification of white blood cells and the numerical taxonomy agreed, although they were based on qualitatively different criteria. This, we felt, was a fundamental test for the clustering algorithm.[24,25]

## Chromosome Classification By Clustering

In a more stringent test, the clustering procedure was used to reconstruct the seven principal groups of human autosomal chromosomes, using pooled mean values of mitotic chromosome arm lengths and centromeric index as they have been accepted in the Denver-London system of classification[2,17] (Fig. 17-6). Detection of homologues was not at issue here. Analyses in Euclidean

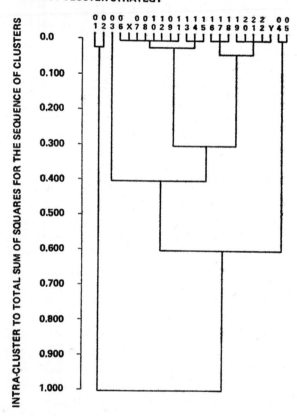

CLUSTER TREE FOR CHROMOSOMES
OF THE DENVER CLASSIFICATION

Figure 17–7. Chromosome classification by cluster synthesis.

a. The conventional chromosome assignments have been reconstituted, with minor exceptions for the largest and smallest chromosomes, using the Denver pooled chromosome measurements in Euclidean two-space with the nearest-neighbor or connectivity-emphasizing merger strategy. Similar arrangements with altered resolution were obtained in infra-Euclidean two-spaces with Minkowski exponents less than 2.

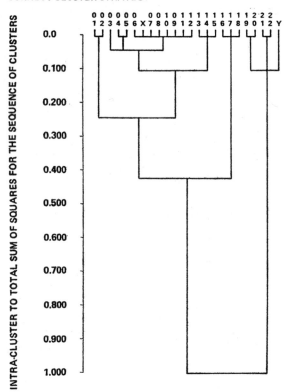

Figure 17–7b. Cluster synthesis applied to the logarithmic transformations of the Denver mean chromosome arm and total lengths in Euclidean space (the "ratio scale") recovers the traditional groupings with chromosome 3, however, maintaining its integrity.

and non-Euclidean two-spaces based on the Denver mean values were performed, and data preprocessing was confined to centering and scaling by range or by standard deviation. Chromosome constellations compatible with the groups enumerated in the Denver classification: A (1–3), B (4–5), C (6–12 and X), D (13–15), E (16–18), F (19–20), and G (21–22 and Y), emerged at low values of the objective measure for a broad range of dissimilarity measures and clustering strategies. For example, using long arm and total chromosome length, scaled by their standard deviations, as parameters in Euclidean space, the conventional associations were reproduced by the nearest-neighbor merger strategy, except that the small autosomes of groups F and G were consolidated; chromosome X was grouped with 6 as expected, but in a discrete subcluster of group C; and chromosomes 1, 2, and 3 were individually discernible (Fig. 17–7a). However, resolution shifted to an arrangement identical with the Denver standard when chromosome parameters were first logarithmically transformed. The conventional seven groups were successfully reconstituted with the minor modification that chromosome 3 was recognized as an additional cluster, closer to Group B than to group A (Fig. 17–7b). Similar experiments using arm lengths hand-measured on an enlarged microphotograph of an actual metaphase, and DNA estimates obtained manually from digitized scans, yielded kindred results plus proper homologue assignments without forced pairing.

### DISCERNMENT OF HEALTH STATE FROM SERUM IMMUNOGLOBULIN PATTERNS: A QUADRATIC PROBLEM

The determination of state of health on the basis of multiple biochemical determinations is a particularly challenging problem in medical decision-making because normalcy and pathology, the two states to be discriminated, are not always sharply defined in the physician's mind, nor clearly indicated by pronounced modes and discontinuities in the data. Medical evaluation usually involves comparison of single-time test results for the various biological or physiological indicators with "normal ranges" derived from similar measurements in "normal" subjects. The "normal range" for a particular variable is traditionally taken as the sample mean ± two standard deviations.[14] The individuality of clinical biochemical patterns is *ipso facto* ignored in diagnosis, since long-term serial measurements on healthy individuals are seldom made. Moreover, since correlation is completely ignored, the sequence of unrelated univariate decisions, assuming erroneously as it does, statistical independence of variables, is more prone to errors of classification than would be a single covariance-sensitive multivariate decision (Fig. 17–8).

The standard deviation of the single-time determinations used to define "normal ranges" consists of four components of variation: (a) an analytical component (random replication and instrumentation errors), (b) an intra-individual or subject-specific

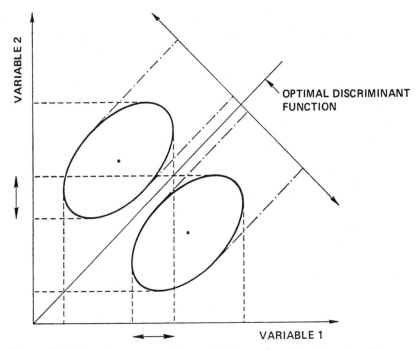

Figure 17–8. Covariance as an element in improving discrimination. For purposes of illustration, two ellipsoidally symmetric distributions differing in location but not in dispersion are represented by probability density isopleths. Orientation, scale, and location are such that ranges of variation in both coordinate directions preclude univariate discrimination. The oblique line, however, is an excellent decision boundary.

component, (c) an inter-individual, intrastate component, and (d) an interstate component. The clinical literature amply attests to the fact that, not only do "normal ranges" shift and dilate with age, but factors such as sex, race, heredity, and environment operate concurrent with disease. Even test values for a healthy individual exhibit wide daily or weekly fluctuations. Normal ranges correlate highly with good health, and outliers with disease in young adults, but aberrant values in older subjects are often less important medically. Uncertain laboratory quality control can further and artifactually distort the distribution of abnormal as well as normal values in both individual and composite group biochemical profiles.

Accordingly, it is appropriate to think, not of two well-defined categories, normal and abnormal, which are to be distinguished in the decision-theoretic manner, but of a stochastic multivariate continuum, in which individual positions continuously vary. The problem for computational diagnosis is to partition this continuum optimally in some sense. In view of the apparent accentuation of biological variation by analytical error and intra-individual variability, delineation of the intermediate zone between "normal" and "abnormal" constitutes the principal challenge to computational diagnosis.

The objective of the immunoglobulin study was to develop algorithms for assessing health state, given single-time clinical observations of serum immunoglobulin concentration and a modicum of ancillary patient information. There were just two diagnostic possibilities: "healthy" and "not healthy."

The immunoglobulin study contrasted with the leukocyte study in four important respects. First, it involved discrete and continuous variates simultaneously. Second, the diagnostic categories consisted of demonstrable (biracial) subcategories. Third, the line of demarcation between health states, as defined by the physician, is "fuzzy" due to correlations of within-state biological variability with age and race. Fourth, class membership requirements were somewhat arbitrary but conservative; the criterion for ill health was inpatient status, while the criterion for good health was physical fitness for employment in the same hospital.

The discriminant function screening procedure for health state, based on laboratory determination of serum immunoglobulin concentration, took some, but by no means all of the forementioned sources of variation into account. Separate tests indicated tight laboratory quality control. Although serial measurements were available for some patients, there were none for controls, and in any case, these were insufficient for statistical studies. We were committed to exploring the possibility of a very general screening test that would be useful under the same conditions that clinical medical evaluations were being made.

For each subject, concentration of gamma globulins Ig G, Ig A, and Ig M were measured by conventional chemical analysis, and total immunoglobulin concentration EG was also obtained by electrophoresis. From these four analytical determinations, five additional variables—relative concentrations—were computed. The subject's medical profile consisted of twelve variables, ten continuous and two nominal, as follows:

1. EG (by electrophoresis)
2. Ig G (by chemical analysis)
3. Ig A (by chemical analysis)
4. Ig M (by chemical analysis)
5. $\Sigma G = Ig\ G + Ig\ A + Ig\ M$
6. $Ig\ G\ /\ \Sigma G$
7. $Ig\ A\ /\ \Sigma G$
8. $Ig\ M\ /\ \Sigma G$
9. $\Sigma G\ /\ EG$
10. race ($+1$ for Caucasian, $-1$ for Negro)
11. sex ($+1$ for male, $-1$ for female)
12. age

There are effectively only 11 degrees of freedom since variables 6, 7, and 8 are linearly dependent.

The decision rules were synthesized using data on 226 patients and controls (67 percent Caucasian, 33 percent Negro), and validated using data on 54 additional subjects (63 percent Caucasian, 37 percent Negro). A deliberate effort was made by the collaborating hematologists to match patients and controls within each racial group with respect to socioeconomic levels and environment.

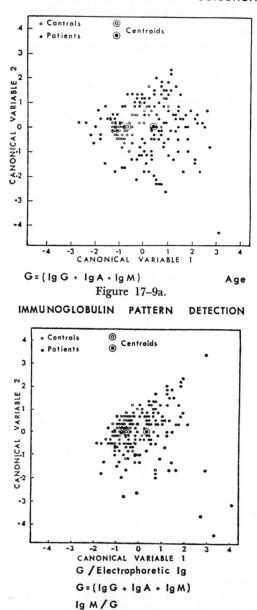

IMMUNOGLOBULIN PATTERN DETECTION

$G = (Ig\,G + Ig\,A + Ig\,M)$      Age

Figure 17–9a.

IMMUNOGLOBULIN PATTERN DETECTION

G / Electrophoretic Ig

$G = (Ig\,G + Ig\,A + Ig\,M)$

Ig M / G

Figure 17–9c.

Figure 17–9. Typical canonical two-spaces for the serum immuno globulin concentration study. Examination of the configurations in conjunction with analysis of dispersion indicates that nonlinear discriminants are appropriate, and furthermore, that a hybrid scheme, consisting of a logical decision tree to adjust for racial characteristics, plus quadratic dis-

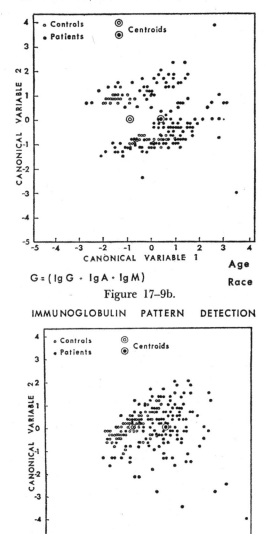

IMMUNOGLOBULIN   PATTERN   DETECTION

G = ( Ig G + Ig A + Ig M )

Figure 17–9b.

IMMUNOGLOBULIN   PATTERN   DETECTION

G / Electrophoretic Ig

G = ( Ig G + Ig A + Ig M )

Ig M / G

Figure 17–9d.

crimination within each tree branch, may provide a useful screening tool. The variables used are in a: total immunoglobulin concentration, $\Sigma G = IgG + IgA + IgM$, and age; in b: $\Sigma G$, plus age and race; in c: the three best parameters, $\Sigma G$, $IgM/\Sigma G$, ıd $\Sigma G/EG$; and in d: $\Sigma G$, $IgM/\Sigma G$, $\Sigma G/EG$, along with age and race.

Patients were hospital inpatients, having a fairly uniform distribution of age from 0 to 78 years, with median and mode coinciding at 42 years. Controls were candidates for hospital jobs, having satisfactory pre-employment health history, physical examination, radiological reports, and the customary hematological, white cell, urological, and serological tests. They had a positively skewed age distribution with mode at 20 years and mean at 27 years.

Canonical transformations using linear combinations of variates facilitated visualization of the data by enhancing within-state clustering and between-state separation. The geometric configurations were similar for virtually all combinations of variates tested. Graphic displays of the best two-dimensional subspaces suggested the presence of strong correlations among the variates, independent of health state, but different covariance properties for the two health states. Healthy subjects comprised a compact cluster core, while patients constituted a more diffuse, asymmetrical halo. There is visual suggestion of overlapping subclusters. Individual plots by race showed similar shapes but different locations, orientations, and scales (Fig. 17–9).

Formal multivariate analysis of dispersion corroborated this. White and nonwhite controls have comparable correlation structures, as do white and nonwhite patients, but mean vectors and standard deviations are racially dependent for each health state. Age was significantly correlated with the immunological factors. In fact, it is the most powerful single indicator of health state, by itself yielding correct evaluations for 79 percent of the controls and 65 percent of the patients. There were significant correlations of different sign among the immunological factors. This indicated that adjustment for covariance was warranted in any feature selection procedure for two reasons: (a) to eliminate redundancy, and (b) to capitalize on those correlations which are contradistinct to inter-group mean differences. Correlation graphs for some of the factors are shown in Fig. 17–10. These preliminary computations implied that separate discriminant analyses for each racial group were warranted, and that, in any case, nonlinear discriminants were more appropriate than linear functions.

The stepwise selection procedure based on maximizing incremental discriminatory power as measured by Wilks' lambda

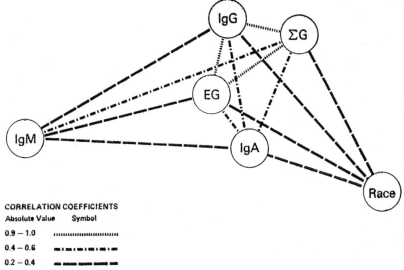

CORRELATION COEFFICIENTS

| Absolute Value | Symbol |
|---|---|
| 0.9 – 1.0 | ,,,,,,,,,,,,,,,,,,,,,,,,,,,,,,, |
| 0.4 – 0.6 | ▬ ▪ ▬ ▪ ▬ ▪ ▬ ▪ ▬ ▪ ▬ |
| 0.2 – 0.4 | ▬ ▬▬ ▬▬ ▬▬ ▬ |

Figure 17–10. Correlation graph for serum immunoglobulins. Line segments proportional to the correlation coefficients link the quantities: EG, Ig G, Ig A, Ig M, and ΣG (see text), and the dichotomous race variable. Keyed bonds indicate very high, high, and moderate degrees of correlation. The tabulated immunoglobulin correlation coefficients were derived from a pool of controls and patients without regard to race.

|  | EG | Ig G | Ig A | Ig M | ΣG | Race | Age |
|---|---|---|---|---|---|---|---|
| EG | 1.00 | | | | | | |
| Ig G | .91 | 1.00 | | | | | |
| Ig A | .56 | .42 | 1.00 | | | | |
| Ig M | .33 | .22 | .25 | 1.00 | | | |
| ΣG | .93 | .96 | .60 | .43 | 1.00 | | |
| Race | −.29 | −.25 | −.25 | −.03 | −.27 | 1.00 | |
| Age | −.08 | −.10 | .16 | −.00 | −.05 | −.04 | 1.00 |

yielded a graded subset of variates. The computer selection included derived variates (namely relative concentrations) not considered by the physician, in preference to primary variates (namely absolute concentrations) that he always uses. Whether or not age and race are ignored, three factors, 5, 8, and 9, best carry the linear discriminatory information, and additional variates are superfluous from the point of view of classification performance. When age and race are considered, variates 5, 7, 8, and 9 best carry the quadratic information.

These variates were used in quadratic discrimination and in a

## TABLE 17–III
### IMMUNOGLOBULIN PATTERN DISCERNMENT
### PERCENT CORRECT DIAGNOSIS FOR LINEAR AND QUADRATIC DISCRIMINANTS

#### LINEAR DISCRIMINANT FUNCTIONS

| | Parameters Included | | | | Fcns | Sample | Percent Correct | | |
|---|---|---|---|---|---|---|---|---|---|
| G | G/EG | Ig M/G | Age | Race | | | $N \to N$ | $A \to A$ | All |
| x | x | x | | | 2 | Entire | 89 | 61 | 70 |
| x | x | x | x | x | 2 | Entire | 83 | 78 | 79 |

#### QUADRATIC DISCRIMINANT FUNCTIONS

| | Parameters Included | | | | Fcns | Sample | Percent Correct | | |
|---|---|---|---|---|---|---|---|---|---|
| G | G/EG | Ig M/G | Age | Race | | | $N \to N$ | $A \to A$ | All |
| x | x | x | | | 2 | Entire | 92 | 73 | 79 |
| x | x | x | x | | 2 | Entire | 89 | 86 | 87 |
| x | x | x | | x | 2 | Entire | 92 | 69 | 77 |
| x | x | x | (x) | | 4 | Entire | 93 | 75 | 81 |
| | | | | | | White | 92 | 71 | 77 |
| | | | | | | Colored | 94 | 87 | 91 |
| x | x | x | x | (x) | 4 | Entire | 89 | 85 | 86 |
| | | | | | | White | 87 | 80 | 82 |
| | | | | | | Colored | 92 | 97 | 95 |

*Note:* Parameters retained in the discriminant analyses are indicated by "x" if used explicitly as a variable, and by " (x)" if used implicitly in the sense that separate analyses were conducted for each racial subgroup.

The number of discriminant functions (= number of categories) is also indicated, along with the percent correctly diagnosed by the computer program in a sample of 280 subjects, of which 75 were judged clinically normal, 205 ill, by attending physicians. "N → N" stands for normals correctly classified, and "A → A" for abnormals correctly classified, whereas "All" stands for the total number correctly classified.

The immunoglobulins involved were G, total concentration; EG, electrophoretically determined concentration; and IgM, immunoglobulin M.

companion set of linear analyses. In each case, the decision rule was the sample analog of the appropriate quadratic or linear Bayes rule, assuming symmetric cost and neglecting prior information.

Consensus between physician and computer evaluations of health state was obtained in 82 to 95 percent of the cases. Results for some of these computer experiments appear in Table 17–III. Race and age were important for sharpening normal bounds. The best diagnostic performance was achieved when separate analyses for each racial group were conducted, with group-specific covariance adjustment for age effects. The superiority of quadratic functions further confirmed the presence of nonlinearity. For purposes of discrimination, controls could be described by a unimodal, ellipsoidally symmetric probability distribution, involving a quadratic function of the variables. Although a similar distribution is inappropriate for patients, the results justify the use of a quadratic pair for contrasting health and disease states.

Originally it had been hoped that one electrophoretic determination could replace three analytical determinations of serum immunoglobulin concentration, and constitute a more rapid and less expensive diagnostic laboratory procedure. The computer experiments, however, showed that, although definitely not independent, each type of assay carried valuable diagnostic information that was not duplicated by the other. Although the effort to justify laboratory economies was frustrated, the complete immunoglobulin profile shows definite promise for inclusion in a multiphasic screening program.

## DELINEATION OF PSYCHIATRIC SYNDROMES BY CLUSTER ANALYSIS

In an application to a nominal data base, hierarchical clustering was used to define and detect psychiatric syndromes in patients admitted by the Community Emergency Mental Health Service of Hahnemann Medical College, Philadelphia.[33] A total of 417 patients were included in the study. The patients resided in urban Philadelphia, mostly in low-income districts, and very few had any education beyond the high school level. Most (47 percent) were referred by a hospital or social agency; some (33 percent) were either self-referred or brought in by family and friends; the remainder (20 percent) were brought in by police.

At the time of admission, each patient was interviewed and rated on a 15-item scale by a psychiatric social worker, and an independent evaluation was made by a psychiatric resident. The 15-item scale used for the emergency patients was derived from an independent factor analytic study of psychiatric inpatients [12,16] and it required evaluation of the following symptoms:

1. somatic concern
2. anxiety
3. emotional withdrawal
4. conceptual disorganization
5. guilt feelings
6. tension

7. mannerisms and postures
8. grandiosity
9. depressive mood
10. hostility
11. suspiciousness
12. hallucinatory behavior
13. motor retardation
14. uncooperativeness
15. unusual thought content.

Rating levels 0–5 were used to represent subjective judgments covering the spectrum from "not present" to "extremely severe," with "light," "moderate," "moderately severe," and "severe" as intermediate states. Although the scales for the various factors have identical ranges, they may have different internal distortions.

A patient's ratings on these 15 items constituted his psychiatric profile. In order to emphasize profile shape and deemphasize amplitude and elevation, the 15 scores for each patient were normalized by elevation and scatter (translated about their mean and scaled by their standard deviation). The cluster analysis was conducted in Euclidean 15-space with the merger strategy emphasizing the evolution of compact clusters. However, because each

**PSYCHIATRIC SYNDROMES STUDY**

patient symptom vectors

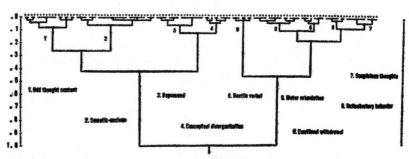

Figure 17–11. Final cluster tree for the psychiatric syndrome study. Each patient was represented in a Euclidean 15 space by profiles extracted from ratings made during the emergency admission interview, and computer-normalized by elevation and scatter. Nine major compact clusters have evolved at the 0.1 level. Names assigned to the clusters correspond to the most prevalent symptom manifest in the members.

profile was normalized initially, there are effectively only 13 degrees of freedom.

Nine syndrome types were found at the 0.1 level of the objective measure (Fig. 17–11). Profiles within each cluster were then analyzed for internal similarities and each cluster was labelled according to the symptom most prevalent among its members. The original sample decomposed as follows:

1. odd-thought content            17 percent
2. somatic anxious               23 percent
3. depression                    28 percent
4. conceptual disorganization     3 percent
5. motor retardation             4 percent
6. emotional withdrawal         4 percent
7. suspicious thought           10 percent
8. hallucinatory behavior        5 percent
9. hostile verbal                 6 percent

Correlations between the diagnostic labels assigned at the time of admission and the computer-generated classification were highly significant (at the 0.001 level). As a result of the preliminary interview, residents had judged the patients to be psychotic (50%), neurotic (20%), suffering from a personality disorder (25%), or otherwise afflicted (mainly with alcoholism) (5%). The four largest syndrome types: odd-thought (1), somatic anxious (2), depression (3), and suspicious thought (7), were covered by the six physician-supplied diagnostic labels:

A. psychosis with organic brain damage    6 percent
B. paranoid schizophrenia           15 percent
C. schizophrenia                  27 percent
D. neurosis                      22 percent
E. personality disorders          22 percent
F. transient or social maladjustment    8 percent

In particular, (a) most (83%) of the odd-thought group were considered to be psychotic or schizophrenic; (b) most (84%) of the suspicious thought group were considered schizophrenic or paranoid schizophrenic; (c) the somatic anxious comprised psychoneurotics with anxiety depression (40%) or personality disorders (28%); and (d) most of the depressed group (73%)

consisted of neurotics, primarily with depression and sometimes with anxiety. Statistically significant correlations were also found between cluster assignment and background variables such as sex, age, source of referral, presence of acute external stress, and diagnostic indications warranting urgent treatment.

A new sample of 300 patients displayed the same distribution of profile types and diagnostic labels, and validated the computer-generated classification of psychiatric syndromes for the catchment area of the hospital. The psychiatric composition of the emergency sample differed from the typical sample composition for psychiatric inpatients, although the same syndrome types were represented. Thus, patient profile type, as determined by the initial emergency interview, can be used to anticipate the type of treatment needed, and to motivate specific fiscal recommendations for apportionment of emergency mental health care resources.

## DELINEATION OF BEHAVIORAL SYNDROMES IN SCHOOL CHILDREN

A predictive application of the clustering algorithm to educational psychology involved delineation of behavioral syndromes in elementary school children, and examination of their relationships to scholastic potential, actual academic achievement, and background variables.[32] The ultimate purpose was to detect and correct incipient learning problems which are influenced by home environment and social pressures before they mature. The approach called for (a) developing reliable and readily applied tools for describing overt classroom behavior, (b) delineating typical behavior patterns at each grade level, and (c) comparing behavior patterns across grade levels from kindergarten through sixth grade. A study of individual behavior profiles in the light of such profile patterns may point out relatively inefficient performance in apparently satisfactory students, as well as confirm suspected correlations between deviant or problem behavior and poor scholastic achievement. The parallels to medical diagnosis and treatment planning are obvious.

The data base for this study consisted of 809 children in seven grades of a suburban Philadelphia public school system in 1968, with 101 to 132 students in each grade. The children were rated by teachers using the independently developed Devereaux Elementary School Behavior rating scale.[31] This method of evaluation involves 47 behavioral items which are scored on nominal scales having either 5 or 7 possibilities. These correspond to teacher impressions of the intensity or frequency of certain types of behavioral displays.

Prior to the computer study, a set of recurring profile types was abstracted from similar data by the collaborating psychologists. They relied on subjective judgments resulting from their own cumulative experience. These categories served as a basis of comparison for the computer-constructed behavioral types. In addition, the psychologists observed high correlations between in-class achievement scores and behavioral aberration, even after statistical adjustment for I.Q. For this purpose, problem behavior was measured by the total number of factor deviants from a plus or minus one standard deviation interval about norms.

In contrast, the computer analysis utilized the entire behavior profile rather than isolated, prominent factors. Using factor analysis, clustering, and correlation techniques, a set of predictors based on academically relevant behavior patterns and a behavioral taxonomy suitable for routine classroom use were derived.

First, from the 47 behavioral items, the following 11 factors were determined for each child:

1. classroom disturbance
2. impatience
3. disrespect-defiance
4. external blame
5. achievement anxiety
6. external reliance
7. comprehension
8. inattentiveness-withdrawal
9. irrelevant responsiveness
10. creative initiative
11. need for closeness to teacher.

When converted to standard scores relative to the norm for the child's grade, these comprise his behavior profile. A final transformation involved translating each standard score by the mean of all 11 standard scores for the individual, and scaling by their standard deviation (normalizing by elevation and scatter). In this way, absolute profile amplitude is suppressed in the delineation of behavioral types, and shape—exaggerated responses relative to a child's entire behavioral complex—is emphasized.

Next, the clustering algorithm was applied, grade by grade. Dissimilarity was defined in terms of distance in a Euclidean 11-space. An iterative search for nearest neighbors generated a hierarchy of compact clusters for each grade. Significant clusters were defined as those which exist at a value of 0.1 for the objective measure.

Finally, accepting the computer-generated grouping, pooled within-cluster correlation coefficients, Wilks' lambda, and F-ratios were computed for ten background variables:

1. sex
2. age
3. mother's and 4. father's age
5. mother's and 6. father's educational level
7. sibling position of child within the family
8. family size
9. race
10. achievement score, measured on a ten-level scale:
    A, A−, B+, B, B−, C+, C, C−, D, F.

F-ratios were used to compare mean values for each cluster pair, and they provided a more sensitive test than lambda. In the absence of other information, the customary distributions were presumed for these statistics, and levels of significance were chosen as customary in biostatistics. In most instances, only prominent differences were of interest, and this procedure was adequate.

In each grade, five or six clusters of varying size were found at the 0.1 level of the objective measure. Virtually the same behavioral prototypes were represented in the clusters for each grade. These computer-generated prototypes matched the previously delineated psychological types well and comprised underachievers, good achievers, very high achievers, normal achievers, acting-out normal achievers, and anxious-dependent normal achievers (Fig. 17–12).

BEHAVIOR PROFILE CLUSTERS: Normalized Cluster Tree

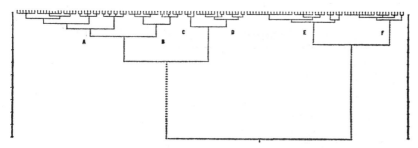

Figure 17–12. Final cluster tree for behavior profiles based on the Devereaux Elementary School behavior rating scale. Eleven-dimensional student profiles were normalized by elevation and scatter, and clustered with the compactness strategy. The tree for fourth grade shows six groups at the 0.1 level of the objective measure. Clusters A, C, and D form the "low-achiever" group, and clusters B, E, and F form the "high-achiever" group. These groups recur in the trees for the other grades. Cluster assignments correlate highly with achievement scores.

The results for fourth grade are illustrative (Fig. 17–13). Whereas the mean profile for this grade is an almost flat response, means of the six computer-generated clusters are quite diverse. A group of three clusters with modest academic performance (averages of C+ to D) was labelled "low achievers." In this group, the cluster of underachievers were reliant, inattentive pupils with low comprehension and abnormally deviant profiles. Acting-out normal achievers showed disruptive and attention-attracting behavior, coupled with normal comprehension. Anxious-dependent normal achievers had normal to high ratings in achievement, anxiety and external reliance, and also had normal comprehension.

A second group of three clusters were called "high achievers" because of above average academic performance (grade averages B– to A). The very high achievers and good achievers alike are generally subdued in class; very high achievers rank somewhat higher in comprehension, but good achievers rank higher in creativity. The cluster of normal achievers was too small for statistical characterization, but members tended to be inattentive and dependent on the teacher.

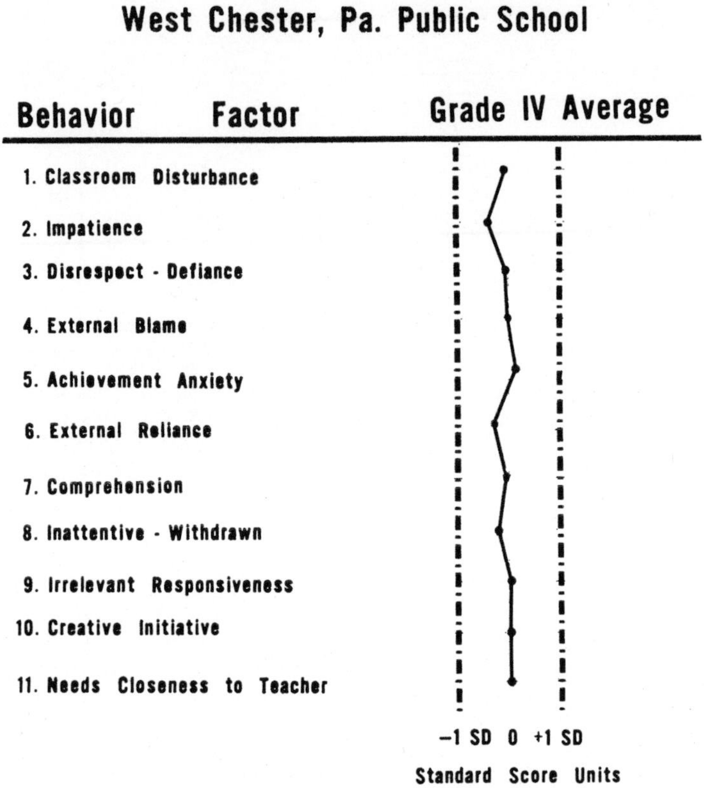

# West Chester, Pa. Public School

Figure 17–13a.

Figure 17–13. Composite behavior profiles for fourth grade. The grade average is an almost flat response, while averages for the six main clusters are highly and differently structured.

    a. The grade average.

    b. The three "low-achiever" profile prototypes.

    c. The three "high-achiever" profile prototypes.

The most pronounced external difference in all grades was in achievement, at the 95 percent significance level. Parental education is highly correlated with cluster assignment in the two highest grades, while the sexual composition of clusters differs at the 90 percent significance level in the lower grades. In grades with high racial mix (11 to 27 percent nonwhite), intercluster racial differences were almost as pronounced as differences in achievement.

BEHAVIOR PROFILE CLUSTERS   :   West Chester, Pa. Public School   Grade IV

**Low Achievers**

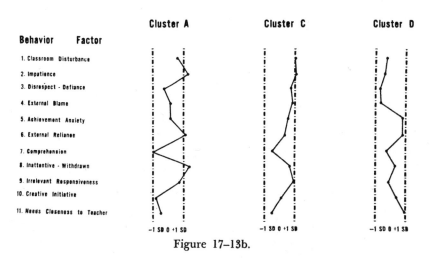

Figure 17–13b.

BEHAVIOR PROFILE CLUSTERS   :   West Chester, Pa. Public School   Grade IV

**High Achievers**

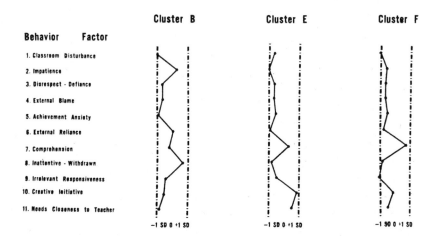

Standard Score Units

Figure 17–13c.

In view of the utility of objective profile analysis, the behavioral study has already been extended to a larger data base of 800 students, and is being broadened to include profile amplitude concurrent with shape.

## SUMMARY AND DISCUSSION

We have described two mathematical approaches—discriminant analysis and cluster synthesis—for emulating diagnostic logic in the areas of disease identification and disease systematics. We have reviewed motivational considerations and shortcomings of these models in the light of realistic complications. Finally, we have illustrated their capabilities in a diverse, nontrivial set of medical and psychological problems. Since the two methods model different diagnostic activities, it should not be surprising that they operate on the basis of different premises and prior information. Both, however, are fundamentally concerned with extracting and characterizing among-class differences and within-class similarities. Discriminant analysis uses statistical techniques, whereas cluster synthesis uses quasi-statistical techniques in pursuing this common theme.

In the decision-theoretic approach to identification, a preconceived disease taxonomy is adopted as an infallible standard. Computer diagnosis involves discriminant function evaluations based on patient profiles—one for each diagnostic possibility. The favored diagnosis ensures that the risks or the probabilities of "error" are constrained, if not minimized. In practice, decisions are based on near-optimal actual rules, not on fully optimal ideal rules, since probabalistic assumptions about the discriminant functions involve unknown population parameters which must be estimated.

The validity of specific diagnostic inferences and extrapolations to future performance should be suspect to the extent that statistical hypotheses are unfulfilled, superfluous variables are included and dilute discriminatory resolution, and sampling deficiencies preclude reliable estimates of the required prior information. Nevertheless, the robustness of linear and quadratic discriminant analyses toward actual departures from theoretical requirements, and their widespread success, can hardly be ignored.

The performance of a decision-theoretic scheme for diagnosis is determined in part by the number and the nature of variables included in the analysis. Retention of relevant but covarying predictors is seemingly inefficient, but intuition suggests that redundancy might provide a corroborative effect and thereby enhance diagnostic prowess, as measured by the "error" rate. On the other hand, it can be shown that retention of correlated variables may sometimes adversely affect the statistical significance of achieved discrimination, so that these variables are extraneous according to this alternative measure.

Design and evaluation of a diagnostic scheme cannot properly be treated independently. The technical error of using the sample of subjects to determine the diagnostic scheme and to predict its performance results in over-optimistic estimates. In order to obtain good schemes and have confidence in predictions of their behavior, the best use must be made of the available sample information. This includes simultaneously optimizing (a) number of subjects, (b) number of variables per subject, (c) measurement resolution of each variable, and (d) apportionment of samples among the diagnostic categories, all in the light of any structural assumptions about the underlying probability distribution of subjects and variables within diagnostic categories, risks or penalties of diagnostic error, the cost of measurement, and the cost of computation.

Thus criteria and strategies of four types enter into the construction of a decision-theoretic algorithm for diagnosis: (a) classification strategies which optimize a performance criterion (such as error rate) ; (b) parameter estimation strategies which provide optimal values in a statistical sense, given the available sample data (such as maximizing sample likelihood) ; (c) feature selection strategies for meeting criteria of effectiveness and conciseness; and (d) experimental design strategies which apportion the available data optimally into learning and test sample, so that predictions of diagnostic performance will be as accurate as possible.

Accordingly, the effectiveness of a statistical algorithm is always operationally limited by both theoretical requirements and practical constraints. The computer can be used to great advantage for the selection of variables, the prediction of diagnostic performance, and the evaluation of competing proposals according to several measures of effectiveness.

In the cluster synthesis approach to classification, a disease taxonomy responsive to patterns detected in the available data is generated in preference to codification based on external information. The notion of cluster is explicated in terms of an admixture of quantitated statistical, psychological, and mathematical concepts such as similarity, connectivity, proximity, tendency, and significance. The hierarchical clustering algorithm which was developed can efficiently accommodate a broad range of cluster shapes and topologies with its repertoire of diverse strategies. Each strategy utilizes a unique recursive modification of the matrix of similarities, within an otherwise fixed basic program structure, and produces a nest of clustered objects. Some of these matrix transformations depend on absolute similarity values, some only on their rank order, so that nominally and ordinally scaled data can be meaningfully examined within a single framework.

The clustering algorithm was initially intended for efficient pattern articulation in fairly well-behaved data bases. It was quickly realized that the original program structure characterized all hierarchical designs, and that, by introducing appropriate mathematical generalizations, its domain could be extended to many other potentially powerful clustering strategies. However, hierarchical clustering is still a limited approach by its very definition. First, a cluster assignment, once made, cannot be reconsidered and revoked. Second, a cluster tree is equivalent to a nest of increasingly coarser partitions into equivalence classes. No provision exists in the current version for assigning a degree of membership in a cluster, or for tolerating multiple membership, that is, for participating in several clusters to varying degrees, except post hoc, although clearly such measures can readily be generated. These restrictions do not seem serious in the light of the useful pattern extraction and trend analysis which has in fact been achieved in noncontrived applications.

Examples for the decision-theoretic approach were drawn from two clinically important problems: (a) the optical discrimination of leukocytes in the context of an automated differential white blood cell count, and (b) the assessment of health state from an analysis of serum immunoglobulin concentrations. In both cases, a preliminary definition of the diagnostic categories by partial extension rather than intension is used to obtain characterizing discriminant functions. Although these two problems are superficially alike—both are classification/diagnosis problems—the data bases are statistically dissimilar. Difficulties arise in interpreting the overlap of hypothetical underlying probability distributions and in defining normalcy. On the one hand, the leukocyte problem involves well-defined polymodal distributions with little ambiguity as evidenced by overlap. On the other hand, the serum immunoglobulin data display no clear-cut evidence of multimodality and suggest no natural criteria for discerning discrete health states.

For the discrimination of normal human leukocytes, linear compounds of four cell descriptors were sufficient, despite pronounced heterogeneity of covariance. Among-class differences apparently dwarf all other relevant phenomena. The four descriptors can be assigned plausible photometric interpretations, and represent four families of cell features: (a) contrast, (b) nuclear-cytoplasmic comparisons, (c) concentration, and (d) size and content.

Health-state screening based on serum immunoglobulin concentration was best performed by a simple hybrid decision algorithm which utilized two pairs of quadratic discriminants, embedded in a two-level logical decision tree. Each discriminant pair involved three independent analytical determinations of the constitutent immunoglobulins, plus an age adjustment. The decision tree itself automatically adjusts for demonstrated ethnic correlations. Although the pure decision-theoretic approach can make the same adjustment, provided that identical variables are used for all groups, the tree approach leaves open the possibility of a better-performing analysis based on group-specific feature selection.

Behavior of the cluster synthesis was tested in a diversified set of problems from medicine and psychology.

The two biomedical applications—human leukocyte and chromosome classification—involved objectively determined, continuous-valued descriptors. Generally accepted morphologically based classifications exist for both leukocytes and chromosomes. Computer-generated cell parameters, however, were not purported analogs of traditional verbalized morphological criteria (such as shape and granularity), although they can be assigned photometric interpretations. On the other hand, chromosomes were characterized by the conventional parameters, length and centromeric index or their DNA content. Preprocessing of parameters, when used, consisted of centering about the mean and scaling by variances or ranges, or else canonical transformation. It is interesting to note that better results were obtained in infra-Euclidean spaces $(p \leq 2)$ than in any other type of Minkowski space. The anticipated five white cell types and the seven chromosome groups were recovered from the data.

In sharp contrast, the two psychological applications—delineation of psychiatric syndromes in adults and behavioral patterns in juveniles—involved subjectively determined, nominally scaled data for which unambiguous, formal classifications are lacking. Trends have been observed, of course, but intension of the nomenclature has not been standardized, hence extensions may be different. External psychiatric criteria abound, but they too are subjective, informal, often controversial, and hard-to-apply. No comparable criteria or even an informal taxonomy had yet been developed for normal behavioral syndromes. Since rating scales are the source of information, monotone invariant clustering is desirable. Finally, internal analysis of individual profiles for subject-specific deviant behavioral or emotional trends is of psychological interest, and warrants preprocessing to emphasize profile shape, a technique peculiar to this type of analysis.

It would be surprising to find even moderate failure reported by the computational diagnosticians, simply because medical expertise and intuition are brought to bear, albeit implicitly, in the analyses. The physician's judgment in selecting variates, and his care in recording patient responses for scrutiny by computer program, determine the properties of the common domain for all proposed algorithms. A specific algorithm will perform well or poorly in this common domain according as its underlying statistical assumptions are realistic or not. No machine can yet replace the physician's knowledge of relevancy, but it can assist him in optimally using what he knows.

Beyond the not-to-be underemphasized impact of the physician's preliminary filtering of variables, the widespread reports of success in computational diagnosis to date are, to some degree, a reflection of the simplicity of the diagnostic problems undertaken, and a commentary on the fortunate robustness of the decision-theoretic and clustering techniques.

Three final points warrant mention. First, it is seldom feasible to implement feature selection in a manner logically consistent with optimal discrimination. The difficulties are in part computational and due to the combinatorics, and in part statistical and due to sampling variation and estimation procedures involved in deriving actual decision rules. Second, standards of acceptable discriminatory performance are ultimately decided by the diagnostician. They may be less stringent than optimal performance in the sense of Bayes, or perhaps more stringent. Third, in the context of the decision-theoretic approach, the operational meaning of the term, "diagnostic error" must be carefully appraised. It should be remembered that the current and perhaps naive standard for evaluation of computer diagnosis is diagnostic coincidence between physician and machine.

It would be irresponsibly naive to expect that one or two computer algorithms could embrace all the complexities of the diagnostic process. By the same token, it would be unduly conservative and pessimistic to ignore those with demonstrated capabilities and the promising avenues of approach to computer-assisted diagnosis which they indicate.

## ACKNOWLEDGMENTS

This research was sponsored by the National Institutes of Health, partially under grant USPHS–1–R01–GM–16913 and conducted at the Department of Radiology, University of Pennsylvania, Philadelphia, Pennsylvania, U.S.A. Supplementary computer time was supported by grant USPHS–RR–515 to the University of Pennsylvania Medical School Computing Facility.

The author also appreciates the continued assistance of the National Institutes of Health and use of facilities of the Division of Computer Research and Technology for completing this manuscript.

The author wishes especially to express appreciation to Dr. Mortimer Mendelsohn, Professor of Radiology, University of Pennsylvania, who encouraged expansion of the methods which grew out of our initial collaborative research on leukocyte discrimination and development of new techniques; to Dr. Harry Hart Wagenheim and to Richard and David Prewitt.

Leukocytes for optical discrimination were provided by Drs. Mortimer L. Mendelsohn and Brian H. Mayall of the Department of Radiology, and serum immunoglobulin concentrations were furnished by Drs. Howard Rawnsley and Dean Arvan of the Pepper Hematology Laboratory, Hospital of the University of Pennsylvania. Dr. George Spivack of the Community Mental Health Center, Hahnemann Medical College, Philadelphia, collaborated on the psychological applications of cluster analysis, joined by Dr. Marshall Swift in the study of behavioral syndromes, and by Dr. Stephen Schwartz in the study of psychiatric syndromes. The author is grateful for their enthusiasm and cooperation.

## REFERENCES

1. Abramson, N. and Braverman, D.: Learning to recognize patterns in a random environment. *IRE Trans Infor Theory, 8:*558–563, 1962.
2. Bergsma, D. (Ed.): Chicago conference: Standardization in human cytogenetics. *Birth Defects: Original Article Series,* Vol. II. New York, The National Foundation, 1966.
3. Chow, C. K.: An optimum character recognition system using decision functions. *IRE Trans Electr Comp, 12:*247–254, 1957.
4. Chu, J. T.: Optimal decision functions for computer character recognition. *J Assoc Comp Mach, 12:*213–226 (No. 2) 1965.
5. Chu, J. T. and Chueh, J. C.: Error probability in decision functions for character recognition. *J Assoc Comp Mach, 14:*273–280 (No. 2) 1967.
6. Cooper, P. W.: Hyperplanes, hyperspheres, and hyperquadrics as decision boundaries. In J. T. Tou and R. H. Wilcox (Eds.) : *Computers and Information Sciences.* Washington, D.C., Spartan Books, 1964, pp. 111–138.
7. Day, N. E.: Linear and quadratic discrimination in pattern recognition. *IEEE Trans Infor Theory, 15:*419–420, 1969.

8. Fisher, R. A.: The use of multiple measurements in taxonomic problems. *Ann Eugenics, 7:*179–188, 1936.
9. Fisher, R. A.: The statistical utilization of multiple measurements. *Ann Eugenics, 8:*376–386, 1937.
10. Highleyman, W. H.: The design and analysis of pattern recognition experiments. *Bell Systems Tech J, 41:*723–744 (No. 2) 1962.
11. John, S.: Errors in discrimination. *Ann Math Stat, 32:*1125–1144 (No. 4) 1961.
12. Lorr, M. and Klett, C. J.: Psychotic behavioral types. *Arch Gen Psychiatry, 20:*592–597, 1969.
13. Morrison, D. F.: *Multivariate Statistical Methods.* New York, McGraw-Hill, 1967.
14. Murphy, E. A.: A scientific viewpoint on normalcy. Perspect Biol Med, Spring, 1968, pp. 333–348.
15. Nilsson, N. J.: *Learning Machines.* New York, McGraw-Hill, 1965.
16. Overall, J. E. and Gorham, D. R.: The brief psychiatric rating scale. *Psychol Rep, 10:*799–812, 1962.
17. Penrose, L. S.: Editorial comment to the report of the Denver Conference, 1960. *Ann Human Gen, 24:*319, 1960.
18. Prewitt, J. M. S. and Mendelsohn, M. L.: The analysis of cell images. *Ann N. Y. Acad Sci, 128:*1035–1053, 1966.
19. Prewitt, J. M. S. and Mendelsohn, M. L.: A general approach to image analysis by parameter extraction. Proc Conf on the Uses of Computers in Radiology. Columbia, Missouri, Univ. of Missouri, 1966.
20. Prewitt, J. M. S.: In progress report for 1967, scanning cytophotometry and digital computers. M. L. Mendelsohn, J. M. S. Prewitt, B. H. Mayall, B. H. Perry, and T. J. Conway. Part IV:1–7, Department of Radiology, Univ. of Pennsylvania.
21. Prewitt, J. M. S.: Machine perception of white blood cell images. In 2nd IEEE Pattern Recognition Workshop, The Hague, Netherlands, August 1968.
22. Prewitt, J. M. S.: Selection of variables and prediction of performance in decision-theoretic approaches to diagnosis. Proc Conf on Computer Applications in Radiology, University of Missouri, Columbia, Missouri, 1970.
23. Prewitt, J. M. S.: A versatile hierarchical clustering algorithm with objective function and objective measure, in preparation (a).
24. Prewitt, J. M. S.: Cytotaxonomics of leukocytes based on photometric properties, in preparation.
25. Prewitt, J. M. S.: Parametric and non-parametric recognition by computer: An application to image processing. In M. Rubinoff (Ed.): *Advances in Computers,* Vol. 12, 1972.
26. Rao, C. R.: The utilization of multiple measurements in problems of biological classification. *J R Stat Soc,* Series B, *10:*159–203 (No. 2) 1948.

27. Rao, C. R.: *Advanced Statistical Methods in Biometric Research*. New York, John Wiley and Sons, 1952.
28. Sampson, P.: Stepwise multivariate linear discrimination. In W. Dixon (Ed.): *BMD Biomedical Computer Programs*. Berkeley, University of California Press, 1965.
29. Sokal, R. R. and Sneath, P. H. A.: *Principles of Numerical Taxonomy*. San Francisco, W. H. Freeman, 1963.
30. Sebestyen, G. S.: *Decision-making Processes in Pattern Recognition*. New York, Macmillan, 1962.
31. Spivack, G. and Swift, M.: The Devereaux Elementary School Behavior Rating Scales: A study of the nature and organization of achievement related disturbed classroom behavior. *J Spec Educ, 1:*71–90, 1966.
32. Spivack, G., Swift, M. and Prewitt, J. M. S.: Syndromes of disturbed classroom behavior: A behavioral diagnostic system for elementary schools. *J Spec Educ,* April, 1971.
33. Spivack, G., Schwartz, S., Goldman, C. and Prewitt, J. M. S.: Symptom syndromes of emergency cases in an urban community mental health center. *Compr Psychiatry,* 1971, in press.
34. Ward, J. H., Jr.: Hierarchical grouping to optimize an objective function. *J Am Stat Assoc, 58:*236–244, 1963.
35. Welch, B. L.: Note on discriminant functions. *Biometrika 31:*218–220, (Parts I and II) 1939.

Chapter 18

# DIAGNOSIS OF THE ELECTROCARDIOGRAM*

HUBERT V. PIPBERGER
JEROME CORNFIELD
ROSALIE A. DUNN

## INTRODUCTION

$D$IAGNOSIS OF THE electrocardiogram (ECG) is considered a two-stage problem. The first stage involves pattern recognition of the ECG record components—P, QRS, and T waves. An accurate delineation of the waveform beginning and endpoints is essential for timing purposes. After a brief discussion of this wave recognition problem, we present an elaboration on the second stage, the diagnostic process.

Recently, attention has been focused on still another aspect of ECG diagnosis, the analysis of cardiac rhythm disturbances or arrhythmias. Algorithms developed for this type of analysis are extensions of wave recognition programs. They deal with waveforms sequence variations. A detailed discussion of this phase is beyond the scope of this presentation.

### Electrocardiographic Wave Recognition

Fig. 18–1 shows a typical ECG record of one cardiac cycle and indicates the beginning and end of the waveforms which must be recognized in the analysis. In routine clinical recording, a substantial amount of noise is superimposed on ECG records. Automatic processing systems cannot deal with this interference as easily as a human interpreter. Noise consists of 60 Hz line interference, muscle potentials, baseline shifts due to movements of the patient or to DC drift, and electronic noise including low and

* Supported in part by Grants # HE 09696 and GM 15004 National Institutes of Health, U. S. Public Health Service.

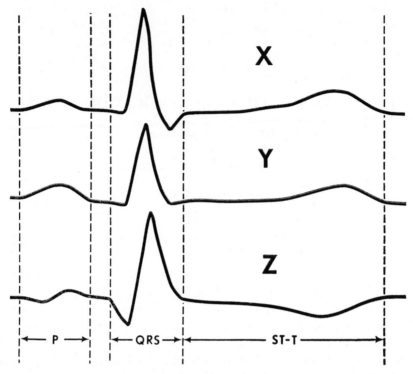

Figure 18–1. Typical ECG record of one cardiac cycle using 3-lead orthogonal system. Dotted lines mark the beginning and end points of the P, QRS and ST-T cycles which are recognized in the computerized pattern recognition analysis.

high frequency components. Both analog and digital filters have been used to eliminate noise, but any filtering process begets new problems since frequency spectra of electrocardiograms and noise overlap. Filters which do not distort electrocardiographic waveforms are difficult to design. Digital notch filters have been proposed to eliminate 60 Hz interference. They can reduce noise in a very small frequency range without substantial wave distortion; but a relatively large amount of computation time is required, which is not always practical in routine clinical use.

The majority of available wave recognition programs are based upon first derivatives of either single scalar leads or curves of spatial magnitude. The latter are obtained from simultaneously

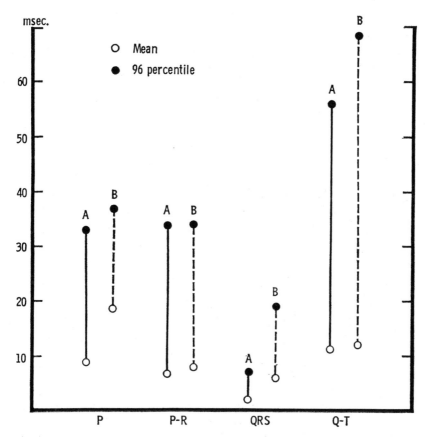

Figure 18–2. Comparison of beat-to-beat variation (BBV) of ECG time meas-urements determined by computer wave recognition (A) with that by visual wave recognition (B). Mean BBV is indicated by white circles; black circles delimit the maximal variation. As compared to visual determination, BBV (mean and maximal) in P and QRS duration and Q-T interval were signifi-cantly reduced by computer wave recognition, whereas the variation in P-R interval remained almost unchanged. (From Ishikawa *et al.*,[1] by permission of the C. V. Mosby Company)

recorded orthogonal leads. Since certain deflections (particularly small ones like P waves) may result in low amplitude projections on scalar leads, the single lead approach is more difficult than the spatial magnitude curve approach. When appropriate threshold values for the rate of change are determined for beginnings and ends of the various waveforms, the majority of the ECG waves

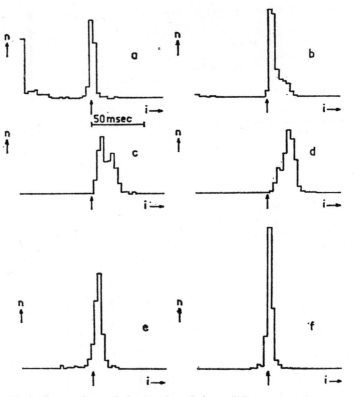

Figure 18–3. Comparison of the results of three different waveform recognition methods. The arrow indicates the point of QRS onset recognized by the cardiologist. The height of the histogram above point $i$ represents the number of automatically analyzed VCGs whose QRS onset was a distance $i$ from the clinicaly determined point. a, b, c and d represent results from the threshold method, with thresholds at 4, 10, 17 and 25 respectively, of the maximum of the spatial velocity; e represents results from the least squares fitting method; f, the template method. (From van Bemmel, *et al.*,[3] by permission of the author)

can be satisfactorily identified. With this relatively simple approach, up to 20 percent of the desired endpoints may be missed, however; more satisfactory results necessary for clinical application hopefully can be derived with additional refinements.

To put the performance of automatic wave recognition programs into proper perspective, visual determinations of wave endpoints and results by computer technics should be compared.

Both inter- and intra-observer variations in ECG wave recognition by human observers are responsible for a major source of disagreement with results from quantitative ECG analysis. Could this source of error be substantially decreased by applying fixed algorithms to this problem? Ishikawa and co-workers [1] recently reported on such a comparison (Fig. 18–2). QRS durations showed a mean variation of 6 msec with a maximum of 19 msec when determined visually from one heart beat to the next over a period of nine cardiac cycles. This variation was reduced to a mean of 2 msec with a maximum of 7 msec when an automatic wave recognition program was applied using a "least square fit" method with standardized waveforms. These results indicate that the physiological variations in wave durations are less than usually assumed by visual methods in clinical practice.[2] Greater consistency in wave recognition would result in greater efficiency in quantitative analysis of the electrocardiogram.

A unique comparison of different wave recognition technics has been reported recently by van Bemmel and co-workers [3] (Fig. 18–3). Histograms a to d represent results obtained by fixed threshold methods which are most commonly used. The arrow underneath the abscissa depicts the point of QRS onset which was identified visually by the cardiologist who analyzed the wave. The height of the histogram at distance $i$ represents the frequency of automatically determined onsets which differ from the preselected point by $i$ units. Although the procedures shown in histograms a and b appear efficient, a good number of cases fall completely out of the range and are erroneous. The data in diagram e (based on a different approach used in our laboratory) are derived from "least square fits" between unknown records and standardized waveforms. Considerable improvement over the simpler threshold procedures results with this method. Histogram f indicates the outcome of a method developed by van Bemmel and his co-workers.[3] They initially constructed a three-dimensional display of spatial velocity amplitude, time, and frequency density from large numbers of tracings. Then, cross-correlation was performed between the template and the unknown records. The result was a "window" defining inflection points which differed only slightly from those defined by the cardiologist. Initial reports indicate a high degree of accuracy is obtainable with this template method; verification is awaited from independent testing.

The ECG pattern recognition problem is complicated because of the great variety of waveforms and the frequent occurrence of poor signal-to-noise ratios. The clinician is unwilling to tolerate even an occasional failure since it may lead to a serious misinterpretation. The more recent studies on performance evaluations of different methods will eventually lead to significant refinements of the presently available computerized procedures.

### Diagnostic ECG Classification

Since the first reports appeared on automatic interpretation of electrocardiograms, a variety of different diagnostic classification procedures has been proposed. Before discussing some of the more pertinent ones, consider the methods commonly used in routine electrocardiographic interpretation. They can be best described as decision trees. To determine whether or not preset normal limits are exceeded, a special subset of ECG amplitudes and durations is utilized. Sometimes, deviations from the norm indicate more than one abnormality; and additional observations are necessary for final classification. As an example, consider a record with an abnormally long QRS duration. In isolation, this finding indicates a ventricular conduction defect. But, is this abnormality caused by a left or a right bundle branch block, or both? The direction of the terminal QRS forces indicates what branch of the decision tree to follow. If the terminal QRS forces are directed toward the left and posteriorly, a left bundle branch block is assumed. Conversely, if these forces point to the right and anteriorly, a diagnosis of right bundle branch block is made. Most computer programs for ECG analysis in common use are based on decision trees where, in effect, the logic of the cardiologist is being simulated. The diagnostic performance of this method will only be as acceptable as the performance of the cardiologist. Since no generally accepted diagnostic criteria for ECG interpretation exist, these programs require adjustments according to individual diagnostic criteria which are variable from one hospital to the next.

Other investigators, having judged that the capacity of computers to handle such complex procedures was not fully exploited in the simple decision tree approach, attempted to improve diagnostic ECG classification through the use of more complex statistical methods. Since a multitude of variables is involved in the analysis simultaneously, the multivariate statistical approach appeared inviting; and consequently, it represents the common denominator of most early attempts in automated ECG analysis.

Without attempting to make an exhaustive review of all the different approaches proposed, we would like to mention some of the more important ones. The first significant attempt to apply multivariate analysis to ECG diagnosis was made by Cady, Woodbury and co-workers.[4] They applied a stepwise linear discriminant function analysis on Fourier coefficients derived from sets of orthogonal leads. This method permitted the separation of 23 normal tracings from 19 abnormal records from patients with left ventricular hypertrophy (LVH). A number of other investigators also applied linear discriminant function technics successfully; Specht[5] was the first to advocate a polynomial discriminant analysis.

An attractive approach to automatic ECG analysis (the "adaptive filter" technic) was suggested by Stark and co-workers[6] and later in a somewhat different form by Specht.[5] Initially, this type of analysis revolves around training sets of records for various diagnostic entities. A cross-correlation is performed between each new, unknown record and the various training sets. The unknown case is then entered into the group of best correlation. The selected training set is updated on the basis of the new material. By using this approach, the computer becomes a "learning" machine continuously adapting itself to new information. From our own experience,[7] this method is efficient when the training sets are comprised of less than 100 records for each group. Increasing the number of records creates a greater overlap between the training sets, and the cross-correlation results become ambiguous. When the number of samples reaches several hundred each, the sets fuse almost completely.

Bayes' Theorem was first applied to ECG diagnosis by Kimura and co-workers.[8] Using 40 ECG measurements from 825 patient records, a disease matrix (essentially a table of conditional probabilities) was formed. Seventeen different disease groups were used for classification. Results were not encouraging. Possibly, the relatively poor definition of the disease groups (which even the authors admit are "quite illogical" yet inevitable in some instances) was caused by the small number of cases. Due to this lack of material, the method probably was not given a fair trial in this early attempt.

Classification results in almost all early reports on the application of multivariate analysis technics were quite good. To a large extent, this can be attributed to disproportionately small record samples in relation to the number of variables used. When more than 40 ECG measurements are applied to samples of 40 records or less, almost perfect separation is expected. Testing initial results obtained from training samples by applying the method to new, independent samples was rarely attempted due to the lack of material in those early days. If such attempts were made and the excellent initial results could not be duplicated, the authors might have abstained from further publication.[9] In more recent years, the general trend in ECG computer analysis has been directed toward simple decision tree approaches based on time-honored criteria with few attempts to improve the present state of the art in ECG classification.

In classification experiments, cases should always be grouped on the basis of independent information; that is, ECG information should not enter into the initial case selection process. This prerequisite makes it extremely difficult to collect sufficiently large record numbers from one hospital or one medical center in a reasonable amount of time. This fact has probably discouraged the majority of investigators who could not expect to see results during their own lifetime.

For this reason, a different approach was selected in the Veterans Administration; and, as early as 1959, a cooperative study with eight participating hospitals was organized. Clinical protocols based on medical history, physical examinations and laboratory data were developed; and the cases were classified strictly on the basis of these data without the use of ECG information. In addition, autopsy reports were collected whenever available.

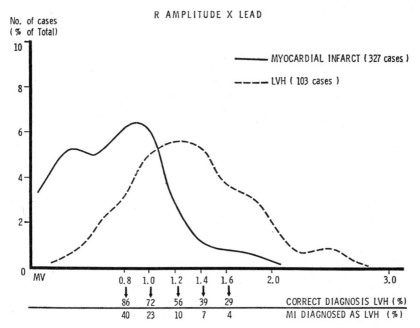

Figure 18-4. Smoothed relative frequency distribution curves for R amplitude in lead X in left ventricular hypertrophy (LVH, broken line) and myocardial infarct (MI, solid line) cases. Below the graph are found two sets of numbers. The upper set indicates the percent of correct classifications of LVH; the lower set, the number of MI misdiagnosed as LVH for the corresponding $R_x$ measurement. Misclassification increases with corresponding increase in correct diagnosis of LVH. (From Kini *et al.*,[10] by permission of the American Heart Association, Inc.)

Record classification for each diagnostic group was begun when the boundaries of the sample ceased to fluctuate. Prior to a critical record number, the addition of new cases leads to substantial changes in the statistical configuration of the samples. The number of records necessary to obtain stable conditions varies from one diagnostic entity to the next. For instance, a sample of normal records becomes reasonably stable when 200 tracings have been collected. For other entities such as left ventricular hypertrophy, the minimal number necessary was approximately 400 records. To test results obtained from the initial core samples, secondary samples of approximately equal size are also necessary. It is obvious that data collection in such studies is an enormous task.

The selection of optimal discriminators between diagnostic entities poses another problem. In the VA Cooperative Study, the first selection of ECG measurements for differentiation between groups was based on 96 percentile ranges where two percent of the cases were cut off on both ends, in order to eliminate "outliers." When these 96 percentile ranges of normals and abnormals are compared, measurements which are potentially good discriminators between groups are identifiable. The substantial overlap between normal and abnormal measurement ranges for patients (a characteristic feature of ECG information which manifests itself quickly) never disappears. A typical example showing the range of overlap for one such measurement between anterior myocardial infarct and left ventricular hypertrophy patients is shown in Fig. 18–4.[10]

As the number of different measurements taken on an ECG

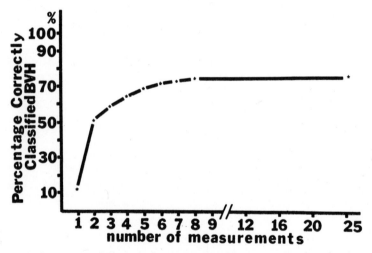

Figure 18–5. Percent of increase in correct classification of biventricular hypertrophy (BVH) ECGs when discrimination is made between normal and BVH cases. The method of diagnosis uses 96 percentile range criteria in conjunction with the likelihood ratio test. With the addition of measurements, percent of correct classifications increases to 73 percent with eight measurements. Thereafter, the curve levels off and no new ECG items, among 25 best discriminators, contribute to increase the percentage. (From Gamboa *et al.*,[11] by permission of the American Heart Association, Inc.)

record increases, a second characteristic of the data set is revealed, that the diagnostic information contained in the ECG data is relatively limited. Fig. 18–5 [11] illustrates such a condition when patients with biventricular hypertrophy (BVH) are distinguished from normal subjects. Seventy-three percent of the BVH patients are correctly classified with eight measurements. Few other BVH

TABLE 18–I

CUMULATIVE PERCENTAGES OF PATIENTS CORRECTLY DIAGNOSED AS HAVING PULMONARY EMPHYSEMA WHEN DISTINGUISHED FROM NORMAL SUBJECTS

|  | *Cases of Pulmonary Emphysema Out of Normal Range (Cumulative) (%)* | *False Positives (Cumulative) (%)* |
|---|---|---|
| QRS measurements | | |
| scalar leads | | |
| $R_x$ | 57 | 2 |
| $R:S_x$ ratio | 63 | 3 |
| $R_x$ peak time | 66 | 6 |
| QT interval (uncorrected) | 71 | 7 |
| $R:S_y$ ratio | 77 | 8 |
| Vectorcardiographic planes | | |
| Maximal $QRS_{xy}$ angle | 80 | 12 |
| Maximal $QRS_{xy}$ amplitude | 81 | 13 |
| Maximal $QRS_{xz}$ amplitude | 82 | 14 |
| Maximal $QRS_{xz}$ angle | 82 | 19 |
| P and T measurements | | |
| scalar leads | | |
| $T_z$ | 84 | 20 |
| $T_y$ | 88 | 21 |
| $P:R_y$ ratio | 89 | 21 |
| Vectorcardiographic planes | | |
| $T_{zy}$ angle | 90 | 22 |
| $T_{xz}$ angle | 92 | 25 |
| $P_{zy}$ angle | 92 | 28 |
| $P_{xy}$ angle | 94 | 29 |

*Note:* Increase in discrimination sensitivity is obtained with the addition of selected measurements from the QRS, P and T components of the ECGs and VCGs. Concurrently, the specificity decreases, i.e. the number of false positives rises at a rate which offsets the sensitivity increase.

patients are detected with the addition of measurements. Even in studies which show increase in discrimination sensitivity with additional measurement data, the gain is usually offset by a concomitant decrease in specificity, i.e. the number of false positives rises. Table 18–I illustrates such a case where discrimination is made between normal subjects and patients with pulmonary emphysema.[12] The percentage of correct classifications of the disease patients is 77 percent using only five measurements with a false positive rate of 8 percent. The addition of four vector QRS measurements increases the correct classifications by 5 percent, but the false positive rate increases to 19 percent. Thus, a small gain in sensitivity is completely offset by the larger loss in specificity. Similarly, addition of seven P and T measurements causes the sensitivity level to rise 12 percent but the specificity level to decline 10 percent. Optimum balance between sensitivity gain and specificity loss is also a crucial problem in automatic diagnosis.

In our own studies on ECG diagnosis, we first started differenti-

TABLE 18–II

TYPICAL SET OF ECG MEASUREMENTS USED TO SEPARATE
MYOCARDIAL INFARCT CASES FROM NORMAL CONTROLS
N/40 vs ANT MI (377)

| | | *Discrim.* | *Product\** |
|---|---|---|---|
| 1. | Max. QRSxz | −0.37 | 468 |
| 2. | Spat. max. QRS | 0.26 | 386 |
| 3. | 3/8 QRSx | 0.46 | 335 |
| 4. | 3/8 QRSxz | −0.21 | 195 |
| 5. | 2/8 QRSxz | 0.44 | 173 |
| 6. | 2/8 QRSx | −0.63 | 144 |
| 7. | Qz | −0.61 | 130 |
| 8. | Tx | 1.00 | 88 |
| 9. | 3/8 QRSz | 0.16 | 46 |
| 10. | 2/8 QRSy | −0.24 | 29 |
| 11. | 2/8 QRSz | −0.50 | 25 |
| 12. | Rz | 0.01 | 9 |
| 13. | 1/8 QRSz | −0.08 | 6 |
| 14. | Qx | 0.10 | 3 |

*Note:* The columns list the discriminant function coefficients, and the products of the coefficients and the averages of the two means of the compared groups. (From Eddleman and Pipberger [13] by permission of the C. V. Mosby Company)
\* Products of mean measurements and discriminant function coefficients (multiplied by 1,000).

ating between normals and various abnormal groups, considering only two groups at a time. Linear discriminant function analysis was used in a previously described manner.[13] Table 18–II shows a typical set of ECG measurements which were used to separate a group of patients with myocardial infarcts from a normal control group of similar age. In addition to the discriminant function coefficients, the products between these coefficients and the average of the two means of the compared groups are shown. These products are relatively good indicators of the contributions made by individual measurements to the differentiation. Large coefficients frequently indicate only that the measurement in question has a small amplitude and vice versa. As can be seen in Table 18–II, the major contributions to differentiation come from the measurements listed on top with negligible contributions from the last ones.

In addition to the linear discriminant function analysis, a likelihood ratio test was used for the classification of individual cases. Since relatively large record numbers had accumulated from the eight hospitals over the last ten years, the results could be tested on independent second samples. These tests were encouraging; for example, 84 percent of a sample of 1002 patients with myocardial infarcts could be correctly diagnosed with a false positive rate of only 6 percent. When the same matrix was applied to 240 cases with myocardial infarcts who had come to autopsy, the recognition rate was even higher, 88 percent. These results were subsequently compared to conventional 12-lead ECG analyses using the Minnesota Code.[14] When the specificity of both methods was kept at the same level with 6 percent false positives each, 49 percent of the same patients with infarcts were correctly classified. The multivariate approach had improved classification by 35 percent (84 percent vs 49 percent).

Differentiation between two groups has a limited significance in a clinical setting. One might ask, "Did patient A suffer a myocardial infarct?" and a simple YES or NO answer is expected from the electrocardiogram. When electrocardiograms are interpreted in the hospital's heart station, it is much more common that such simple YES or NO questions cannot be asked because little or no

TABLE 18-III

**PERCENTAGE DISTRIBUTION OF PATIENTS IN DIFFERENT CLINICAL CATEGORIES BY CATEGORY TO WHICH ASSIGNED ON THE BASIS OF STATISTICAL CHARACTERISTICS OF THE ECG**

| Category by Clinical Protocol | Statistically Assigned Category Percent | | | | | | | Total No. of Patients |
|---|---|---|---|---|---|---|---|---|
| | (1) | (2) | (3) | (4) | (5) | (6) | (7) | |
| Normal (1) | 89.9 | 0.7 | 1.5 | 0.0 | 2.7 | 0.8 | 4.4 | 597 |
| Anterior myocardial infarction (2) | 6.7 | 65.7 | 3.9 | 3.1 | 11.6 | 0.5 | 8.5 | 388 |
| Posterior myocardial infarction (3) | 3.8 | 4.8 | 81.5 | 1.1 | 3.4 | 1.9 | 3.4 | 525 |
| Lateral myocardial infarction (4) | 0.9 | 21.6 | 0.9 | 70.7 | 1.7 | 0.0 | 4.3 | 116 |
| Left ventricular hypertrophy (5) | 20.4 | 11.9 | 6.9 | 0.9 | 50.8 | 3.7 | 5.5 | 437 |
| Right ventricular hyperthropy (6) | 26.9 | 3.0 | 4.5 | 0.0 | 5.2 | 50.0 | 10.4 | 184 |
| Pulmonary emphysema (7) | 10.6 | 8.9 | 7.9 | 2.0 | 4.4 | 4.0 | 62.2 | 405 |
| | | | | | | | | 2602 |

additional information is available about the patient in question. In this situation, all ECG diagnoses have to be considered simultaneously. A method had to be developed where all of the most common ECG diagnoses are taken into consideration. The method now in use and undergoing further development at the Veterans Administration Hospital involves a maximum likelihood procedure which considers seven possible diagnostic categories simultaneously for each ECG analysis.

Table 18–III indicates the seven categories and the number of patients in each for the trial run. For each of the 21 pairwise comparisons, approximately 10 to 15 apparently most discriminating ECG variables were selected on the basis of inspection of the 96 percentile ranges. This led to a total of 76 variables appearing in one or more pairwise comparisons of which 14 were azimuthal (angular measurements in the horizontal plane). For the latter 14, rather than using the angular measurement itself, $\theta$, the following transformation is used:

$$y = \cos(\theta - \overline{\theta}_1) - \cos(\theta - \overline{\theta}_2) \tag{1}$$

where $\overline{\theta}_1$ and $\overline{\theta}_2$ are the smallest and largest of the seven vector means.[15] Thus, difficulties that can arise in averaging azimuthal angles directly are avoided.

For each of the seven diagnostic categories, the 76 variables are assumed to have a multivariate normal distribution with possibly differing means, but with the same variance-covariance matrix. Denoting the 76-dimensional variable by the single symbol x and the assumed distribution of x for the $i^{th}$ category by $f(x|i)$, the posterior probability that an individual with the vector value x falls in category i is the following (see Chap. 6, Equation 2.3):

$$P(i \mid x) = \left[ \sum_{j=1}^{7} f(x \mid j))g_j / f(x \mid i)g_i \right]^{-1} \tag{2}$$

where the $g_i$ have been taken as proportional to the numbers of patients in the last column of Table 18–III. With the assumptions stated, the likelihood ratio for category j relative to category i is given by the following: [16]

$$\frac{f(x \mid j)}{f(x \mid i)} = \exp \left[ \sum_{k=1}^{76} \lambda_k \left( x_k - \frac{\bar{x}_{kj} + \bar{x}_{ki}}{2} \right) \right] \qquad (3)$$

where $\bar{x}_{kj}$ = mean of the $k^{th}$ variable in the $j^{th}$ diagnostic category;

$\lambda_k$ = the discriminant function coefficient = $\sum_{l=1}^{76} s^{kl} (\bar{x}_{lj} - \bar{x}_{li})$

and $s^{kl}$ = the element in the $k^{th}$ row and $l^{th}$ column of the inverse of the pooled variance-covariance matrix.

Each individual has been assigned to the category for which his posterior probability as given by Equation 2 was greatest. The matrix showing the percent of agreement and disagreement in ECG classification between the cardiologist and probability method is given in Table 18–III.

## DISCUSSION

How do results obtained by multivariate analysis compare with those obtained in routine clinical electrocardiography? Such comparisons are extremely difficult because sensitivity and specificity rates are frequently not available for conventional diagnostic criteria. This situation is somewhat improved for the diagnosis of myocardial infarct where Kurihara and co-workers [14,17] have reported on false positive and false negative rates from large autopsy samples using the Minnesota Code.

Eighty-three percent of the infarcts were correctly diagnosed using the likelihood ratio method and combining the location categories (anterior, posterior, and lateral) since the medical diagnosis for each of the 1029 infarct cases (Table 18–III) was based on clinical information which does not permit verification of the exact location of the infarct. Only 2 percent of the normals were misclassified as infarcts. This compares favorably with the correct classification rate of 49 percent with Minnesota Code criteria at a false positive rate of 6 percent. Multivariate analysis still exceeds conventional 12-lead analysis by 34 percent. An additional 3 percent, 1 percent, and 4 percent of the normal subjects were misclassified as left ventricular hypertrophy, right ventricular hypertrophy (RVH), and pulmonary emphysema respectively, which are tolerable since a small percentage of the normal control subjects are assumed to have cardiac disease which may remain clinically silent. The results for RVH with 50 percent correct classifications are least encouraging. This can be explained, however, by the type of cases which formed the core RVH sample; 134 cases with mitral stenosis. This disease entity is relatively rare in a population of veterans since such cases are usually eliminated at the time of induction. The sample material is composed of cases with mild lesions that were overlooked at the time of induction or those that developed rheumatic heart disease either in the military service or later (relatively uncommon). Classification results for RVH are expected to improve when case material from a general hospital population becomes available as a core sample.

Overall, the classification results are considered to be quite satisfactory, with 74 percent correct classifications, when compared to other studies. Simonson and co-workers [18] reported a correct classification rate between 50 and 55 percent for 12-lead electrocardiograms and vectorcardiograms when all ECG abnormalities were considered simultaneously. These results were obtained in a cooperative study with a number of outstanding electrocardiographers participating. The most important feature of the multivariate analysis described is the high degree of specificity. Only 10 percent of the normals were misclassified; whereas, Gunnar and co-workers [19] found a false positive rate of more than 30 percent for the most common VCG criteria for myocardial infarct when they studied an autopsy sample. Fleischli and co-workers [20] reported false positive rates between 30 and 50 percent when two of the most popular computer programs were used. This study was based, however, on relatively small samples of 238 abnormals and 545 normals. More studies comparing various systems are needed in order to arrive at more reliable data.

The results in Table 18–III, gratifying though they are, may understate the error in diagnosis that will occur when the method is applied to new cases. The prior probabilities used are those calculated to minimize classification error in the test material. But these probabilities will be less precisely known for new cases; and because of this, classification error will increase. Similarly, classification error is usually greater in new material than in the material from which the decision rule was derived. On the other hand, a more systematic selection of discrimination variables and a relaxation of the multivariate normality assumption, both of which we hope to investigate in the future, may decrease classification error.

By far the most important lesson learned from these studies is the realization of the need for large data bases. More than ten years and the cooperation of eight hospitals were needed to collect the material used in our study in order to arrive at the results presented. Diagnostic studies in electrocardiography can serve as a model for other studies in clinical medicine. Whenever possible, such studies should be based on a cooperative effort of several hospitals in order to accumulate sufficiently large amounts of material which is necessary when computers are to be used with greater advantage and to their full capacity to handle multiple variables and large record samples. In the past, it has been disappointing that so many promising beginnings in ECG computer analysis were not pursued because of a lack of material. Such efforts need to be well coordinated, and much detail work has to go into these studies. In the final analysis, improvement in diagnosis compensates for all the sweat and tears which have to be shed on the way.

## REFERENCES

1. Ishikawa, K.; Batchlor, C. and Pipberger, H. V.: Reduction of electrocardiographic beat-to-beat variation through computer wave recognition. *Am Heart J, 81:*236, 1971.
2. Fischmann, E.; Cosma, J. and Pipberger, H. V.: Beat-to-beat and observer variation of the electrocardiogram. *Am Heart J, 75:*465, 1968.
3. van Bemmel, J. H.; Duisterhout, J. S.; van Herpen, G.; Bierwolf, L. G.; Hengeveld, S. J. and Versteeg, B.: Statistical processing methods for recognition and classification of vectorcardiograms. Proceedings, XI International Symposium on Vectorcardiography, New York, 1970. Amsterdam, North-Holland Publishing Company (in press).
4. Cady, L. D., Jr.; Woodbury, M. A.; Tick, L. J. and Gertler, M. M.: A method for electrocardiogram wave-pattern estimation. Example: Left ventricular hypertrophy. *Circ Res, 9:*1078, 1961.
5. Specht, D. F.: Vectorcardiographic diagnosis using the polynomial discriminant method of pattern recognition. *IEEE Trans Biomed Eng, BME–14:*90, 1967.

6. Stark, L.; Okajima, J. and Whipple, G. H.: Computer pattern recognition techniques: Electrocardiographic diagnosis. Communications of the ACM, 5:527, 1962.

7. Stallmann, F. W. and Pipberger, H. V.: Unpublished observations.

8. Kimura, E.; Mibukura, Y. and Mirua, S.: Statistical diagnosis of electrocardiogram by theorem of Bayes. *Jap Heart J, 4:*469, 1963.

9. Pipberger, H. V.; Schneiderman, M. J. and Klingeman, J. D.: Love-at-first-sight effect in research. *Circulation, 38:*822, 1968.

10. Kini, P. M.; Eddleman, E. E., Jr. and Pipberger, H. V.: Electrocardiographic differentiation between left ventricular hypertrophy and anterior myocardial infarction. *Circulation, 42:*875, 1970.

11. Gamboa, R.; Klingeman, J. D. and Pipberger, H. V.: Computer diagnosis of biventricular hypertrophy from the orthogonal electrocardiogram. *Circulation, 39:*72, 1969.

12. Kerr, A., Jr.; Adicoff, A.; Klingeman, J. D. and Pipberger, H. V.: Computer analysis of the orthgonal electrocardiogram in pulmonary emphysema. *Am J Cardiol, 25:*34, 1970.

13. Eddleman, E. E., Jr. and Pipberger, H. V.: Computer analysis of the orthogonal electrocardiogram and vectorcardiogram in 1002 cases with myocardial infarction. *Am Heart J, 81:*608, 1971.

14. Kurihara, H.; Kuramoto, K.; Terasawa, F.; Matsushita, S.; Seki, M. and Ikeda, M.: Reliability of abnormal Q and QS patterns classified by the Minnesota Code for the diagnosis of myocardial infarction in aged people. *Jap Heart J, 8:*514, 1967.

15. Batschelet, E.: *Statistical Methods for the Analysis of Problems in Animal Orientation and Certain Biological Rhythms,* Section 8. Washington, D. C., The American Institute of Biological Sciences, 1965.

16. Truett, J.; Cornfield, J. and Kannel, W.: A multivariate analysis of the risk of coronary heart disease in Framingham. *J Chronic Dis, 20:* 511–524, 1967.

17. Kurihara, H.; Kuramoto, K.; Murata, K.; Terasawa, F.; Seki, M. and Ikeda, M.: Incidence of abnormal Q and QS patterns classified by the Minnesota Code in 74 autopsied cases of myocardial infarction in the aged. *Jap Heart J, 8:*419, 1967.

18. Simonson, E.; Tuna, N.; Okamoto, N. and Toshima, H.: Diagnostic accuracy of the vectorcardiogram and electrocardiogram. A cooperative study. *Am J Cardiol, 17:*829, 1966.

19. Gunnar, R. M.; Pietras, R. J.; Blackaller, J.; Dadmum, S. E.; Szanto, P. B. and Tobin, J. R., Jr.: Correlation of vectorcardiographic criteria for myocardial infarction with autopsy findings. *Circulation, 35:* 158, 1967.

20. Fleischli, G. and Stratbucker, R.: Comparative evaluation of scalar and vector computerized EKG systems. Exhibit #S116, 19th Annual Scientific Sessions of the American College of Cardiology, New Orleans, La., 1970.

## Chapter 19

# ALGORITHMIC DIAGNOSIS: A REVIEW WITH EMPHASIS ON BAYESIAN METHODS*

JOHN A. JACQUEZ

## INTRODUCTION

Medical diagnosis has long been one of the more dramatic examples of human problem solving. The hero of one of the dominant legends of medicine is the great clinician who quickly scans the patient and with some mysterious ability picks out the relevant information to make an immediate diagnosis, while the lesser clinicians stand around and applaud in awe. That great exemplar of inductive detective ability, A. Conan Doyle's Sherlock Holmes was modeled on the great Scots clinician Bell. But "how physicians diagnose" is not the main problem under discussion here although it is closely related to our main subject. We are concerned with inductive methods of diagnosis which can be formalized in algorithmic form for use with modern digital computers. A number of such algorithms have been used in the past decade with Bayes' Theorem getting the main attention. In fact it is just over a decade since Ledley and Lusted [1] first proposed that Bayes' Theorem provided the theoretical basis for computer-assisted diagnosis in medicine. And indeed many of us believe that the Bayesian approach provides a general theoretical basis for diagnostic algorithms. Whether or not physicians operate in the same way as any one or a mixture of diagnostic algorithms is relevant for questions about the performance of humans as diagnosticians. However, our main concern for the moment is to formulate and test diagnostic algorithms and to compare their performances

* This work was supported by grant #GM 892–08 from the U.S. Public Health Service.

as well as to compare their performances with those of physicians.

My purpose in this paper is to review the work which has been done on computer-assisted diagnosis. Rather than try to carry out an exhaustive review I would like to highlight some of the important problems by examining a series of models of the patient sample which is used as a data base and of its relation to the population being studied. It is in this context that I would like to review some selected studies which illustrate particular problems or which forcefully make important points.

## TERMINOLOGY, BAYES' THEOREM AND LIKELIHOOD

I use the notation $S_i$ to stand for a sign, symptom or other finding and use the generic term "attribute" for any $S_i$. The notation $A_k$ will designate a subset of attributes which includes, of course, subsets consisting of one attribute. $D_j$ represents the $j^{th}$ diagnostic class which, for simplicity, we can call a disease. For the sake of completeness and for those who do not use these concepts daily, I would like to review Bayes' Theorem in the context of diseases and attributes, to illustrate its meaning, and to present some of the standard nomenclature. Those who are well acquainted with the basic concepts can skip this section.

Suppose we are given a classification of a population in terms of a set of mutually exclusive and exhaustive categories—the *diseases*. Fig. 19–1 illustrates the situation diagrammatically, the population being divided into mutually exclusive subsets. By analogy, think of the area of each subset in Fig. 19–1 as a measure of the number of individuals in that subset. Note that the subsets $D_1$, $D_2$, . . . need not represent individual diseases, some may consist of more than one disease present simultaneously; the important point is that this division of the population should be a division into mutually exclusive diagnostic categories and each member of the population fall into one of the categories.[2] Now suppose that we can also classify the individuals of this population in terms of another set of features—the *attributes*. The attributes are not mutually exclusive and in fact any one individual may have many of the attributes. Basically, we want to know how the distribution of attributes in the population is related to the classification by diseases and in particular, given one individual from

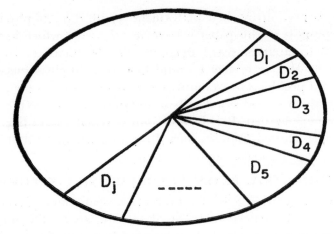

**Figure 19–1.** Classification of a population by mutually exclusive diagnostic categories.

the population and his attributes, what inferences can one make about his disease classification. Consider those individuals which have the subset of attributes $A_i$. This subset is shown in Fig. 19–2, it overlaps a number of the subsets of diseases. The cross-hatched area in Fig. 19–2 represents the number of individuals

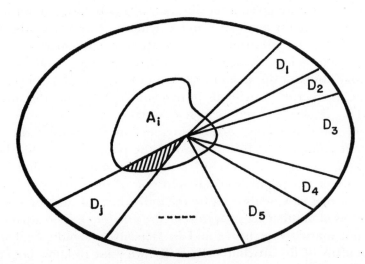

**Figure 19–2.** Overlapping of classification by mutually exclusive diagnostic categories and by (not mutually exclusive) attributes.

which have both disease $D_j$ and the subset of attributes $A_i$, i.e. $D_jA_i$. Let N be the total number of individuals in the population and let $N(D_j)$ be the number in subset $D_j$, $N(A_i)$ the number in subset $A_i$ and $N(A_iD_j)$ the number in subset $A_iD_j$. Then the equation for the frequency of individuals which are both in $A_i$ and $D_j$, $P(A_iD_j)$ can be factored in two ways, as is shown in Equations 1 and 2.

$$P(A_iD_j) = \frac{N(A_iD_j)}{N} = \frac{N(A_iD_j)}{N(D_j)} \cdot \frac{N(D_j)}{N} \qquad (1)$$

$$P(A_iD_j) = \frac{N(A_iD_j)}{N} = \frac{N(A_iD_j)}{N(A_i)} \cdot \frac{N(A_i)}{N} \qquad (2)$$

Note that $N(D_j)/N$ and $N(A_i)/N$ are simply the frequencies of $D_j$ and $A_i$ respectively, $P(D_j)$ and $P(A_i)$. $N(A_iD_j)/N(D_j)$ is written $P(A_i/D_j)$ and is the *conditional probability* of $A_j$ given $D_i$, that is, it is the probability that a patient who is known to have $D_j$, also has $A_i$. Similarly, $N(A_iD_j)/N(A_i)$ is $P(D_j/A_i)$, that is, the probability that a patient known to have $A_i$ also falls in $D_j$. Combining Equations 1 and 2 gives us 3.

$$P(D_j/A_i) = \frac{P(A_i/D_j)P(D_j)}{P(A_i)} \qquad (3)$$

$N(A_i)$ can also be written as the sum over disease subsets, $D_k$, of all individuals who have both $D_k$ and $A_i$. Hence Equation 4 holds.

$$P(A_i) = \frac{N(A_i)}{N} = \sum_k \frac{N(A_iD_k)}{N(D_k)} \cdot \frac{N(D_k)}{N} = \sum_k P(A_i/D_k)P(D_k) \qquad (4)$$

Substituting 4 in Equation 3:

$$P(D_j/A_i) = \frac{P(D_j)P(A_i/D_j)}{\sum_k P(D_k)P(A_i/D_k)} \qquad (5)$$

Equations 3 and 5 are Bayes' Theorem [3] in general form. Suppose $A_i$ is the subset of attributes $S_{i1}S_{i2} \ldots S_{ip}$. If the $S_{ir}$ are mutually independent, that is, if the occurrence of one is not in any way dependent on the occurrence of any of the others for any one or all disease states, then Equations 6 and 7 hold, otherwise 6 and 7 are not true.

$$P(A_i) = P(S_{i1}) \cdot P(S_{i2}) \ldots P(S_{ip}) \qquad (6)$$

$$P(A_i/D_j) = P(S_{i1}/D_j) \cdot P(S_{i2}/D_j) \ldots P(S_{ip}/D_j) \qquad (7)$$

Then Bayes' Theorem assumes the special form given by Equation 8.

$$P(D_j/A_i) = \frac{P(D_j) \prod\limits_{r=1}^{p} P(S_{ir}/D_j)}{\sum P(D_k) \prod\limits_{r=1}^{p} P(S_{ir}/D_k)} \qquad (8)$$

This is the form which has been used in most studies in diagnosis but it is applicable only if the attributes are distributed independently within diseases and this is rarely true. Furthermore it is not desirable for it is the correlation between attributes within diseases which gives us highly diagnostic subsets of attributes.

In Equation 3, $P(D_j)$ is the incidence of $D_j$ in the population. It is also called the prior probability of $D_j$, the probability of $D_j$ occurring before one knows anything about the attributes. $P(D_j/A_i)$ is called the posterior probability of the disease $D_j$ given the occurrence of the attribute subset $A_i$. $P(A_i/D_j)$, the conditional probability of $A_i$ given that $D_j$ occurs, is also called the *likelihood*.

The posterior probability can be updated sequentially as more information is obtained. If a patient has the attributes in subset $A_i$ and $A_k$ is a different subset of attributes and we find he has $A_k$ as well as $A_i$, then we can write Equation 9 for $P(D_j/A_kA_i)$

$$P(D_j/A_kA_i) = \frac{P(D_j) \cdot P(A_iA_k/D_j)}{P(A_iA_k)} \qquad (9)$$

This may also be written as in Equation 10:

$$P(D_j/A_iA_k) = \frac{P(D_j/A_i)P(A_k/A_iD_j)}{P(A_k/A_i)} \qquad (10)$$

In Equation 10 the posterior probability is updated in terms of the previous estimate and the new information about the occurrence of the attributes $A_k$.

The above derivations need to be modified slightly if some of the attributes come from multinomial rather than binomial distributions.

## SOME MODELS OF THE DATA BASE
### Model 1. The Data Base as Universe
### (The fully specified universe)

In some of the early studies the performance of a method was tested only on the data base which was used to obtain the frequencies. The model for this situation is obvious. Assume a fixed population for which disease incidences and conditional probabilities are known and are identical with those of the data base. Then to test the performance of any method, draw random samples from the data base with replacement; in the long run this is equivalent to examining performance on the data base, i.e. using each individual of the data base once. This approach has been criticized as not giving a good measure of performance on a real population. Although there is point to this criticism, I would rather emphasize the importance of testing each method on the data (a Model 1 study) because this does provide some very important information.

Given that exact frequencies present in the data base are used, the performance of any method on the data base measures the best performance obtainable from this method in the long run on random samples from a population which has the given distribution of diseases and attributes. Furthermore it should be obvious that for a given distribution of diseases and attributes in a population there must be a limit to the diagnostic power of any method and that this limit is set by the relation of the attribute structure to the disease structure of the population. Thus if one has an optimal method, its performance in this test measures the best you can do with this population and attribute structure! Bayes' Theorem, Equation 2, has this optimal property. As a point of reference recall that the maximum number of exclusive subsets that can be formed from n binary nonexclusive attributes is $2^n$, the number of different combinations of the different attributes. The maximum number of diseases that can be differentiated by n binary attributes is obtained if each of the $2^n$ subsets corresponds to one diagnostic category.

The data base rarely consists of more than 1000–2000 patients with perhaps 50 diseases and 50–100 attributes included. Two of the major problems in applying Bayes' Theorem are easily solved. The requirement of a mutually exclusive classification by diseases is solved by fiat in the choice of diseases which are studied and in the choice of data base. The data base is usually small enough so that the data can be stored and the frequency of any subset of attributes for a disease can be calculated directly. Surprisingly, most studies which have been reported have used Bayes' Theorem with the assumption of independence of conditional probabilities and in some cases a study of correlation between attributes has been used to eliminate some attributes which are correlated with others in the population. In most papers in this field performance has been reported in terms of percent correct diagnoses. As Lusted (see Chap. 3) has pointed out, a better measure is given by the percent true positives and percent false positives for each disease.

Scheinok and Rinaldo [4,5] worked with a data base of 300 patients with six diseases and 11 attributes and compared the performance of Bayes' Theorem with that of multiple discriminant analysis. The six diseases used accounted for 97 percent of all diagnoses at the GI clinic at Henry Ford Hospital and were hiatus hernia, gallbladder disease, cancer, duodenal ulcer, gastric ulcer, and functional disorders. With Bayes' Theorem they used the assumption of independence of the conditional probabilities and also used Bailey's [6] modification for the calculation of probabilities. The latter is appropriate when the data base is viewed as a sample from a larger population and is one of the ways of getting around the assignment of conditional probabilities of 0 or 1 when using estimates from finite samples. Its use in Model 1 will degrade the performance of Bayes' Theorem. So one would expect Bayes' formula not to perform optimally in this application. Nonetheless it did as well as discriminant analysis in the diagnosis of three of the diseases, did better in one, and less well than discriminant analysis in two. The authors introduce the interesting idea of using the data base to generate a lexicon of symptom complexes and the associated diagnoses predicted from the data base. The problem with this in practice is that the number of combinations increases as $2^n$ for binary attributes where n is the number of attributes.

Overall and Williams [7] examined the differential diagnosis of hypo-, eu-, and hyperthyroidism with 21 attributes and a data base of 450 patients. They reported that Bayes' Theorem with the assumption of independence gave 93 percent correct diagnoses.

An interesting study on the diagnosis of congenital heart disease is that of Reale *et al.*[8] in which a data base of 1184 patients with 94 diseases but only 46 attributes was used. They report 82 percent correct diagnoses with use of Bayes' formula with the independence assumption. This is partly explained by the fact that 967 of the 1184 patients fell into only 14 disease categories which were relatively well discriminated; with these, 85 percent of the diagnoses were correct. Of the 94 diseases, 65 were represented by only 104 patients. For comparison they also tried using Bayes' formula with equal prior probabilities (incidences) for all diseases; this is equivalent to using the *likelihood* for diagnosis. The overall accuracy then fell to 70 percent; as might be expected there was actually an improvement in the accuracy of diagnosing the rarer diseases but this was more than compensated for by the decreased accuracy of diagnosis of the more common diseases.

Templeton *et al.*[9] presented one of the rare studies in which the independence problem is attacked directly. In a study of the diagnosis of pulmonary lesions, using a data base of 242 patients with nine diseases and 19 attributes, they took into account first order interactions between attributes by tabulating and using the conditional probabilities of all pairs of attributes. This led to a marked improvement in performance; Bayes' Theorem with the independence assumption gave only 67 percent correct diagnoses; inclusion of first order interactions improved this to 95 percent correct diagnoses. I think many of us would conjecture that most of the improvement obtainable from including the interactions is probably obtainable from inclusion of the first order interactions.

Finally I would like to point to Burbank's [10] recent retrospective study of six liver diseases in 52 patients in which he used 144 attributes. Using Bayes' equation with the independence assumption he got 92 percent correct diagnoses on the data base.

## Model 2. The Data Base as a Sample from a Stationary Universe

If the data base is a sample which provides estimates of the probabilities in some stationary but unknown universe, a number of new problems arise. In applying any diagnostic method to new patients one no longer has any guarantee that a patient must fit into one of the diagnostic categories and it is possible that a patient may fit into more than one category. Only experience will tell us how important this problem is. For this model it is important to include a modification such as Bailey's corrections, or better still the estimates of experts, to avoid using estimates of conditional probabilities of 0 or 1. The problems of estimating conditional probabilities of subsets of attributes has rarely been faced squarely, except in the study of Templeton et al.[9] The most frequently used approach has been to examine the correlations between attributes and to eliminate attributes so as to make the assumption of independence of the conditional probabilities, $P(S_i/D_j)$, more realistic. This tactic actually discards information unless an attribute which is discarded is so highly correlated with one which is retained that it is practically redundant.

Probably one of the most frequently quoted studies is that of Warner's group [11,12,13] on the diagnosis of congenital heart disease. The data base consisted of 1,035 patients and included 35 diseases and 53 attributes. The results of a Model 1 type of study were not reported. Their estimates of probabilities were not obtained solely from their data base but included components of expert judgment derived both from a review of the literature and their thinking in terms of the pathophysiology of the diseases involved. They reported results on 84 new patients. An interesting facet of the study was a comparison of the performances of an expert cardiologist, a clinical physiologist, and a third year resident. Each of the physicians collected his own data for his diagnosis and then the data collected by each one was used for a computer diagnosis with use of Bayes' Theorem with independence of conditional probabilities, $P(S_i/D_j)$, assumed. Not only did the third year resident do less well than the others but the computer diagnoses based on his data were not as accurate as the computer diagnoses based on the data of the others, suggesting that one reason a less experienced individual does not perform as well as an expert is that he does not collect as much relevant information. Unfortunately no comparison was given of the performance on the original data base (Model 1) and on the new patients.

In the study of Reale *et al.*[8] such a comparison is available. Recall that he reported 82 percent correct diagnoses on the data base; this fell to 62 percent on 125 new cases which were not in the data base.

Boyle *et al.*[14] compared the performance of Bayes' Theorem (with the independence assumption), with that of the likelihood in the differential diagnosis of 88 new cases of simple goiter, Hashimoto's disease, and thyroid carcinoma. The incidence data came from 300 cases and the conditional probabilities were estimated from 155 cases; 30 attributes were used. The authors' expert judgement was used to replace entries of 0 in the table of conditional probabilities with entries in the range .0001–.02. They concluded that the likelihood method was better; the difference between the two methods was in three cases of thyroid carcinoma which the Bayes' formula missed as a first diagnosis.

In the study of Templeton *et al.*[9] they also drew 51 cases randomly from their data base of 242 cases and then used the remaining 191 as their data base. The percentage of correct diagnoses for the 51 cases was then 40 percent and 27 percent respectively for Bayes' formula with the independence assumption and with the first order interactions included. As might be expected, when the random sample of 51 was examined it was found that two diagnoses were considerably overrepresented in comparison with the sample of size 191 which was used as data base.

In Burbank's study [10] of 52 cases of liver disease, besides examining the performance of Bayes' formula in a Model 1 situation he also successively removed each individual to use as a test case and used the remaining 51 as a data base. This sort of test is commonly known as a jacknife in the jargon of statistics. He apparently used no method to remove entries of 0 from the table of conditional probabilities. The percentage of correct diagnoses then fell to 58.5 percent, the majority of the errors being for cases which fell in the low-incidence groups.

These results raise the question of how large should a data base be. Intuitively one might answer that the data base should be large enough to give in some sense, "stable" estimates of probabilities. A related question is, how many attributes are needed? The two are not independent and the number of attributes required obviously depends on the size of the data base, the number of diseases, and the distributions of the attributes over the diseases. Mount and Evans [15] reported the results of an interesting simulation in which they used 20 diseases and a maximum of 100 independently distributed attributes with an average attribute frequency in the population of 0.1. They then generated samples of size 100, 300, 1000 and 3000 to use as data bases for the calculation of the incidences and the conditional probabilities, $P(S_i/D_j)$. They also generated samples of size 500 from the same parent population and used Bayes Theorem to calculate the posterior probabilities of the various diseases for the different data bases as well as with the known true probabilities and all of this for increasing numbers of attributes. They found that they needed approximately 40 attributes to get a 95 percent diagnostic accuracy with Bayes' Theorem with use of the true probabilities. If the probabilities were estimated from data bases of size 1000 or 3000 they did almost as well but performance was considerably poorer when the probabilities estimated from the data bases of size 100 or 300 were used. The results shown in Fig. 19–3 give the percent correct diagnoses for the probabilities calculated from data bases of different sizes as a function of the number of symptoms used.

The results of Mount and Evans, as well as other considerations, suggest that Bayes' Theorem be used sequentially as the attributes are collected. In fact one of the distinctive features of Bayes' Theorem is that it incorporates the inductive idea of updating one's opinion as new data are collected. In the sequential decision tree approach, the idea of choosing the next set of attributes to be collected so as to minimize some cost is added. The intuitive idea is that it should seldom be necessary to collect all attributes on each patient; as the attributes are collected the search for a diagnosis begins to narrow down to some more likely candidates. At such a point one wants to run the tests which offer the most potential gain; this is measured in terms of a cost function. Gorry and Barnett [16] used a sequential decision tree method with a

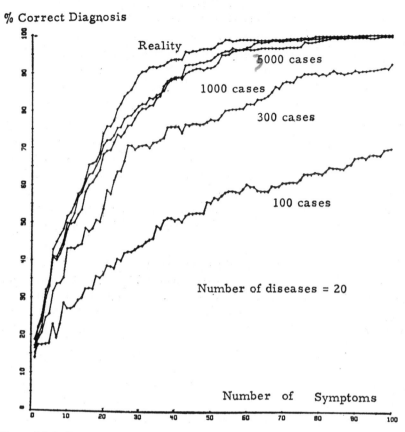

% Correct Diagnosis

Reality

5000 cases

1000 cases

300 cases

100 cases

Number of diseases = 20

Number of Symptoms

Figure 19–3. Percentage of correct diagnoses for 500 cases as function of number of symptoms used in making the diagnoses. The number of cases used to calculate incidences and conditional probabilities are given for each curve. For the top curve, labeled Reality, the true incidences and conditional probabilities were used. (From Mount and Evans [15])

probability matrix for the diagnosis of congenital heart disease and some test cases supplied by Warner and his associates. They reported that the sequential decision tree approach required far fewer attributes per patient to reach the same diagnostic accuracy as the single application of Bayes' Theorem after collecting all attributes on the patients.

## Model 3. The Data Base as a Sample from a Time-varying Universe

Many have pointed out that there may be seasonal and long-term changes in the incidences of some diseases. For some diseases there may even be sudden, large and short-term changes, epidemics. One which shows all three is the incidence of the complex pneumonia-influenza. Serfling *et al.*[17] have shown that the death rate due to pneumonia-influenze shows a small linear trend in time, a seasonal cycle which is well described by a sum of two cosine functions plus superimposed bursts associated with major epidemics of influenza. Fig. 19–4 shows how dramatic these fluctuations are in mortality. Presumably the conditional probabilities are much less subject to such variation but one might expect some long-term trends in the conditional probabilities of attributes in some syndromes and diseases as these diseases become more clearly defined with increase in medical knowledge.

Although one can point to these problems, I have no examples of work on algorithmic diagnosis in which they clearly are important. The major change that would be required is that estimates of incidence data be "current"; this implies that the data base used for incidences be updated frequently and that "older cases" be dropped from it. New estimation problems result because of the trade off between size and accuracy of the data base and its sensitivity to recent changes. Because we have little experience with real problems in this area it might be worthwhile to carry out a simulation such as that of Mount and Evans but with time-dependent probabilities for the disease incidences and then examine the performance of some diagnostic algorithms with use of a number of different sizes of data bases and different rates of updating.

### Reprise. Problems in the Application of Bayes' Theorem

Most of the difficulties met in the use of Bayes' Theorem have been encountered in the last section. I would like to review them and emphasize some of the important points.

### Multiple Diseases

This is no problem in many special areas where the number of diagnoses is small and they are in the main mutually exclusive. It

## PNEUMONIA-INFLUENZA DEATH RATES
## BY MONTH, UNITED STATES

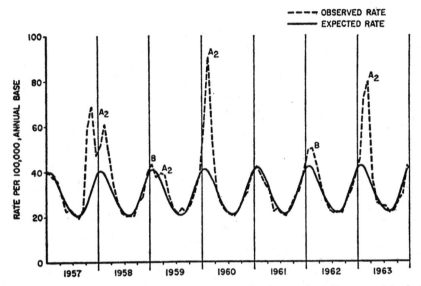

Figure 19–4. Monthly pneumonia—influenza death rates for all ages and both sexes combined for the period 1957–1963. The solid line is the calculated rate which includes a secular trend and seasonal fluctuation. The dashed line is the observed rate: the peaks labeled A2 and B correspond in time with epidemics of influenza A2 and B respectively. (From Serfling, Sherman and Houseworth [17])

is not a problem in a Model I type of study. For large disease classifications this is not so. For a set of m diseases that are not mutually exclusive, the number of possible combinations of diseases is $2^m$. These do form a mutually exclusive diagnostic classification. Even if only all pairs are included, the total number of diagnostic categories becomes $m(m+1)/2$ (all singles plus all pairs). For m even of moderate size, it seems unreasonable to attempt to tabulate all incidences for all possible combinations or even for all pairs. The reasonable approach would be to include only combinations of diseases which appear at greater than some given frequency in practice and to disregard the rare combinations for the time being. I am not aware of any studies of multiple diseases which focus on the question of whether or not the combined attributes of commonly accurring disease combinations mimic other diseases. However, Brodman and his co-workers [18,19] report that multiple diagnoses are common in practice. They report an average of 2.9 diagnoses per patient in the practice of a group of internists and an average of 2.4 diagnoses per patient in the practice of a busy general practitioner.

### Estimation of Conditional Probabilities

An attempt to estimate the conditional probabilities of all possible combinations of attributes again gets us in trouble with the combinatorial possibilities. For n binary attributes and m mutually exclusive diagnostic categories there are $2^n$ different attribute combinations per disease and so one would have to estimate $m.2^n$ conditional probabilities, $P(A_i/D_j)$. This is why the assumption of independence of the conditional probabilities has been used so frequently. One reasonable alternative which avoids some of the worst consequences when the attributes are not independently distributed is to take into account first order interactions by directly estimating the conditional probabilities for all pairs of attributes as well as for the individual attributes, as was done by Templeton *et al.*[9] However, the tactic used most frequently has been to examine the correlations between attributes and to discard attributes so as to make the independence assumption more reasonable. As pointed out before this is the wrong thing to do because it throws away information. It should be done only when attributes are very highly correlated so that one really carries all of the information. The more reasonable thing to do is to use correlation studies to identify those subsets of attributes for which the conditional probabilities should be estimated directly without use of the independence assumption. Furthermore, as the data base increases the correlation studies should be repeated at intervals to see if new correlations become obvious as the information increases. Some attributes may carry little discriminatory information and may in fact act more like noise. Our aim should be to eliminate such attributes. Thus studies similar to that of Mount and Evans should be done with real data bases and the usefulness of different attributes tested on real populations in Model 1 and Model 2 type studies.

For some diseases our knowledge of the pathophysiology of the disease process tells us that certain attributes should be correlated but sufficient data are not available to give us good estimates of the conditional probability for the combined attributes. For example, suppose $A_1$ and $A_2$ are two distinct subsets of attributes for which we have estimates, $P(A_1/D_j)$, $P(A_2/D_j)$. It is possible to use the judgement of experts to obtain good estimates of $P(A_1A_2/D_j)$ by providing the estimators with appropriate reference points. If subsets $A_1$ and $A_2$ contain no common attributes then relation 11 must hold.

$$\text{Max. } \{0, \ P(A_1/D_j) + P(A_2/D_j) - 1\} \leq P(A_1A_2/D_j) \leq \text{Min.}$$
$$\{P(A_1/D_j), P(A_2/D_j)\} \tag{11}$$

Of course if $A_1$ and $A_2$ are independent, $P(A_1A_2/D_j) = P(A_1/D_j) \cdot P(A_2/D_j)$. For example, if $P(A_1/D_j) = 0.7$ and $P(A_2/D_j) = 0.4$, $P(A_1A_2/D_j)$ must lie between .1 and .4, and is 0.28 if $A_1$ and $A_2$ are independent. Thus in asking an expert's opinion it would be important to provide him with these reference points and to point out that $P(A_1A_2/D_j)$ must lie between .28 and .4 if $A_1$ and $A_2$ are positively correlated, and between .1 and .28 if they are negatively correlated.

### Data on Incidences

The data base from which incidence data are obtained may well be considerably smaller than that from which conditional probabilities are obtained because of the requirement that *local* incidences be used. Thus we can expect that estimates of incidences will be less good than the estimates of conditional probabilities. Intuitively, I would guess that the conditional probabilities are more important and that we can put up with more error in the estimation of incidences. It might be useful to examine this question with use of simulation or with some real data bases and testing to see how introduction of error into the various probabilities affects diagnostic accuracy.

### Updating the Probabilities

In all but a Model 1 type of study the data base is only a sample, so one should include provision for adding new patients to the data base. Hence, one has to specify how a diagnosis is to be validated for addition of new patients to the data base. As a general rule one would want to validate a diagnosis with use of tests which are not available in the attribute set, such as autopsy or operative findings. As a result, the rate of expansion of the data base may be small in comparison with the rate of entry of test cases into the study.

The aim of expanding the data base is stable estimation with high diagnostic performance. The jacknife used by Burbank, that is, successively removing each patient from the data base and using that patient as a test case for the reduced data base is a remarkably good test of the performance of a diagnostic method based on that data base. I would recommend its use as a test for stability of estimation as the data base is expanded.

### Use of Bayes' Theorem in a Sequential Decision Tree

Bayes' Theorem incorporates the idea of a sequential addition of data. It seems only natural to add the concept of costs for deciding what tests to use next. The major problem is the practical one of how to obtain estimates of costs acceptable for general use. However, Ginsberg (see Chap. 13) has shown that costs can be obtained and also that it is a long and arduous process.

### CONCLUSIONS

In conclusion I would like to give you my estimates of the future of computer-assisted diagnosis. Discussions of the usefulness of algorithmic aids to diagnosis have too often been obscured by arguments about its utility in the daily practice of medicine. From the experience accumulated in the past decade I would list four significant areas of use for algorithmic diagnosis.

1. *Studies of Differential Diagnosis.* One remarkable function of algorithmic methods of diagnosis in general and of Bayes' Theorem in particular has been developing so slowly we have failed to recognize it. Bayes' Theorem, used with a collection of cases in a Model 1 type of study is a new paradigm for the presentation of studies of the differential diagnosis of a group of related diseases. It provides the theoretical framework for examining the diagnostic capability of the "attribute" structure of a set of pa-

tients in terms of the "disease" structure! And it is this application which provides the rationale and basis for examining the contributions of the different attributes to the differential diagnosis of a set of diagnostic categories.

2. *Teaching Diagnosis.* Models 1, 2 and 3 and the use of Bayes' Theorem in a sequential decision mode provide a new and better way to teach diagnosis and this aside from the use of computer assisted instruction in the usual sense.

3. *Computer Programs as Consultants.* I believe that diagnostic programs will be used as consultants in certain specialties. For example, developments in computer diagnosis of the ECG have reached the stage that it is safe to predict that computer diagnosis of the ECG will be available as a routine in the near future.

4. *Computer Diagnosis and the Delivery of Medical Care.* In the past many physicians have pointed out that most problems seen in daily practice are so routine that the use of computers would be superfluous. This limits the usefulness of computer-assisted diagnosis, if the patterns of medical practice remain as they are today. However, the increasing demands for health services have put serious strains on the old methods of delivering health care. The demands of our society may well lead to marked increase in large group practices patterned in part on the Kaiser-Permanente program.[20] In that case, nonemergency cases may have a history taken and a series of laboratory tests and perhaps even some parts of a physical examination before they even get to see the physician. The results of the preliminary work-up may then be processed by a diagnostic program which would provide the physician with a summary of the work up, a list of significant findings and perhaps some suggestions for further work-up as part of a differential diagnosis.[21,22] At the moment this seems to me the least important of the four.

## REFERENCES

1. Ledley, R. S. and Lusted, L. B.: Reasoning foundations of medical diagnosis. *Science, 130:*9–21, 1959.
2. Woodbury, M. A.: Inapplicabilities of Bayes' Theorem to diagnosis. Proc. 5th Intern. Conf. on Med. Electronics, Liege, Belgium, 1963, pp. 860–868.

3. Kendall, M. G. and Stuart, A.: *The Advanced Theory of Statistics*, 2nd Ed., Vol. 1. New York, Hafner Publishing Co., 1963.

4. Scheinok, P. A. and Rinaldo, J. A., Jr.: Symptom diagnosis: optimal subsets for upper abdominal pain. *Comp Biomed Res, 1:*221–236, 1967.

5. Scheinok, P. A. and Rinaldo, J. A., Jr.: Symptom diagnosis: A comparison of mathematical models related to upper abdominal pain. *Comp Biomed Res, 1:*475–489, 1968.

6. Bailey, N. T. J.: Probability methods of diagnosis based on small samples. In *Mathematics and Computer Science in Biology and Medicine*. London, Her Majesty's Stationary Office, 1965, pp. 103–107.

7. Overall, J. E. and Williams, C. M.: Conditional probability program for diagnosis of thyroid function. *JAMA, 183:*307–313, 1963.

8. Reale, A.; Maccacaro, G. E.; Rocca, E,; D'Intino, S.; Gioffre, P. A.; Vestri, A. and Motolese, M.: Computer diagnosis of congenital heart disease. *Comp Biomed Res, 1:*533–549, 1968.

9. Templeton, A. W.; Jansen, C.; Lehr, J. L. and Hufft, R.: Solitary pulmonary lesions. Computer-aided differential diagnosis and evaluation of mathematical methods. *Radiology, 89:*605–613, 1967.

10. Burbank, F.: A computer diagnostic system for the diagnosis of prolonged undifferentiating liver disease. *Am J Med, 46:*401–415, 1969.

11. Warner, H. R.; Toronto, A. F.; Veasey, L. G. and Stephenson, R.: A mathematical approach to medical diagnosis. *JAMA, 177:*175–183, 1961.

12. Toronto, A. F.; Veasey, L. G. and Warner, H. R.: Evaluation of a computer program for diagnosis of congenital heart disease. *Progr Cardiovasc Dis, 5:*362–377, 1963.

13. Warner, H. R.; Toronto, A. F. and Veasey, L. G.: Experience with Bayes' theorem for computer diagnosis of congenital heart disease. *Ann NY Acad Sci, 115:*558–567, 1964.

14. Boyle, J. A.; Greig, W. R.; Franklin, D. A.; Harden, R. McG.; Buchanan, W. W. and McGirr, E. M.: Construction of a model for computer-assisted diagnosis: application to the problem of non-toxic goitre. *Q J Med*, New Series, *35:*565–588, 1966.

15. Mount, J. R. and Evans, J. W.: Computer aided diagnosis. A simulation study. Proc. 5th IBM Med. Sympos, 1963, pp. 113–128.

16. Gorry, G. A. and Barnett, G. O.: Experience with a model of sequential diagnosis. *Comp Biomed Res, 1:*490–507, 1968.

17. Serfling, R. E.; Sherman, I. L. and Houseworth, W. J.: Excess pneumonia-influenza mortality by age and sex in three major influenza A2 epidemics, United States, 1957–58, 1960 and 1963. *Am J Epidemiol, 86:*433–441, 1967.

18. Brodman, K. and van Woerkom, A. J.: Computer-aided diagnostic screening for 100 common diseases. *JAMA, 197:*901–905, 1966.

19. Brodman, K. and Goldstein, L. S.: The medical data screen. An adjunct for the diagnosis of 100 common diseases. *Arch Environ Health, 14:*821–826, 1967.

20. Garfield, S. F.: The delivery of medical care. *Sci Am, 222:*15–23, 1970.

21. Collen, M. F.; Rubin, L. and Davis, L.: Computers in multiphasic screening. In R. W. Stacey and B. O. Waxman (Eds.): Computers in Biomedical Research. N. Y., Academic Press, 1965, pp. 339–52.

22. Collen, M. F.: Periodic health examinations using an automatic multitest laboratory. *JAMA, 195:*830–833, 1966.

# INDEX